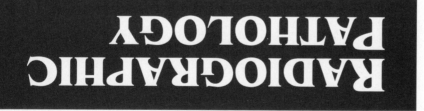

RADIOGRAPHIC PATHOLOGY

RADIOGRAPHIC PATHOLOGY

TerriAnn Linn-Watson, MEd, RT, RDMS
Associate Professor
Health Sciences Department
Chaffey College
Rancho Cucamonga, California

SAUNDERS
An Imprint of Elsevier

SAUNDERS
An Imprint of Elsevier

The Curtis Center
Independence Square West
Philadelphia, Pennsylvania 19106

RADIOGRAPHIC PATHOLOGY   ISBN 0-7216-4129-6

Printed in the United States of America.

Last digit is the print number: 9   8   8   6

To
Kendrick Kale and Kamden Edward
Mom can shoot hoops with you now

Preface

In this exceedingly hurried world, our endeavors to condense and include tremendous amounts of material into radiologic technology school curricula are beset by many difficulties. With most radiologic technology school courses limited to 24 months and a tremendous amount of didactic material to cover in certain areas, particularly pathology, only the surface can be scratched.

Radiologic technology is one of the most rapidly growing and changing professions in the health-care field. It is now formally listed as a profession. Great trust, responsibility, professionalism, and technical knowledge are now necessary to perform the work of a radiologic technologist. This move to professionalism makes the radiologic technologist responsible for acquiring more knowledge and understanding of pathologic conditions so that she or he is able to perform responsibly the duties specific to the profession.

This textbook grew from an accumulation of 11 years of lecture notes that needed to become somehow manageable. Those notes grew to accommodate the changing role of radiographers from the perception of being "button pushers" to that of being a critical member of the diagnostic health-care team. Each member of this health-care team must have more knowledge, more skills, and more cross-training than ever before. The radiologic technologist cannot afford to be content with just "taking x-rays." The technologist must strive to have the skills to become indispensable to the busy imaging department.

The purpose of the textbook and student workbook is to guide the student technologist through material that need not be as difficult as some portray it. The book is arranged so that the basics are covered first, with the more difficult areas at the end of the book. This allows the reader to build a pathology foundation. The goals and objectives and detailed outline in the front of each chapter allow the reader to become familiar with the chapter's contents. The table at the end of the chapter summarizes the content of the chapter, and the review questions address each one of the objectives. These two areas are designed to reinforce the reader's learning.

The entire project was born out of a love for teaching the challenging topic of pathology. It is my hope that the student will find this text to be a useful tool in preparation for becoming that indispensable technologist in the ever-changing world of health care.

talw

Acknowledgments

Writing a textbook such as this is not an individual task. In the preparation of this book, I had occasion to call on the talents and efforts of people without whose assistance it could not have been brought to completion.

Leslie and Christen Linn, my parents, who sat up with me on those 32-hour typing sprees—proofreading, sorting radiographs, and making coffee.

Dr. Robert Stevenson for his support and invaluable help with various pathological conditions and for allowing me to use many radiographs from his teaching file.

Linda Lewis for her photographic expertise and very late nights trying to get those last-minute photos done.

Drs. David Berry, Patrick Bryan, Saba El Yousef, and Arvind Kumra for answering my many questions and putting up with the nuisance I often became.

All of the evening technologists with whom I work at San Antonio Community Hospital Department of Radiology for helping me collect the many pathologies seen in this text.

Helaine Barron who "mothered" me to get the project completed—God bless—we did it!

Lisa Biello and Bill Norcutt for the emotional support and allowing me to cry on their shoulders on more than one occasion.

The 1995 graduating class of Chaffey College who became the guinea pigs for a trial run.

To all, I extend my sincerest thanks and profound appreciation.

Brief Contents

Detailed Contents

CHAPTER I

Pathology Principles

Goals

1. To review the basic terminology related to general principles of pathology.
2. To learn the difference between structural and functional diseases.
3. To learn the causes of diseases.
4. To become familiar with the different types of injury and inflammation.
5. To recognize the different types of growth disturbances.
6. To review the types of tissue and how tissue repairs itself.

Objectives

At the completion of the chapter, the radiographer will be able to:

1. Define the various terms used in general pathology.
2. Define structural disease and explain its formation.
3. Define functional disease and give examples.
4. List and define the causes of disease.
5. Describe acute and chronic injury.
6. Explain the various aspects of inflammation and how inflammation heals.
7. List the different types of fundamental tissue and give examples.
8. Explain growth disturbances and give examples of benign and malignant types.

I. Disease
  A. Pathology
  B. Etiology
  C. Disease
  D. Pathogenesis
  E. Diagnosis
  F. Prognosis
  G. Procedure
  H. Test
  I. Manifestations
    1. Symptoms
      a. History
    2. Signs
    3. Syndrome
  J. Frequency
  K. Incidence
  L. Prevalence
  M. Morbidity Rate
  N. Mortality Rate
II. Classification of Diseases
  A. Structural Disease
    (Organic)
    1. Lesion
    2. Genetic and
      Developmental
      a. Congenital
      b. Hereditary
    3. Acquired Injury and
      Inflammatory
      a. Necrosis
      b. Sublethal Cell Injury
        (Degeneration)
    4. Hyperplasia and
      Neoplasia
  B. Functional Disease
    1. Pathophysiologic
    2. No Lesion
III. Causes of Diseases
  A. Exogenous
    1. Physical
      a. Trauma

    2. Chemical
    3. Microbiologic
      a. Infections
  B. Endogenous
    1. Vascular Diseases
      (Insufficiency)
      a. Anoxia
      b. Ischemia
      c. Infarct
      d. Myocardial Infarct
    2. Immunologic Diseases
      a. Autoimmune
    3. Metabolic Diseases
  C. Idiopathic
  D. Iatrogenic
  E. Nosocomial
IV. Injury
  A. Acute
    1. Hypoxia/Anoxia
    2. Thrombus
    3. Embolus
  B. Chronic
    1. Atrophy
      a. Senile
      b. Disuse
      c. Pressure
      d. Endocrine
V. Inflammation
  A. Phagocytosis
  B. Acute
    1. Cardinal Symptoms
      a. Red Skin
      b. Swelling
      c. Heat
      d. Pain
    2. Loss of Function
    3. Congestion
  C. Chronic
    1. Necrosis Uncommon
    2. Sublethal Degeneration

  D. Fluids
    1. Transudates
    2. Exudates
      a. Purulent (Pus)
        1. Suppurative
          Inflammation
        2. Abscess
        3. Empyema
VI. Repair
  A. Regeneration
  B. Granulation Tissue
  C. Wound
    1. Primary Union
    2. Secondary Union
VII. Fundamental Tissue
  A. Epithelial
  B. Connective
  C. Muscle
  D. Nerve
VIII. Altered Tissue Growth
  A. Hyperplasia
    1. Hypertrophy
  B. Metaplasia
  C. Neoplasm
    1. Benign
    2. Malignant
      a. Invasion
      b. Metastasis
        1. Seeding
        2. Lymphatic
        3. Hematogenous
      c. Carcinoma
      d. Sarcoma
      e. Lymphoma
      f. Leukemia
      g. Differentiation
        1. Grading
      h. Staging

An understanding of basic principles of pathology and an awareness of the radiographic appearances of specific diseases are essential goals in the training of a radiologic technologist. A technologist is aided in the selection of proper modalities and in determining the need for a repeat radiograph when he or she properly understands disease processes. Many types of diseases exist, and many conditions can be demonstrated radiographically. The role of the radiologic technologist is to display visually the changes in normal anatomy and tissue density that are caused by disease.

Before the various components of disease processes and healing mechanisms can be fully understood, a review of basic terminology is essential. A good foundation in medical terminology will be most helpful in digesting the somewhat difficult information presented in this and following chapters.

DISEASE

Pathology is, in the broadest sense, the study of disease processes. **Etiology** is the study of the cause of a disease and is often misused as a synonym for the actual cause of the disease.

Disease is any abnormal change in the function or structure within the body. It is a morbid process, usually having specific characteristic symptoms and, in some cases, physical signs. A disease can primarily affect one or more organs, or can target one organ and affect another one secondarily. Pathology is also concerned with the sequence of events that leads from the cause of a disease, to abnormalities, and finally to manifestations. This sequence of events that renders the disease apparent is called **pathogenesis.** A **diagnosis** is the determination of the disease an individual is believed to have, and a **prognosis** is the predicted course of a disease and the prospects for the patient's recovery. In order to determine the diagnosis and prognosis, a number of factors are considered. Clinical manifestations may point to a specific diagnosis. If not, the patient is evaluated by various **procedures** such as a barium enema or an arthrogram. An analysis of specimens taken from the patient, such as blood or excrement, can also help determine the disease process. These are known as **tests.**

The term **manifestations** refers to observed changes in the patient that are caused by the disease, namely symptoms, signs, and syndrome. A **symptom** is the patient's perception of the disease, such as a headache or abdominal pain. Symptoms are subjective, and only the patient can identify them. A written description of symptoms in a patient's record is referred to as the **history. Signs** are objective manifestations that are physically observed by the health examiner. A mass, rash, and abnormal pulse rate are all examples of signs. A cluster of findings that characterize a specific abnormal disturbance is known as a **syndrome.**

All disease processes are measured by frequency, incidence, and prevalence. **Frequency** is the rate of occurrence of a pathologic process that is measured over a given period of time, normally 1 year. **Incidence** is the number of newly diagnosed cases of a disease in 1 year. **Prevalence** is the number of people who have any given disease at any given point in time. Two other definitions that will be encountered are morbidity rate and mortality rate. **Morbidity rate** refers to the ratio of sick to well persons in a given area. **Mortality rate** is the ratio of actual deaths to expected deaths.

CLASSIFICATION OF DISEASES

All diseases of the body are produced by an alteration either in structure or in function of an organ or system. Since disease is an abnormal change within the body, the two classifications of diseases are structural and functional.

Structural disease, also known as **organic** disease, involves physical and biochemical changes within the cell. These changes are known as **lesions.** For a disease to be considered of a structural nature, the organ involved must be altered in some way as to present a pathologic entity. Three broad categories classify most structural diseases, although some diseases fall into more than one category and some are difficult to classify.

Genetic and developmental diseases are caused by abnormalities in the genetic makeup of the individual or abnormalities due to changes in utero.

The range of abnormalities in this category is very broad, extending from deformities present at birth, known as **congenital** abnormalities, to changes caused by genes but influenced by the environment so that they are not manifested until later in life. **Hereditary** diseases result from developmental disorders genetically transmitted from either parent to the child and are derived from ancestors.

Acquired injuries and **inflammatory diseases** are diseases caused by internal or external agents that destroy cells or cause the body to injure itself by means of inflammatory processes. External agents of injury include physical and chemical substances and microbes (see the section on causes of diseases). The major internal mechanisms of injury are vascular insufficiency, immunologic reactions, and metabolic disturbances. **Necrosis** occurs when the direct effects of an injury kill the cells in the injured area. Any injury to a cell that does not cause the cell to die is known as a **sublethal cell injury.** Also known as **degeneration,** this is the initial cell response following injury. An inflammatory disease results from the body's reaction to a localized injurious agent. Types of inflammatory diseases include infective diseases, toxic diseases, and allergic diseases.

Hyperplasias and neoplasias are categories used to describe diseases characterized by increases in cell populations. **Hyperplasia** is a proliferative reaction to a prolonged external stimulus and usually regresses when the stimulus is removed. **Neoplasia** is presumed to result from a genetic change that produces a single population of new cells, which can proliferate beyond the degree that is considered normal. Both hyperplasia and neoplasia are discussed later in this chapter.

Functional diseases are those diseases in which the function of the organ may be impaired, but its structural elements are unchanged. The basic change is a physiologic or functional one and is referred to as a **pathophysiologic change.** The onset begins without the presence of any lesions, such as those diseases triggered by psychic or psychophysiologic factors. Many mental illnesses are considered functional disorders. The most common functional disorders are tension headache and functional bowel syndrome, disorders that are caused by unconscious stimulation of the autonomic nervous system.

CAUSES OF DISEASES

Diseases are initiated by injury, which may be external or internal in origin. Causative agents that are external in nature are called **exogenous;** internal agents are called **endogenous** agents.

External causes of disease are divided into **physical, chemical,** and **microbiologic.** Direct physical injury by an object is called **trauma.** Other physical agents causing disease include extreme heat and cold, electricity, atmospheric pressure, and radiation. Chemical injuries are generally subdivided by the manner of injury into poisoning and drug reactions. Microbiologic injuries are usually classified by the type of organism (such as bacteria or fungi) and are termed **infections.**

Internal causes of disease fall into three large categories. **Vascular diseases** may involve obstruction of blood supply to an organ or tissue, bleeding, or altered blood flow such as occurs with heart failure. Vascular insufficiency is the leading internal cause of structural disease and results in tissue necrosis due to **anoxia** (lack of oxygen). Without sufficient oxygen to feed the tissue, the muscle dies. Deficiency of oxygen and nutrient-laden blood in the muscle is termed **ischemia,** and an area of necrotic tissue is called an **infarct.** Ischemic infarct occurring in the heart is known as **myocardial infarct** and is the leading cause of death from vascular insufficiency. **Immunologic diseases** are those caused by aberrations of the immune system and affect the body's ability to fight disease. If the body produces agents that actually attack it, the process is known as **autoimmune disease.** Overreaction or unwanted reactions of the immune system causes allergic diseases. **Metabolic diseases** encompass a wide variety of biochemical disorders and will not be discussed further in this text.

Diseases of unknown cause are termed **idiopathic.** Adverse reactions resulting from treatment by a health professional produce **iatrogenic** disease. **Nosocomial** diseases are those acquired while the patient is in a hospital environment.

INJURY

There are two types of injury: acute and chronic. **Acute injury** has a sudden onset and is severe although short-lived. Acute injury can involve **hypoxia** (reduced oxygen supply to tissue) or even anoxia. Such injuries can lead to necrosis. When an acute injury occurs, a **thrombus** (a blood clot that adheres to a vessel wall) may accompany it. Thrombi can narrow the vessel, causing vascular insufficiency. If the thrombus dislodges and moves through the blood stream, it is called an **embolus.** Any particulate matter that moves through a vessel is an embolus. Examples of common emboli after a severe fracture of a long bone, particularly the femur, are fat and bone marrow. Emboli and thrombi are dangerous and should be treated promptly.

Chronic injury is one of a recurring nature,

such as a shoulder that dislocates repeatedly. With chronic injury, atrophy is usually involved. **Atrophy** is an acquired process that is regressive. It results from a decrease in cell size or cell numbers or both. It is actually a progressive wasting away of any part of the body, causing impairment or loss of function. There are four types of atrophy.

1. **Senile:** This type of atrophy occurs with age and involves shrinkage of the brain tissue. Memory is impaired, but senile atrophy is *not* Alzheimer's disease.
2. **Disuse:** When a body part is not used it will atrophy. An example is a casted leg in which the muscle tissue shrinks considerably in the 6 to 8 weeks of disuse.
3. **Pressure:** Atrophy as a result of steady pressure on tissue is not uncommon. Bedsores are an example of pressure atrophy.
4. **Endocrine:** This type of atrophy is caused by decreased hormonal production. For example, when a woman goes through menopause, estrogen and progesterone are no longer produced. The lack of these hormones causes the uterus and ovaries to shrink.

INFLAMMATION

As with injury, there are acute and chronic inflammations. When an injury occurs, the body responds by becoming inflamed at the site of injury. Inflammation is what actually allows the healing process to begin. The inflammatory response serves a protective and defensive purpose in that it attempts to neutralize and destroy injurious agents. Leukocytes attack the cellular debris and clean the site. This process is known as **phagocytosis.**

Acute inflammation has four clinical cardinal symptoms:

1. red skin (rubor)
2. swelling (edema)
3. heat at site (calor)
4. pain (dolor)

A fifth symptom may be loss of function; however, this depends on the site and the extent of injury. Loss of function is not usually considered a cardinal symptom because of its variable occurrence. Both heat and redness of the skin are caused by increased vascularity at the site of injury. The blood vessels become dilated and there is increased permeability of the capillary walls. Vasodilation allows an increase in blood supply to be delivered to the injured area; resulting in **congestion.** Congestion manifests itself by heat and redness of skin and becomes apparent within minutes after an injury.

Swelling and pain occur as a result of exudate increasing interstitial fluid, which then presses on nerve endings.

Chronic inflammation lasts for extended periods of time and is often associated with sublethal degeneration. Tissue necrosis is uncommon. Examples of chronic inflammation are asthma, hay fever, and other allergies. Many are environmental.

Fluids that are results of inflammation are called transudates or exudates, which should be distinguished from one another. As capillaries dilate and become permeable, passage of fluid from one side of the vessel wall to the other becomes possible. A **transudate** is a collection of fluid in tissue or in a body space caused by increased hydrostatic or decreased osmotic pressure in the vascular system without loss of protein into the tissue. Thus transudates are watery, with low protein content. **Exudates** are the result of increased osmotic pressure in the tissue because of high protein content and are caused by inflammation or obstruction of lymphatic flow. Exudates tend to be more localized than transudates because most inflammations are localized, whereas the effects of increased hydrostatic pressure or depleted serum proteins are usually generalized.

Purulent exudate (also called **pus**) is an exudate that is loaded with live and dead leukocytes. An inflammatory reaction with a lot of purulent exudate is called **suppurative inflammation.** A localized collection of pus is an **abscess.** When pus fills a body cavity such as the pleural cavity, the term **empyema** is used.

REPAIR

Regardless of the cause or the type of inflammation, the sequence of events that occur in an inflammation is:

1. Alteration in vascularity and capillary permeability
2. Spread of white blood cells (leukocytes) to the site of inflammation
3. Phagocytosis
4. Repair of injury

When the body attempts to heal itself and return to its normal status, repair is being accomplished. There are two primary types of repair, **regeneration** of normal parenchymal cells that are identical to the original cells, or proliferation of **granulation tissue** and eventual scar formation. In the latter case, the original structure and function of the tissue is not restored. Since regeneration allows the original structure and function to be duplicated and restored, this is the most desired form of repair.

The repair process of wounds is separated into **primary union** and **secondary union,** depending on whether the wound edges are placed together or left separated. The best example of repair by primary union is that which follows a clean surgical incision of the skin in which there is minimal tissue damage and the edges of the wound are closely approximated by tape or sutures.

Repair by secondary union utilizes the same basic process as primary union, except there is greater injury, with consequent greater tissue damage and more inflammation to resolve. To fill the void left by tissue damage, there is a tremendous proliferation of capillaries and fibroblasts. This is a long process that leaves scars in the form of fibrous connective tissue.

FUNDAMENTAL TISSUES

The cells of the body are derived from one cell, the fertilized ovum. The cells of the developed organism can be divided into germ cells (normally confined to the gonads) and somatic cells. Somatic cells are classified under four major categories: epithelial cells, connective tissue cells, muscle tissue cells, and nervous tissue cells.

Epithelial cells are generally those that arise from the embryonic ectoderm and endoderm. Different forms of epithelial cells have different functions. Some create tissue to form the lining of body spaces, while others become a protective layer and cover surfaces of the various glands and organs.

Connective tissue cells, which are mostly derived from mesoderm, are the most widespread in the body. They lend support wherever the body needs it, such as tendons and ligaments. Their main purpose is to connect and bind.

Muscle tissue cells are also derived from mesoderm but resemble epithelial cells in their close approximation to each other. Muscle tissue cells are long and slender and are called fibers. The fibers decrease in length and increase in thickness to cause contraction and provide movement. Muscle tissue plays a role in vital body functions. There are three types of muscle tissue: voluntary (striated), involuntary (smooth), and cardiac (involuntary, striated).

Nerve tissue cells are derived from ectoderm and include nerve cells (neurons) and their supporting cells (neuroglia). Nerve tissue is the most highly specialized tissue in the body. It activates and integrates the body as a whole. Neurons have very long processes, known as axons, which carry electrical impulses to the brain and spinal cord, causing all conductivity in the body.

ALTERED TISSUE GROWTH

The tendency of cells to undergo a growth alteration is related to their involvement in physiologic replacement. The proliferative capacity of cells relates to the process of maturation from a nonspecific cell type to a specialized cell. There is a direct relationship between the reproductive capability of the cell and the occurrence of disease. Two cell types that undergo continuous replacement are epithelial and endothelial. As such, these cells are the most susceptible to growth changes. Muscle tissue has limited ability to reproduce; therefore, growth alterations are uncommon. Alterations in growth are very rare in nerve tissue in that neurons and neuroglia are incapable of reproduction.

Altered tissue growth, also known as **growth disturbance,** can be defined as a departure from normal tissue growth caused by the multiplication of cells. Since hyperplasias and neoplasms are both characterized by proliferation of cells that increase tissue mass, these can be classified as the two categories of growth disturbances. Hyperplasias and neoplasms differ on the basis of cause and growth potential.

Hyperplasia is an exaggerated response to various stimuli in the form of an increase in the number of cells in the tissue. Hyperplasia may recede if the stimulus is removed, provided permanent structural changes have not occurred. Hyperplasia typically involves tissues that undergo physiologic replacement, but it may involve stable tissue. Hyperplasia may be caused by a wide variety of stimuli, such as a remote response to inflammation, hormone excess or hormone deficiency, chronic irritation, or unknown factors. Hypertrophy should be distinguished from hyperplasia; both frequently occur together. **Hypertrophy** refers to an increase in cell size, whereas hyperplasia refers to an increase in cell numbers. The term hypertrophy is best applied to muscles, as the muscle fiber (cell) enlarges as a response to increased workload rather than undergoing hyperplasia. **Metaplasia** occurs when a normal cell becomes abnormal. This is unlike hyperplasia in that metaplasia is an abnormality of growth in an individual cell. As such, it has not taken on tumor characteristics.

Neoplasms are growths that proliferate with varying degrees of independence from normal cellular control mechanisms. Neoplasms are presumed to arise by mutation or altered genetic control. They behave as if they were an independent parasitic organism. A neoplasm continues to grow after the agent is removed.

Most neoplasms can be classified as benign or malignant. **Benign** neoplasms are single masses of cells that remain localized at their site of origin and limited in their growth. Examples of benign tumors include adenoma, angioma, cystadenoma, fibroma, lipoma, and myoma. **Malignant** neoplasms are defined by their potential to invade and metastasize at some point in their life history. **Invasion** refers to direct extension of neoplastic cells into surrounding tissue without regard for tissue boundaries.

Metastasis means transplantation of cells to a new site. There are three ways for metastasis to occur:

1. **Seeding:** This is a diffuse spread of tumor cells. The tumor invades a body cavity by penetration. An example is a gastrointestinal tumor in which cells penetrate the peritoneum and travel to the bladder.
2. **Lymphatic:** This is the most common way tumor cells are spread. The cells travel through the lymph system to other areas.
3. **Hematogenous:** This occurs when cells penetrate blood vessels and are then sent into the circulatory system. When the large cells get trapped in the small vessels, they pass through the vessel wall and into the tissue, where they multiply.

The term carcinoma or sarcoma is added to the name of the tissue when malignant neoplasms are defined. If the neoplasm is from the epithelium, **carcinoma** is used; if it is from nonepithelial tissue, such as connective tissue, **sarcoma** is used. **Lymphoma** is cancer of the lymphatic system, whereas **leukemia** is malignancy of the blood and related organs.

Currently, in the United States, the leading cause of death due to cancer in women is endometrial carcinoma. Breast and lung carcinoma follow closely. In males, heart disease and prostate cancer are the leading causes of death. Bronchogenic carcinoma has fallen to 3rd place in recent years.

When a malignant tumor reproduces the normal structure it is said to be **differentiated.** The more highly differentiated the tumor, the less the degree of malignancy. The process of determining the degree of differentiation, and thus the degree of malignancy, is expressed as **grading.** Grade 1 tumors are the most differentiated and least malignant. Grade 4 are the most malignant and least differentiated. The size of tumors at the primary site and the presence of any metastasis are evaluated through a process known as **staging.** Staging is critical, as the choice of treatment relies on this assessment.

Throughout the remaining chapters of this book, it will be helpful to refer to this chapter as well as to the glossary. The pathologic conditions that are about to be studied are not easily memorized. There are many "classic signs" seen on the radiograph that will need to be remembered, and the reader is encouraged to take the time necessary to fully understand the processes and not simply memorize them.

Review Questions

1. Define functional and structural diseases. What is the major difference between the two? Give two examples of each type of disease.
2. List the three major forms of organic disease. What are the fundamental characteristics of each of these forms?
3. Name the six major types of causes of disease. Which causes are external and which are internal in origin?
4. Name the four types of atrophy encountered and define each. What type of injury is atrophy usually associated with?
5. List the three ways that malignant neoplasms disseminate to distant sites of the body. Explain how each of these happens.
6. What are the characteristics of acute and chronic injury?
7. Define growth disturbance. Name the two categories and explain the difference between the two.
8. Define repair. List the two primary types of repair and explain each.
9. Define the following terms.

Pathogenesis	Idiopathic
Syndrome	Prognosis
Sign	Procedure
Necrosis	Thrombus
Neoplasia	Embolus
Infection	Diagnosis
Nosocomial	Symptom
Manifestation	Congenital anomaly
Degeneration	Hyperplasia
Anoxia	Malignant
Etiology	Iatrogenic
History	Phagocytosis
Lesion	Test
Inflammation	Ischemia
Benign	Pathology

10. List the four clinical cardinal symptoms of acute inflammation. How does inflammation allow healing to begin?
11. Name four types of fundamental tissues and give an example of each.
12. Describe how acute injury can be associated with vascular insufficiency.

CHAPTER II

Contrast Media

Goals

1. To learn the three classifications of contrast media.
2. To be able to list the characteristics of the contrast media used in radiography.
3. To recognize the uses and contraindications of contrast media and the treatment for reactions to contrast media.

Objectives

At the completion of the chapter, the radiographer will be able to:

1. List commonly used contrast media with their indications, contra-indications, and use in special procedures.
2. Define the classifications of contrast media and give examples of each.
3. List the characteristics of radiopaque and radiolucent contrast media.
4. Explain the composition of positive contrast media.
5. Describe the difference between ionic and nonionic contrast media.
6. List the adverse reactions possible to contrast media and what treatment should be given.
7. Explain how contrast media are chosen for a procedure.

I. Classifications
  A. Radiolucents
    1. Air
    2. Oxygen
    3. Carbon Dioxide
    4. Nitrous Oxide
  B. Radiopaques
    1. Insoluble
      a. Barium
    2. Water-Soluble
      a. All Others
  C. Radionuclides
    1. Emit Radiation
    2. Used in Nuclear Medicine
II. Characteristics
  A. Radiolucent (Negative)
    1. Low Atomic Weight
    2. Decreases Organ Density
    3. Decreases Absorption of Radiation
    4. Increases Film Density
    5. Radiolucent
    6. Absorbed by the Body
  B. Radiopaque (Positive)
    1. High Atomic Weight
    2. Increases Organ Density
    3. Increases Absorption of Radiation
    4. Decreases Film Density
    5. Radiopaque
    6. Excreted Unchanged by Liver or Kidneys
    7. Relatively Nontoxic
III. Composition of Radiopaques
  A. Iothalamate
    1. Methylglucamine (Meglumine) Salts
    2. Sodium Salts
    3. Combination of 1. and 2.
  B. Diatrizoate
    1. Methylglucamine (Meglumine) Salts
    2. Sodium Salts
    3. Combination of 1. and 2.
  C. Cation (Positive Charge)
    1. Either Meglumine or Sodium Salts
  D. Anion (Negative Charge)
    1. Other Side Chain
IV. Nonionic versus Ionic Contrast Media
  A. Chemical Structure
  B. Osmolality
V. Selection of a Contrast Medium
  A. Viscosity
  B. Type of Ionic Salt
  C. Iodine Content
  D. Miscibility
  E. Persistence
  F. Toxicity
  G. Osmolality
VI. Procedures and Contrast Media
  A. Biliary
    1. Telepaque (Iopanoic Acid)
    2. Oragrafin (Ipodate)
      a. Sodium
      b. Calcium
    3. Cholografin (Meglumine Salt of Iodipamide)
    4. Hypaque (Sodium Diatrizoate)
    5. Renografin (Meglumine Diatrizoate)
    6. Conray (Meglumine Iothalamate)
    7. Cholecystagogues
  B. Gastrointestinal
    1. Barium Sulfate
    2. Hypaque
    3. Gastrografin (Meglumine Diatrizoate)
  C. Genitourinary
    1. Hypaque
    2. Renografin
    3. Conray
  D. Neurogenic
    1. Pantopaque (Iophendylate)
      a. Disadvantages
      b. No Longer Used
    2. Amipaque (Metrizamide)
    3. Isovue (Iopamidol)
    4. Omnipaque (Iohexol)
  E. Respiratory
    1. Dionosil (Propyliodone)
  F. Salivary Ducts
    1. Lipiodol (Iodized Oil)
    2. Ethiodol (Ethiodized Oil)
  G. Reproductive
    1. Water-Soluble
      a. Salpix (Meglumine Diatrizoate)
      b. Sinografin (Meglumine Diatrizoate)
    2. Oily
      a. Lipiodol
      b. Ethiodol
  H. Lymph System
    1. Localizing Dye
      a. Evans Blue
      b. Azurine Blue
      c. Patent Blue Violet Dye
    2. Contrast Medium: Ethiodol
VII. Reactions to Contrast Media and Their Treatment
  A. Minor
    1. Nausea
    2. Vomiting
    3. Hives
    4. Urticaria
      a. Antihistamine
      b. Subcutaneous Epinephrine
      c. Intravenous Line
  B. Intermediate
    1. Hypotension
    2. Respiratory Distress
      a. Bronchospasm
        1. Epinephrine
        2. Oxygen
        3. Bronchodilator
      b. Laryngospasm
        1. Epinephrine
        2. Oxygen
      c. Angioedema
        1. Subcutaneous Epinephrine
        2. Intravenous Line
  C. Major
    1. Increased Pulse
    2. Drop in Blood Pressure
      a. Intravenous Infusion of 5% Dextrose in Water
      b. Antihistamine
      c. Adrenalin (Epinephrine) Mixed with Sterile Water
      d. Oxygen
      e. Solu-Cortef (Hydrocortisone Sodium Succinate)
  D. Vasovagal
    1. Pallor
    2. Cold Sweats
    3. Rapid Pulse
    4. Near Syncope
      a. Trendelenburg Position
      b. Intravenous Line

CLASSIFICATIONS

Contrast agents are used in radiography because some organs and tissues do not have sufficient density or provide adequate contrast with adjacent tissues to be visualized without the aid of a contrast medium. In radiography, contrast means density difference.

Contrast media are classified as pharmaceuticals by the Federal Food and Drug Administration. There are three classifications of contrast materials: radiopaques, which absorb radiation; radiolucents, which decrease density; and radionuclides, which emit radiation and are used in nuclear medicine. Radionuclides will not be discussed further in this text; however, the radiographer should be aware that they are considered contrast agents and that they emit radiation.

CHARACTERISTICS

Radiolucents are also called negative contrast agents. There are four: oxygen, air, nitrous oxide, and carbon dioxide. Of these four, two of them are dangerous because they can cause a gas emboli. Those two are air and oxygen.

Characteristics of negative contrast media are:

1. low atomic weight—therefore it will
2. decrease the organ density—because it
3. absorbs less radiation—which causes a
4. greater film density
5. radiolucent (can see through it)
6. rapidly absorbed by the body

Procedures utilizing negative contrast include pneumoarthrography and pneumocolon (air-contrast barium enema). Most other procedures that utilized negative contrast media, such as pneumoventriculography, pneumoencephalography, and retroperitoneal pneumography, have become outdated with the advent of computed tomographic and magnetic resonance imaging technology.

Radiopaques are also called positive contrast agents. There are two categories of positive media: insoluble, of which barium is the only one, and soluble, which are all the others. Barium does not dissolve in water to any significant degree but is merely suspended. Mixing is necessary so that the barium crystals remain dispersed in water. If the container is allowed to stand, the barium crystals settle to the bottom.

The soluble agents contain iodine in some form. Iodine is used because it is readily available, has a nonmetallic atomic number, and is easily exchangeable with other ions. Water-soluble contrast agents are not without their disadvantages. These agents are hypertonic, causing water and electrolytes to be drawn into the bowel. The high tonicity also causes dilution and reduces the degree of contrast.

Characteristics of positive contrast agents are:

1. high atomic weight—therefore they
2. increase the organ density—because it
3. absorbs more radiation—which causes
4. decreased film density
5. radiopaque (can't see through it)
6. readily excreted unchanged through the liver or kidneys
7. relatively nontoxic

COMPOSITION

Differences in radiopaque contrast media can cause significant changes in radiodensity of tissue substance, which is related to the amount of iodine in the contrast medium. Two common iodinated substances are iothalamate and diatrizoate. Each of these contains methylglucamine (meglumine) salts or sodium salts or a combination of the two. Meglumine compounds are less toxic but are more viscous than sodium compounds. All positive contrast media are made up of a cation (a positive charge) and an anion (a negative charge). The cation is either the sodium or the meglumine compound. The anion is basically the same in all media, with the exception of one side chain, and determines the rest of the makeup of the contrast agent.

NONIONIC VERSUS IONIC CONTRAST MEDIA

The development of radiopaque, iodinated intravascular contrast media of lower osmolality (LOCM), both ionic and nonionic in nature, has made better and safer contrast media available. A great deal of research into the chemistry and molecular structure, toxicity, and solubility of contrast materials has resulted in the development of iodinated compounds that can be safely used in intravascular diagnostic radiology. The express purpose of these agents is to provide contrast enhancement and improved diagnostic images. The currently available contrast media can be divided into four major groups according to their chemical structure: ionic monomers, ionic mono-acid dimers, nonionic monomers, and nonionic dimers. An example of an ionic monomer is iothalamate. The nonionic monomers include iohexol (Omnipaque), iopamidol (Isovue), and others. Ioxaglate meglumine and ioxaglate sodium (Hexabrix) is an ionic dimer. This compound provides the same ratio of atoms to ionized particles as do LOCMs. The lower osmolality, reduced toxicity, and high interaction with water (hydrophilicity) of the LOCM offer an increased safety factor for patients, especially those with known risk factors.

The chemical structures of nonionic and ionic contrast media differ significantly. A common error is made in thinking that nonionic means noniodinated, which is untrue. It must be remembered that both ionic and nonionic compounds contain iodine.

In the 1960s, all water-soluble contrast media were salts of iodinated benzoic acid derivatives. These compounds became the mainstay of radiographic and computed tomography imaging. Be-

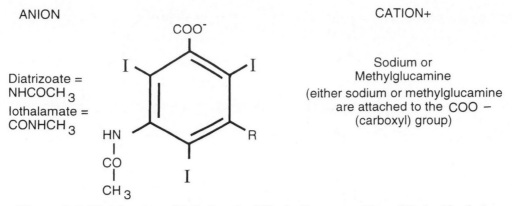

ANION

Diatrizoate = NHCOCH$_3$

Iothalamate = CONHCH$_3$

COO$^-$

CATION+

Sodium or Methylglucamine (either sodium or methylglucamine are attached to the COO – (carboxyl) group)

Figure 2–1. Diatrizoate and iothalamate differ in the composition of their side chain.

cause they are salts, they consist of a positively charged cation and a negatively charged anion. Typically, they are organic acids with three hydrogen atoms replaced by iodine atoms and three hydrogen atoms replaced by simple side chains. These salts are strong acids and are completely dissociated (ionized) in solution. For every three iodine atoms in solution for contrast, two particles for osmolality exist—one anion and one cation. The cation most often used is sodium or a sodium and methylglucamine combination. Examples of these ionic monomers include diatrizoate sodium-meglumine (Renografin and Hypaque) and iothalamate sodium or meglumine (Conray). Figure 2–1 shows a triiodinated fully substituted benzene ring compound. Diatrizoate and iothalamate differ only in the composition of their side chains at the 3-carbon position (R). Either sodium or methylglucamine (meglumine) is attached to the carboxyl (COO-) group at the 1-carbon position.

The late 1960s brought about a significant advance in iodinated radiopaque contrast agents with the concept of a ratio between the imaging effect of the contrast medium and the osmotic effect of the contrast medium. In other words, attention was focused on the ratio between the number of iodine

atoms present and the number of particles in solutions. These are the osmolality and ionicity of contrast agents, which have a bearing on the toxicity of agents. The cation was eliminated from the ionic media because cations contain no iodine and give no diagnostic information. However, it was responsible for as much as 50 percent of the osmotic effect of an agent, which increases the risk for adverse reactions. The ionizing carboxyl group (COO-) of high osmolality contrast media is replaced with a nondissociating group such as amide or glucose. When dissolved in water, a nonionic compound forms a molecular (nonionizing) solution. Each dissolved molecule contains three iodine atoms and only one particle in solution, a ratio of three to one. Figures 2–2 and 2–3 show nonionic monomeric configurations such as iopamidol or iohexol. Notice that there are five hydroxyl (OH) groups found in iopamidol and that there are six in iohexol. Since the carboxyl groups have been eliminated and hydroxyl groups have been added, these are low in osmolality. Finally, in Figure 2–4, an ionic dimer, Hexabrix, is shown. This compound contains six iodine atoms but it dissociates in solution into an anion and cation. Sodium and meglumine are

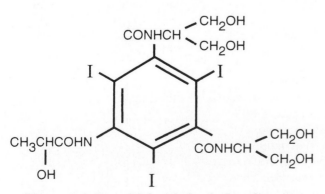

Figure 2–2. Iopamidol with five hydroxyl groups.

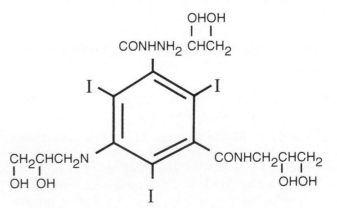

Figure 2–3. Iohexol contains six hydroxyl groups.

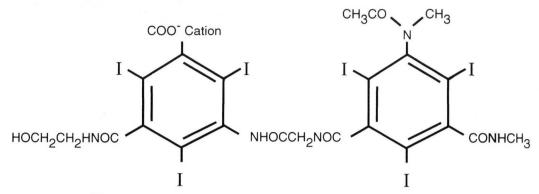

Figure 2–4. Hexabrix is a nonionic dimer with six iodine atoms.

attached to the carboxyl (COO-) group. Because Hexabrix contains six iodine atoms and two ionized particles, it still retains the three to one ratio of the low osmolality contrast agents.

Osmolality of a contrast agent is a significant factor to consider when side effects may cause severe complications. Conventional ionic agents are significantly hyperosmotic to body fluids such as blood because they dissociate into separate ions in solution. This can cause adverse effects, such as cardiac problems, vein cramping and pain, and abnormal fluid retention. Nonionic contrast agents have an osmolality that is significantly closer to human plasma than a corresponding ionic agent at a similar iodine concentration because of the three to one ratio explained earlier. Nonionic monomeric compounds are only one to three times the osmolality of human serum. Nonionic dimeric compounds can approach a hypo-osmolar or iso-osmolar state with human serum and still remain viscous with high iodine concentrations. Contrast agents that have less osmolality than body fluid will result in fewer and less severe side effects. Thus nonionic contrast agents are advantageous in this respect; however, there is no appreciable difference in image quality with nonionic media.

Table 2–1 compares the iodine concentration and the osmolality of the various types of contrast media.

THE SELECTION OF CONTRAST AGENTS

When choosing a contrast medium, there are certain characteristics to look for.

1. Viscosity: The resistance of fluid to movement (how thick it is) is known as viscosity and depends on molecular size and concentration, as well as the friction of the component molecules in solution. In general, viscosity varies proportionately with the concentration of iodine. As iodine content rises, so does viscosity. The viscosity is largely controlled by the composition of the side chain on the molecule. Meglumine compounds are more viscous than are sodium salt compounds. The more viscous a material, the harder the injection is to give. There are several methods to reduce the difficulty of the injection. The contrast agent can be heated to reduce the viscosity; a needle with a larger bore or a catheter with a larger diameter can be used; the injection can be made under pressure; the injection can be delivered over a longer period of time.

2. Type of ionic salt: The two ionic salts most commonly used in ionic contrast media are sodium and meglumine. Each is associated with characteristics that can influence properties of the compound. Sodium salts permit high iodine con-

Table 2–1.

Iodine Concentration and Osmolality for Ionic and Nonionic Contrast Agents as Related to the Human Plasma

Substance	Iodine Concentration, % (mg/mL)	Osmolality
Hexabrix	32 (320)	600
Iopamidol	30 (300)	616
	37 (370)	796
Iohexol	30 (300)	672
	35 (350)	844
Meglumine diatrizoate Sodium diatrizoate injection 60%	29.2 (292)	1420
Meglumine diatrizoate Sodium diatrizoate injection 76%	37 (370)	1940
Human plasma	—	300

centrations without high viscosity and are recommended for urography. Contrast media that contain a greater amount of meglumine salt deliver a smaller amount of iodine per second to the patient because of the increased weight of the meglumine ion. To illustrate this concept, Hypaque 50% and Conray 60% are compared. The Hypaque contains 100 percent sodium salt and Conray contains 100 percent meglumine salt. Yet the iodine content of Hypaque is 300 mg/mL as compared with 282 mg/mL found in Conray. Contrast agents containing meglumine salts are used in procedures such as peripheral arteriography.

3. Iodine content: It is the volume distribution of iodine in the contrast agent that provides the contrast enhancement for imaging. The more iodine content there is in the contrast agent, the more attenuation of the radiographic beam. Contrast agents may have a high, moderate, or low iodine concentration; however, 300 mg of iodine is needed to produce adequate opacity on radiographs. For example, Renografin 60% contains 292 mg of iodine and is acceptable for the renal system. However, for visualization of the blood vessels, Renografin 76%, which contains 370 mg of iodine, is needed. Higher concentrations of iodine are necessary to overcome dilution and the speed with which the contrast agent travels.

4. Miscibility: The ability of the medium to mix with other fluids is called miscibility. Oily contrast media have either a very low or a zero miscibility factor, whereas water-soluble agents have a very high factor. Media with a high miscibility factor have less of a chance of causing an emboli; however, these contrast agents become diluted with the fluids they are injected into.

5. Persistence: Persistence refers to the amount of time the contrast agent stays in the body. Negative contrast media are rapidly absorbed, so the radiographs have to be taken relatively quickly.

6. Toxicity: An obvious consideration in the selection of a contrast medium is whether the compound is lethal when injected. Methylglucamine salt compounds are less toxic than sodium salts. The more meglumine salt, the lower the iodine content that is actually delivered to the body. Because the meglumine salt ion weighs more, the iodine delivered per second is less. However, if a contrast medium with a high iodine concentration delivery is needed, thereby causing the choice of sodium over meglumine, calcium and magnesium can be added to reduce the toxicity of the sodium salt agents.

7. Osmolality: The osmolality is a measure of the number of dissolved particles, whether ions, molecules, or compounds, in a solution. Solutions may be hyperosmolar (greater osmolality than body fluids), hypoosmolar (lower osmolality than body fluids), or isoosmolar (equal osmolality as body fluids). The closer the osmolality of a contrast medium is to the osmolality of body fluids, the less potential there is for adverse reactions caused by differences in osmolality. Hyperosmolar compounds cause more direct endothelial damage. The agents with high osmolality may cause more abrupt or severe hemodynamic changes, such as decreased cardiac output, changes in pulmonary artery pressure, and changes in heart rate. All contrast agents have a greater osmolality than body fluids, but they differ in the degree of their hyperosmolality.

Of course, the ultimate choice is left up to the radiologist, but the radiologic technologist needs to be aware of why certain media are used.

BODY SYSTEMS, PROCEDURES, AND CONTRAST AGENTS

The contrast agents discussed in this section are the media most often used for the indicated study. The names listed are trade names, and the compound is in parentheses.

Biliary

Contrast agents used in the biliary examination are known a cholecystopaques. Several of these are oral contrast media that require a specific time frame to highlight the gallbladder.

Telepaque (iopanoic acid) comes in capsule form and is administered the night before the examination. Usually six tablets are taken, one at a time, with a small amount of water. The patient must not consume any fat until after the examination, as a fatty meal will cause the gallbladder to contract and thus excrete the contrast agent.

Another oral cholecystographic agent is **Oragrafin** (sodium or calcium ipodate). **Sodium Oragrafin** is absorbed slowly and affords visualization about 4 hours after it has been ingested. **Calcium Oragrafin** is absorbed quickly, allowing the bile ducts to be seen as early as 20 minutes after ingestion. The gallbladder is usually seen about 12 hours later.

Visualization of the gallbladder with Telepaque depends on its conjugation with glucuronide in the liver, the flow of the bile into the gallbladder, and the concentrating ability of the mucosa of the gallbladder. If the gallbladder is unable to concentrate the compound, there will be essentially no visualization. The action of Oragrafin is different in that visualization of the gallbladder by the use of this material depends on rapid absorption from the bowel and thus an increased amount of contrast medium in the biliary system, which gives more density. This permits visualization of the gallbladder even in the presence of gallbladder disease. Nonvisualization of the gallbladder with both Telepaque and Oragrafin indicates obstruction of the cystic duct, provided liver functions are normal. Nonvisualization of the gallbladder with Telepaque alone does not preclude a patent cystic duct system.

When the gallbladder cannot be visualized with the use of either Telepaque or Oragrafin, an intravenous compound can be used, the most common being **Cholografin** (methylglucamine salt of iodipamide). Cholografin has the same action as Oragrafin, but there is less enterohepatic circulation. One must remember that if the serum bilirubin is over the level of approximately 3 mg per 100 mL, the possibility of visualization with any intravenous or oral compound is highly remote, and an examination is not usually indicated.

The drugs used for the biliary system are excreted and secreted through the biliary system into the gallbladder and then into the feces. A small amount is also excreted by the kidneys, and one may see a faint nephrogram or calyceal effect when using intravenous cholangiographic materials.

If the value of the serum bilirubin and serum alkaline phosphatase is increasing, a percutaneous puncture of the biliary system can be obtained and contrast material substituted for bile. Soluble contrast materials such as **Hypaque** (sodium diatrizoate), **Renografin** (meglumine diatrizoate), and **Conray** (meglumine iothalamate) are used for this type of procedure. If the serum bilirubin is *decreasing* in value, it is generally safer to wait and do an oral or intravenous study.

Cholecystagogues are not contrast media but are gallbladder stimulants and include such agents as Neo-Cholex and Bile-Evac. These do not change the density of the organ. Rather, they cause it to empty to demonstrate function.

Although ultrasonography has, for the most part, replaced cholangiographic procedures, the radiologic technologist must be familiar with the different types of contrast agents used for the various procedures of the biliary system. There are still many physicians who request an oral cholecystogram as a complementary procedure to the ultrasonographic examination.

Gastrointestinal

The contrast medium used most often in any examination of the gastrointestinal system is **barium sulfate.** Barium is an insoluble opaque powder of high atomic weight, which allows increased absorption of the x-ray beam. This produces a white image on the radiograph.

Barium by itself is essentially inert, but barium mixed with fecal material produces severe peritonitis and formation of a granuloma. It is, therefore, standard procedure not to use barium when there is a chance of communication between the bowel and the peritoneal space or the pleural space. Any barium that enters either of these two spaces must be removed surgically.

Water-soluble compounds such as Hypaque and **Gastrografin** (meglumine diatrizoate) are used to examine the gastrointestinal tract when the presence of barium in the gastrointestinal tract may be deleterious to the patient, when there is a possibility of occlusion of the colon, or when surgery is anticipated in the near future. The principal contrast materials are compounds of methylglucamine or sodium salts of diatrizoate. The atomic weight of the iodine-containing or soluble compounds does not give as good a radiodensity as the higher atomic weight of barium, however. Also, as the oral soluble compound passes through the small bowel, it is diluted with small bowel juice, creating an even fainter image on the radiograph. Soluble compounds also create an osmotic load to the bowel, accentuating dehydration.

The use of carbon dioxide or air as a double-contrast material with barium is common in all radiology departments. This combination causes no pharmacologic problem.

Genitourinary System

Three commonly used ionic contrast media for visualization of the kidneys, ureters, and bladder are Hypaque, Renografin, and Conray. Isovue is the nonionic contrast agent used most frequently. All four may be given intramuscularly, intravenously, or intra-arterially. Intravenous injection is the most common method.

Good visualization of the renal collecting system is provided with 20 to 25 mL of the agent injected slowly, as recommended by the pharmaceutical companies. It is common practice to use 75 to 100 mL and inject rapidly; however, it must be remembered that there are more side effects, such as nausea and vomiting, with rapid injection than with slow injection. The technologist should also alert the radiologist if the blood urea nitrogen (BUN) level is above 25 mg per mL of serum, as good visualization of the kidneys usually is then not likely, even with the use of a large amount of contrast medium. A drip-infusion technique generally shows the kidneys even when the BUN level is as high as 100 to 110 mg per 100 mL of serum.

The contrast medium disseminates throughout the body and is rapidly excreted unchanged through the kidneys, primarily by glomerular filtration. The contrast material has an osmotic diuretic effect that can be harmful, particularly in dehydrated elderly and infant patients; therefore, the technologist must be alert to any physiologic changes that the patient demonstrates.

Neurogenic Examinations

For many years, **Pantopaque** (iophendylate injection) was used to demonstrate the spinal canal. This very oily compound had an absorption rate equal to approximately 1 mL per year. It therefore had to be removed as completely as possible from the spinal column after completion of the examination. Its use was also accompanied by side effects such as headache, backache, and fever.

Amipaque (metrizamide), developed in 1968 and marketed in 1975, replaced Pantopaque for myelography. Now even metrizamide has given way to nonionic and safer ionic compounds for water-soluble myelography. Two such compounds are **Isovue** (iopamidol) and **Omnipaque** (iohexol). The iopamidol and iohexol provide equal diagnostic quality to that of metrizamide; however, metrizamide produces more side effects, notably nausea and vomiting. The advantages of a water-soluble contrast agent over oily mediums are many. The low viscosity of the compound allows use of a smaller bore needle than that used with iophendylate. The smaller hole provides fewer chances of seepage of cerebrospinal fluid. Also, since the compound is water soluble, there is no need for its removal after the procedure; therefore, the needle can be removed immediately after injection, eliminating the worry about damage to the spinal cord by a needle sticking into the patient's back during the entire procedure. The water-soluble contrast media are absorbed in 24 to 48 hours and are eliminated primarily through the kidneys.

Salivary Ducts

Oily contrast agents such as **Lipiodol** (iodized oil) and **Ethiodol** (ethiodized oil) are instilled in the excretory ducts of the salivary glands through a blunt needle or catheter. The agent is removed by the placement of lemon or other sour juices in the patient's mouth, which increases the flow of saliva from the salivary glands and expels the contrast material. Water-soluble contrast media are not usually used in sialography because of the possibility of adhesive fibrous changes that could obscure and obliterate the ducts.

Reproductive System

Examination of the uterus and uterine tubes has been accomplished by ultrasonography for many years; however, a contrast medium instilled into the uterus through the cervix to perform a hysterosalpingogram is still a common practice. The contrast medium eventually spills into the abdomen, giving visualization of the uterine tubes and the body of the uterus.

Water-soluble and oily contrast agents are both used, but the oily compounds are favored by some examiners because of a tendency of the water-soluble compounds to create adhesions and possible obliteration of the lumen of the tubes. **Sinografin** (meglumine diatrizoate) and **Salpix** (meglumine diatrizoate) are water-soluble contrast agents; Lipiodol is an oily agent.

Lymph System

The lymph channels must be identified before any contrast agent is injected into them. Small amounts of Evans blue, Azurine blue, or patent blue violet dye are injected between the webs of the first three toes. The localizing dye is picked up by the lymph and concentrated in the lymph channels. An oily contrast medium, Ethiodol, can then be injected slowly under pressure into the lymph channels to the lymph nodes.

REACTIONS TO CONTRAST MEDIA AND THEIR TREATMENT

There are essentially three different types of reactions to contrast materials. The American College of Radiology has classified these three categories of adverse reactions as minor, intermediate, and major. These three, plus a fourth reaction caused by fear, are discussed here along with the treatment most often indicated for the various reactions. All treatments to reactions must be administered by a physician or a nurse acting under the orders of a physician. It is now within the scope of a technologist to administer drugs; however, unless the technologist is properly schooled in pharmacology and venipuncture, it is best to allow a radiologist or radiology nurse to inject contrast media and drugs.

Before the injection of contrast material into a patient, the technologist must always question the patient about the presence of an allergic history, since it has been noted that an instance of adverse reaction is more likely to occur in a patient who has an allergic history. A negative history does not guarantee that the patient will be reaction-free, however. Medicolegally, a test dose should be given to every patient.

During any injection of a contrast medium, the patient should be monitored closely for abnormal response or reaction, and emergency drugs, equipment, and medical personnel should be immediately available. The technologist must be watchful for extravasation of the medium into the arm. If this occurs, the application of a warm wet cloth will help reduce the pain.

A **minor** reaction includes nausea, vomiting, hives, and urticaria. Dermal reactions are usually the least significant of adverse effects associated with contrast media and may not require treatment. Although most dermal reactions are self-limiting, antihistamines are chosen if treatment is indicated. Drowsiness is a frequent side effect of the drug. If urticaria is severe, an antihistamine is probably not adequate. In that event, subcutaneous administration of epinephrine is the recommended treatment. If the reaction is serious enough to require epinephrine, an intravenous line to manage possible further complications is advisable. As stated earlier, most minor reactions do not require treatment. Usually, reassurance by the technologist is all that is needed. It is important, however, to recognize that a minor reaction may be followed by a more severe one.

Intermediate reactions include all of the minor reactions plus hypotension and respiratory distress. Respiratory distress can result from bronchospasm, laryngospasm, or angioedema of the upper airway. Angioedema involves subcutaneous tissue; therefore, subcutaneous administration of epinephrine is the course of treatment. Of course every patient and each clinical situation is different. If Benadryl is given, it should be administered in the arm opposite to that in which the contrast medium was injected. Some antihistamines, particularly Benadryl, create a precipitate with the contrast medium, and care must be taken so that such a precipitate is not injected into the patient. In the event the angioedema is not quickly arrested, an intravenous line is advisable.

Epinephrine is also indicated for bronchospasm or laryngospasm. The patient should also be given oxygen. If epinephrine and oxygen are unable to control the respiratory distress, a bronchodilator can be added to control wheezing. Again it must be noted that a patient's condition may deteriorate rapidly and, if bronchospasm or facial and laryngeal edema persist or progress, the emergency team should be alerted. The patient whose reaction is this severe would best be treated as an in-patient, probably in the intensive care unit.

Major or **severe** reactions require immediate treatment, as they are life threatening. Such reactions are caused by a combination of osmotoxic and chemotoxic properties of the contrast medium molecule as well as the ionic composition of the agent when in solution. All reactions described under "mild" and "intermediate" will manifest themselves, in addition to a change in the pulse rate and the blood pressure. Shock, respiratory wheezing, edema, convulsions, and cardiac arrest are all examples of the severe reactions that can occur. Although cardiovascular reactions are the least common, they carry the most risk. Drug intervention depends almost exclusively on whether the patient has bradycardia or tachycardia. Tachycardia represents an anaphylactoid response. Peripheral vasodilatation and increased capillary permeability result in diminished circulating blood volume, falling blood pressure, and rising heart rate. An intravenous line of 5 percent dextrose in water should be started by a qualified individual while the patient's physician is notified. Once the intravenous line has been started, the sequence of drug administration is the same as noted previously, in that some type of antihistaminic should be administered intravenously. Two to 3 minutes later, epinephrine mixed with sterile saline should be administered as indicated. Oxygen must also be given. Quite often, Solu-Cortef (hydrocortisone sodium succinate) must be given to avoid cardiac arrest.

A fourth reaction, called a vasovagal reaction, is not caused by contrast agents but rather by fear of the examination itself. This type of reaction manifests itself as pallor, cold sweats, rapid pulse, and near syncope. Bradycardia and hypotension together are true indicators of a vasovagal reaction. The patient should be placed in the Trendelenburg position, and, if warranted, an intravenous line should be begun for infusion with isotonic fluids. If the response is inadequate, then intravenous atropine can increase the heart rate.

Most reactions will occur within 5 minutes after injection of the contrast medium, but they may occur much later, after the patient has left the department. The patient's physician must always be alerted in the case of a reaction, as the symptoms of a minor reaction may disappear, but later a more severe reaction may take place. It is not unusual for a reaction to occur 2 to 5 hours after injection.

Review Questions

1. List the three categories of adverse reactions to contrast media as defined by the American College of Radiology. Explain fully the symptoms of each and the progressive treatment each would require. List any possible effects

from the treatment drug. Describe the symptoms of the fourth category of reactions and explain its treatment. How do you know that it is a reaction of the fourth type and not of the three types you listed above?

2. Name the four radiolucent contrast agents. Give examples of examinations that would use these agents. List the two radiolucent contrasts that are considered to be dangerous and explain why.

3. Name the types of radiopaque contrast agents used in radiography. Give one example of each type. What are radionuclides? What modality uses radionuclides?

4. Explain the three reasons that iodine is used in soluble contrast materials.

5. List the seven characteristics of contrast media that are considered before a choice is made as to selection of a particular agent. Define what each means.

6. Explain the composition difference between nonionic contrast agents and ionic contrast agents. How does the composition of the nonionic agents affect the reactions to the agent a patient may experience?

7. List the characteristics exhibited by both radiopaque and radiolucent contrast agents.

8. Explain how the high viscosity of a contrast agent can be overcome for injection.

9. Describe the difference between sodium and calcium Oragrafin. How does either type of Oragrafin differ from Telepaque in the manner by which they enter the gallbladder?

10. Explain why water-soluble compounds would be used to examine the gastrointestinal tract. What side effects might these produce?

11. Explain the difference between the two ionic salts most commonly used in ionic contrast media.

12. Explain the composition of positive contrast media.

CHAPTER III

Skeletal System

Goals

1. To review the anatomy and physiology of the skeletal (osseous) system.
2. To learn theories to perform special radiologic procedures on the skeletal system of the body.
3. To learn the basic pathologic conditions of the skeletal system.

Objectives

At the completion of the chapter, the radiographer will be able to:

1. Define the classifications of the skeleton.
2. List and give examples of the five types of bones in the body.
3. List, define, and give examples of the three classifications of joints in the body.
4. Describe the structure of bones.
5. Describe the physiology and function of bones.
6. List and describe four different special radiologic procedures for the skeletal system.
7. Describe arthrography.
8. List and describe the different types of congenital anomalies discussed.
9. Describe nonneoplastic and neoplastic bone changes and give examples of each.
10. Describe and define the different types of fractures discussed.
11. Describe the six types of arthritis listed.
12. List other joint diseases.

I. Anatomy
  A. Classification of Bones
    1. Skeleton
      a. Axial
      b. Appendicular
    2. Bones
      a. Long
        (Miniature Long)
      b. Short
      c. Flat
      d. Irregular
      e. Sesmoid
  B. Structure of Bones
    1. Periosteum
      a. Outer—Dense Fibrous
        Tissue
      b. Inner—Osteoblasts
    2. Compact (Cortical)
    3. Spongy (Cancellous)
      a. Red Bone Marrow
    4. Medullary (Marrow)
      Cavity
      a. Endosteum
      b. Yellow Bone Marrow
  C. Classification of Joints
    1. Fibrous (Synarthrodial)
    2. Cartilaginous
      (Amphiarthrodial)
    3. Synovial (Diarthrodial)
  D. Structure of Joints
    1. Gliding (Plane)
    2. Hinge
    3. Condylar (Ellipsoidal)
    4. Saddle
    5. Pivot
    6. Ball and Socket
II. Physiology and Function
  A. Ossification
    1. Osteoblast
  B. Growth
    1. Length
      a. Osteoblast
    2. Diameter
      a. Osteoblast
      b. Osteoclast
  C. Functions
    1. Support
    2. Protection
    3. Movement
    4. Production of Blood Cells
    5. Storage
III. Special Radiographic
  Procedures
  A. Tomography
  B. Angiography
  C. Computed Tomography/
    Magnetic Resonance Imaging
  D. Nuclear Medicine

  E. Arthrography
  F. Cardinal Rule of any
    Examination
    1. Right Patient/Right
      Examination
    2. Letter Markers
    3. View Whole Film
    4. Take Two Views
    5. Include One Joint
    6. Best Quality Possible
IV. Pathology
  A. Congenital Anomalies
    1. Extra Sesmoid Bones
    2. Transitional Vertebrae
      a. Cervical Ribs
      b. Transitional
        Lumbosacral Vertebrae
      c. Sacralization
    3. Osteogenesis Imperfecta
    4. Osteopetrosis
    5. Achondroplasia
  B. Nonneoplastic Bone Changes
    1. Osteoporosis
    2. Osteomalacia
      a. Rickets
    3. Renal Osteodystrophy
      a. Brown Tumor
    4. Osteomyelitis—Osteitis
      a. Brodie Abscess
    5. Osteitis Deformans
      (Paget Disease)
      a. Acromegaly
    6. Legg-Calvé-Perthes
      disease
  C. Neoplastic Bone Changes
    1. Benign
      a. Fibrous Dysplasia
      b. Bone Cyst
      c. Chondroma
        1. Exostosis
          (Osteochondroma)
        2. Enchondroma
        3. Chondrosarcoma
          (see Malignant)
      d. Osteoclastoma (Giant
        Cell Tumor)
      e. Osteoid Osteoma
    2. Malignant
      a. Chondrosarcoma
      b. Ewing Sarcoma
      c. Multiple Myeloma
      d. Osteogenic Sarcoma
        (Osteosarcoma)
  D. Fractures
    1. Types of Fractures
      a. Complete
      b. Incomplete (Fissure)

      c. Closed
      d. Compound (Open)
      e. Simple
      f. Comminuted
      g. Transverse, Spiral,
        Oblique, Longitudinal
      h. Stellate
      i. Impacted
      j. Displacement
      k. Distraction
      l. Dislocated
      m. Subluxated
      n. Delayed Union
      o. Malunion
      p. Nonunion
    2. Common Fractures
      a. Plastic
      b. Greenstick
      c. Torus
      d. Epiphyseal
      e. Fatigue (March,
        Stress)
      f. Pathologic
      g. Avulsion
      h. Compression
      i. Galeazzi
      j. Monteggia
      k. Colles
      l. Smith
      m. Bennett
      n. Boxer's
      o. Bimalleolar/
        Trimalleolar
      p. Pott
  E. Joint Pathology
    1. Arthritis
      a. Gout
      b. Osteoarthritis
        (Degenerative Joint
        Disease, Hypertrophic
        Arthritis)
      c. Rheumatoid
      d. Tuberculous
        1. Pott Disease
      e. Ankylosing Spondylitis
        (Rheumatoid
        Spondylitis)
      f. Reiter Syndrome
    2. Bursitis
    3. Spondylolisthesis
      a. Spondylitis
      b. Spondylosis
    4. Disk Herniation
  F. Dislocations
    1. Shoulder
      a. Chip Fracture
    2. Hip

ANATOMY

Classification of Bones

The skeletal system, composed of 206 bones, is commonly divided into the axial skeleton, which contains 80 bones of the skull, spine, ribs and sternum, and the appendicular skeleton, which contains the remaining 126 bones of the extremities pectorial and pelvic girdles. There are five classifications of bones:

1. long bones, such as the femur

2. short bones, as in the carpal bones
3. flat bones, like the parietal bones found in the skull
4. irregular bones, such as the vertebrae
5. sesamoid bones, like the patella

Structure of Bones

Bone is a type of connective tissue, but it differs from other connective tissue because of its calcified matrix. All bones, except articular surfaces that are covered with articular cartilage, are covered with two layers of **periosteum.** The outer layer is made up of dense, fibrous tissue and the inner layer is made up of cells called **osteoblasts** that are associated with the production of bone.

Beneath the inner layer of periosteum is a layer called **compact,** or **cortical,** bone. This is a dense, closely knit bone. The **spongy,** or **cancellous,** bone is below the cortical layer. This is porous, loosely knit bone with a honeycomb appearance.

The **medullary,** or **marrow,** cavity is the open canal that runs down the center of the diaphysis (shaft) of long bones and contains the bone marrow. A layer of **endosteum** lines the marrow cavity. Figure 3–1 shows coronal and cross sectional slices through a long bone, indicating the various structures within it.

Two types of tissue are found in the cavities of bones. Red bone marrow is found in the open areas of spongy bone and forms red blood cells. Yellow bone marrow contains predominantly fat and is found in the marrow cavity of long bones.

Classification of Joints

Joints are a part of the skeletal system and must be considered along with the bones. There are three classifications of joints:

1. fibrous joints are immovable and are also called **synarthrodial**
2. cartilaginous joints are only slightly movable and are termed **amphiarthrodial**
3. synovial joints are freely movable and are called **diarthrodial**

Structure of Joints

Fibrous joints have a layer of fibrous tissue that is between the bones. The sutures of the skull are an example of this tissue. Later in life, the tissue atrophies and disappears, and the bone ends become fused.

Cartilaginous joints have cartilage on the bone ends. Between the two bone ends of a cartilaginous joint is a disk made of cartilage and fibrous tissue. The intervertebral joint spaces are called cartilaginous joints, and the intervertebral disks are the firbocartilaginous plates.

Synovial joints have a space between the ends of the bones. The bones are held together by a capsule. Synovial joints get their name from the fluid found in the joint space. This fluid acts as a lubricant and nourishes the hyaline cartilage that lines the articular surface of the joint. Nerve endings are located in the joint capsule to transmit to the brain the movement of the joint. There are six types of synovial joints:

1. Gliding, also called plane: These have flat surfaces that glide over each other. An example is the vertebrae (Fig. 3–2).
2. Hinge: These joints allow angular motion in one direction, as in the elbow (Fig. 3–3).
3. Condylar, or ellipsoidal: These joints have a head-shaped bone that fits into a concave surface that allows motion of flexion, extension, abduction, adduction, and circumduction. A good example is the wrist (Fig. 3–4).
4. Saddle: These joints have one bone end that is convex, which fits into a concave bone end. This allows all motion, as in a condylar joint. The thumb is a saddle joint (Fig. 3–4).
5. Pivot: The head of one bone is surrounded by a ring of cartilage or bone so that there can be rotation. The joint of C-1/C-2 is a pivot joint (Fig. 3–5).
6. Ball and socket: This type of joint has a head-shaped bone end that fits into a cup-shaped socket, as in the hip (Fig. 3–6).

PHYSIOLOGY AND FUNCTION

It is beyond the scope of this text to provide an indepth description of the formation of bones; however, a general overview is needed in order to understand certain pathologic conditions.

When a baby is still an embryo, the skeleton is really a fibrous membrane or hyaline cartilage. **Ossification** is the process of bone replacing these membranes and begins with the appearance of **osteoblasts,** which are bone-forming cells. The osteoblasts form bone matrix, which is composed of large amounts of mucopolysaccharide substance accumulated around each osteoblast and embedded with bundles of collagenous fibers. As soon as bone matrix is formed, complex calcium salts are deposited in it that calcify the matrix, making it hard.

Bones grow longer as a result of cells multiplying in the epiphyseal cartilage. Ossification then occurs in this new cartilage. Bones grow in diameter by

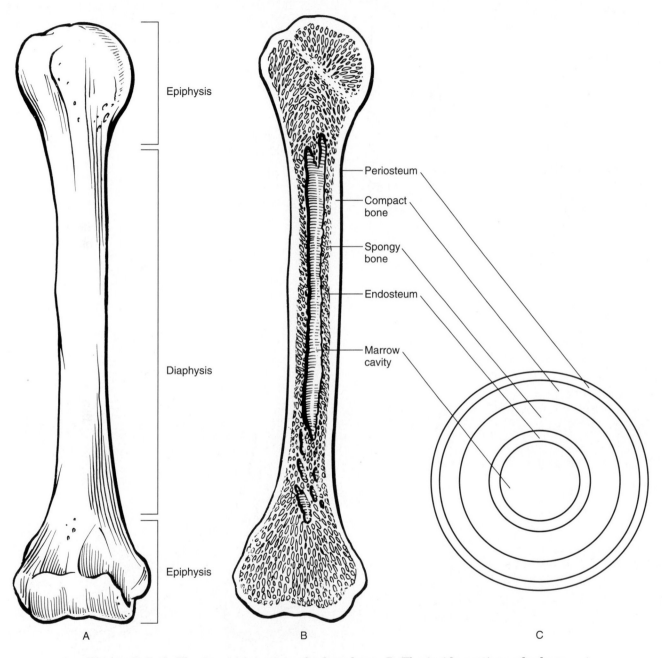

Figure 3–1. *A,* The two major areas of a long bone. *B,* The inside portions of a long bone, including the marrow or medullary cavity. *C,* A cross section of a long bone.

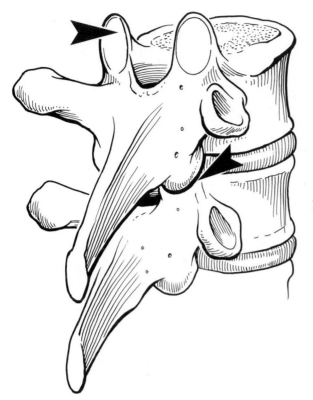

Figure 3–2. The superior and inferior articulating facets meet to form a gliding joint.

Figure 3–3. The humerus and the ulna meet to make a hinge joint.

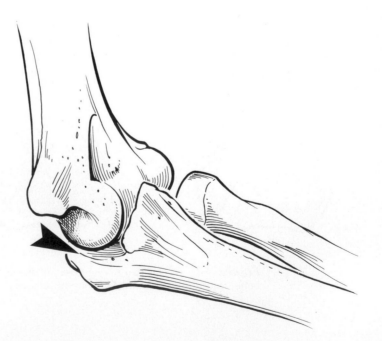

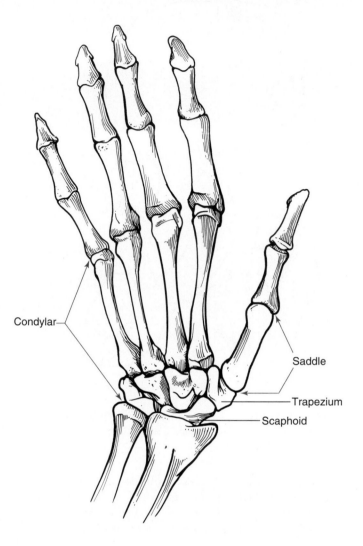

Figure 3–4. The first metacarpophalangeal joint and the carpometacarpal joints are examples of saddle joints. The wrist and metacarpophalangeal joints are condylar joints.

Condylar

Saddle

Trapezium

Scaphoid

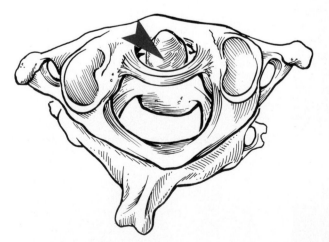

Figure 3–5. The ring of cartilage between the dens and C-1 forms a pivot joint.

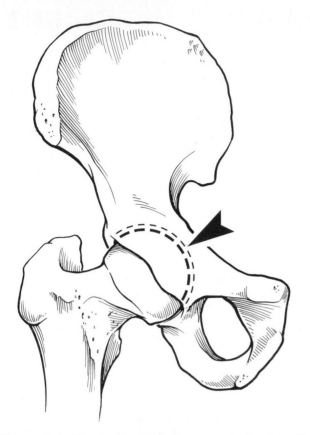

Figure 3–6. The head of the femur as it fits into the acetabulum is a ball-and-socket joint.

the action of two cells. **Osteoclasts** are associated with the absorption and removal of bone. They eat away the inside of the marrow cavity while osteoblasts build up the outside of the bone.

Functions of the skeletal system are as follows:

1. **Support:** The body and the surrounding tissue are supported by the body's skeleton.
2. **Protection:** The organs housed within the body are protected from trauma by the framework surrounding them.
3. **Movement:** The bones and joints are levers and the muscles are the applied force. When a muscle contracts, the bone moves.
4. **Production of blood cells:** The red bone marrow manufactures new blood cells.
5. **Storage:** Important mineral salts such as phosphorous and calcium are stored in the skeletal system.

SPECIAL RADIOGRAPHIC PROCEDURES

Usually, excellent-quality conventional radiography of the skeletal system is sufficient to adequately demonstrate bone lesions and most fractures. However, there are times when more than a routine radiograph is necessary to demonstrate a condition. The following procedures are used to visualize anatomy to determine pathology.

Tomography can be helpful in seeing facial fractures by blurring out the unwanted areas above and below the suspected site of pathology.

Angiography is a good method to determine the extent of lesions. By arteriography, the area can be studied to determine whether it is a neoplasm, whether it is malignant, what the blood supply is (arterial versus venous), whether a biopsy is

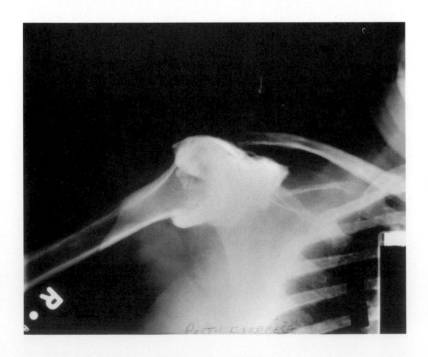

Figure 3–7. Arthrogram of the shoulder.

needed, and if so, where the best needle placement would be. **Computed tomography** and **magnetic resonance imaging** are used extensively to see lesions, fractures, and bone mineralization. Soft-tissue involvement of lesions is seen accurately with computed tomography.

Nuclear medicine isotope uptakes of the skeletal system utilize technetium-labeled bone-seeking pharmaceuticals, which provide high-resolution images. Nuclear medicine will remain clinically and diagnostically useful despite the advancements made in computed tomography and magnetic resonance imaging, as the bone scan provides earlier diagnosis and demonstrates more lesions than other imaging procedures.

Arthrograms are an excellent way to study the joint spaces of the shoulder (Fig. 3–7), wrist, hip, ankle, and most commonly, the knee. Even the temporomandibular joint can be evaluated with arthrography. It is essential for the radiographer to be familiar with this procedure, as it is an examination that can be called almost routine in most radiology departments.

Arthrography is used to demonstrate not only the joint space with the menisci, ligaments, and articular cartilage, but also the surrounding tissue for traumatic damage, disease, and congenital problems (Fig. 3–8). The contrast medium of choice is usually a 30 percent positive contrast solution. A negative contrast agent, such as air, is sometimes used with the positive medium for a double contrast study. If the patient has a history of allergic reactions to iodine, air can be used alone; however, air causes distention of the joint and there is a possibility of an air emboli. Also, the quality of the study is not as good as with positive contrast media or the double contrast method. Positive contrast agents, on the other hand, can obscure the pathology.

The examination is performed under sterile conditions with the radiologist injecting an anesthetic into the joint space and withdrawing synovial fluid. A contrast medium is then injected into the joint space. After the needle has been removed and the joint manipulated to spread the contrast material, spot films under fluoroscopy are taken. Later, several overhead films may be requested. It should be remembered that when any overhead radiographs are made on a double-contrast examination, a horizontal beam should be utilized to demonstrate air fluid levels within the joint.

No matter what type of examination is performed to obtain the diagnosis, six cardinal rules must be remembered.

1. Make sure the correct patient is undergoing the correct examination.

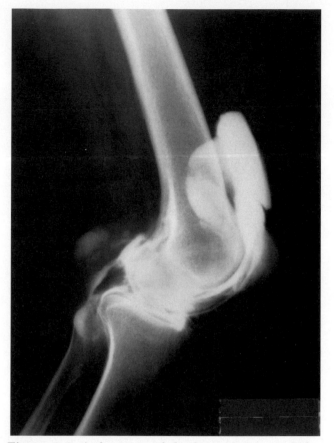

Figure 3–8. Arthrogram of the knee showing a Baker cyst.

2. Make sure the letter markers are on the correct side of the body.
3. View the whole film, not just the areas of interest.
4. Always take two views of a part, at right angles to one another if possible.
5. Always include at least one joint when radiographing extremities.
6. Always take the best quality radiograph that is honestly possible.

PATHOLOGY

Congenital Anomalies

There are some congenital anomalies that are so slight and nonharmful that they are considered nothing more than a variance of the normal skeleton. For example, a small sesamoid bone is sometimes found at the base of the fifth metacarpal. Others are more significant and demonstrate specific radiographic qualities.

A **transitional vertebra** is one that takes on the characteristics of the vertebrae on either side of it. This usually occurs at the junction between the thoracic and lumbar spine or between the lumbar and sacral spine. The L-1 vertebra may have rudimentary ribs articulating with the transverse process, similar to those found at T-12. Another form of transitional vertebra is seen at the C-7/T-1 junction. **Cervical ribs** project off of C-7 (Fig. 3–9) and are of more concern than ribs found at L-1, as they may exert pressure on nerves or arteries and require surgical removal. **Sacralization,** can occur at the L-5/S-1 junction (Fig. 3–10). This happens when L-5 partially or totally *fuses* with the sacrum. If no fusion takes place between the sacrum and L-5, the anomaly is known as transitional lumbosacral vertebrae (Fig. 3-10).

Osteogenesis imperfecta (OI), or "brittle bone" disease, occurs when the skeleton does not ossify properly because of a lack of osteoblastic activity and abnormal collagen formation. The abnormal collagen production also leads to deformed, hypoplastic teeth. The bones are characterized by thin cortices, allowing for fracture with minimal trauma. Fractures can even occur in utero. Multiple fractures in the newborn can result in limb deformities

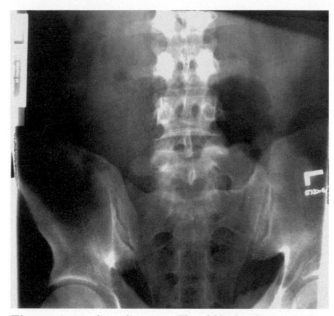

Figure 3–10. Sacralization. The fifth lumbar vertebra demonstrates a transitional transverse process on the patient's left side that is in contact with the sacrum.

and dwarfism (Fig. 3–11). Often, deafness is associated with this disease, since the small ossicles can easily fracture. The connective tissue that surrounds the ossicles may be abnormal as well. The condition of osteogenesis imperfecta becomes less severe with age.

When there is a deficiency of osteoclasts, there is faulty bone resorption. This causes a generalized *increase* in bone density (Fig. 3–12). This condition is known as **osteopetrosis.** This increased density of bone leads osteopetrosis to be called "marble bone" disease. In severe forms, there is obliteration of the marrow cavity and a deformed skull. Patients who suffer from osteopetrosis are prone to osteomyelitis. Radiographically, the bones appear very dense and require an increase in exposure factors to adequately demonstrate the anatomy.

Achondroplasia is the failure of the cartilage that becomes bone to form properly, thus not allowing ossification to proceed as it should (Fig. 3–13). Achondroplasia is the most common cause of dwarfism, since the bones cannot grow in length as they normally would. In contrast to the short arms and legs, the trunk and skull are of normal size. Other malformations include lordosis of the lumbar spine, bow legs, and a bulky forehead with a saddle nose. It is important to remember that the intelligence of achondroplastic dwarfs is not impaired even though the cranium is deformed.

Nonneoplastic Bone Changes

Osteopenia is an umbrella process under which diseases that create decreased bone density fall. When

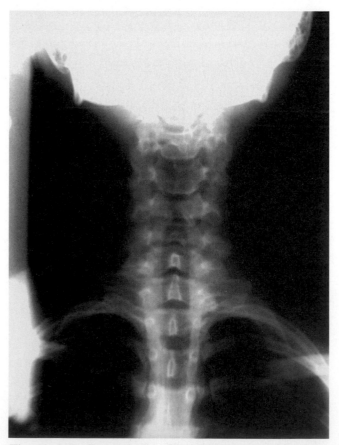

Figure 3–9. Cervical ribs. The patient presented with progressive neck discomfort and tingling of the arms. Cause of symptoms was found to be bilateral rudimentary ribs off the seventh cervical vertebra.

as in Cushing syndrome, are also more susceptible, as the hormone increases the body's ability to reabsorb bone. Pathologic fractures are common in those who suffer from this disease, particularly compression fractures of the thoracic spine causing kyphosis. Other common fractures include fractures of the hip. Radiographs show lack of density due to loss of calcium in the bones and thin cortices with fewer trabeculae. In known cases of osteoporosis, the technical factors should be decreased so as not to overexpose the film and cause a repeat radiograph.

Osteomalacia also falls under the classification of osteopenia because it is an abnormal decrease in bone density caused by a lack of calcium and phosphorus. This defect of mineralization leads to softening of the bone in an adult, even though a normal amount of osteoid is present. This condition is the reverse of osteoporosis, in which there is deficient bone formation. In osteomalacia, there is insufficient calcification of bone. Vitamin D deficiency is a cause of osteomalacia. Pregnancy is another cause, owing to the drain on the calcium in a woman's bones that occurs.

If osteomalacia occurs before the growth plate at the epiphysis closes in children, it is known as **rickets.** Rickets is often called infantile osteomalacia, since the bones lack hardening. In the infantile

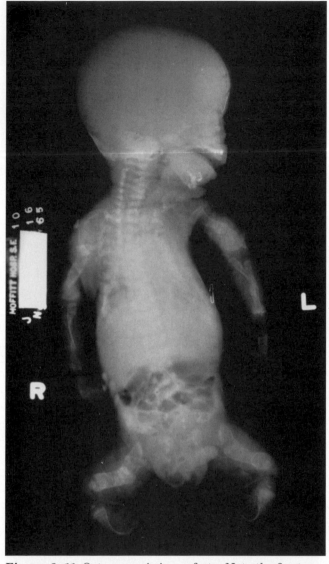

Figure 3–11. Osteogenesis imperfecta. Note the fractures of the femurs and the malformed tibia-fibula. These fractures occurred in utero.

osteoblasts fail to lay down sufficient amount of bone matrix, an abnormal decrease in bone density called **osteoporosis** occurs. There is a lack of osteoid (bone formation), but calcium deposition is normal. The calcium that would normally go to the bone is drained and secreted through urine. Because of this, kidney or bladder stones may be associated with osteoporosis. Osteoporosis may occur in a variety of clinical conditions. Disuse atrophy, as seen in cases of paralysis, causes the bone formation to be diminished and calcium to be drained away. Postmenopausal women are more prone to osteoporosis because of a deficiency in the gonadal hormone level, which leads to decreased bone formation (Fig. 3–14). People who have prolonged use of steroids or suffer from adrenocortical hormone hyperactivity,

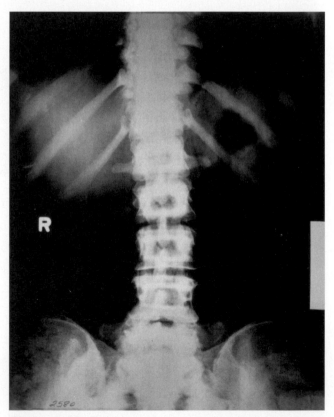

Figure 3–12. Osteopetrosis causes generalized increase in bone density.

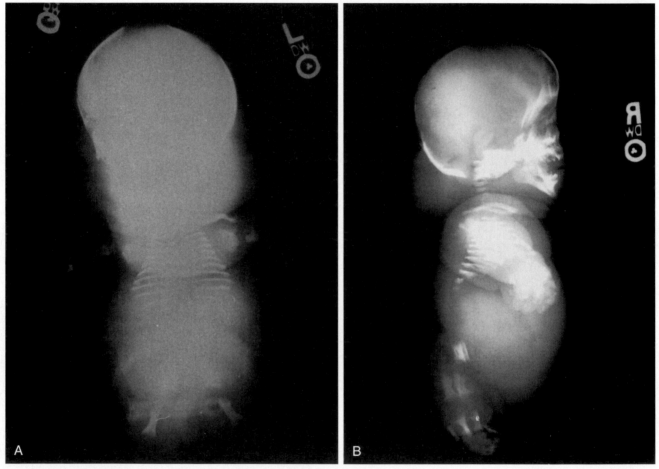

Figure 3–13. Anteroposterior *(A)* and lateral *(B)* views of a stillborn achondroplastic infant. Note the severe soft tissue swelling of the head.

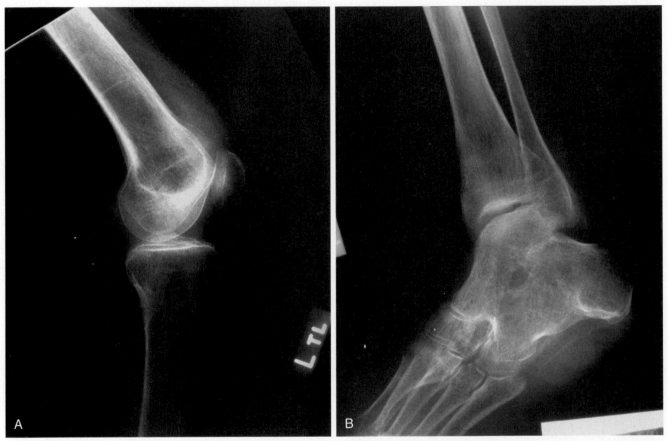

Figure 3–14. Knee *(A)* and ankle *(B)* of a woman with osteoporosis.

form, the osteoid tissue in growing bones is not calcified or hardened, and deformities of the skeleton result. Bowing of the lower legs is a common manifestation (Fig. 3–15).

Osteodystrophy is a disturbance in the growth of bone. Some disturbances are caused by a lack of vitamins, as in osteomalacia, and others are a result of renal failure and are known as **renal osteodystrophy.** Associated **brown tumors** (Fig. 3–16A) are caused by large amounts of osteoclasts eating away from the inside of the bone, causing a lesion. Heightened osteoclastic activity results in subperiosteal bone resorption. This results in a highly characteristic lace-like pattern of the outer cortex of the digits (see Fig. 3–16B), femur, and humerus. In addition to subperiosteal resorption, there is trabecular bone resorption. This leads to a fuzzy, motheaten appearance of the skull known as the "salt and pepper" skull. When renal osteodystrophy occurs in the spine, it causes a "rugger jersey spine." The spine has spaced areas of osteosclerosis (light stripes) and areas of osteolysis (dark stripes), giving it the appearance of a striped polo shirt.

Infection of the bone and bone marrow is termed **osteomyelitis. Osteitis** is infection of only the bone. The infection is most commonly caused by

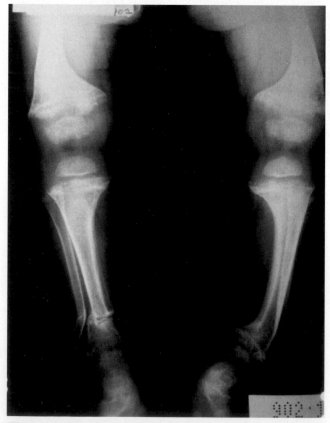

Figure 3–15. Osteomalacia in the form of rickets. Note the pseudofracture of the right tibia and fibula. There is bowing of the bones, a classic sign of rickets.

staphylococci bacteria carried through the blood, but it can be caused directly if bacteria enter the bone from such conditions as a compound fracture. The usual site for development of osteomyelitis is the long bones of the lower limbs (Fig. 3–17).

In the acute stages, the inflammation causes a rise in pressure within the bone, but the periosteum constricts this buildup. This causes the vessels in the bone to become compressed. Within 24 to 48 hours the bone will die. This dead bone is called sequestrum and causes a linear opacity on a radiograph. Unfortunately, radiography is not a very sensitive means of diagnosing this disease, since approximately 50 percent of the bone is destroyed before the changes are visible on a radiograph. The first radiographic abnormality occurs in about 2 weeks and is a poorly defined area of lucency at the site of infection. If sequestra are seen, it is highly suggestive of osteomyelitis as opposed to a neoplasm. A more reliable and faster means of demonstrating the bone destruction is a nuclear medicine bone scan. Areas of increased uptake, or "hot spots," identify the infected site, allowing an early diagnosis. An associated **Brodie abscess** is a focal infection with surrounding dense hardening of the bone and a radiolucent center.

Osteitis deformans, or **Paget disease,** is overproduction of bone. It is an idiopathic disease but appears to be associated with an increased blood flow to the affected bones. This disease is more common in men over 40 and occurs principally at the skull, tibias, and vertebrae (Fig. 3–18). The bones become softened because of the overaction of osteoclasts removing calcium. When the bones become sufficiently soft, they bow. This is particularly true of the tibias. After the period of softening, the bones become hard, causing the deformities to be permanent.

As the bone tries to repair itself, ossification takes place at the outside of the bone (recall the discussion of bone diameter growth). This constant destruction of the inside of the bone with simultaneous production at the outside of the bone, leading to enlargement, is known as **acromegaly** (Fig. 3–19). Since the destruction and production are occurring simultaneously, radiographs demonstrate mixed areas of radiolucent osteolysis and radiopaque osteosclerosis known as the "cotton wool" appearance (Fig. 3–20). This characteristic appearance is evident before any deformity is outwardly evident.

Legg-Calvé-Perthes disease is a common lesion of the head of the femur. It is most often found in young boys around the age of 5 to 10 years. This ischemic necrosis is usually unilateral. The head of the femur at the center of the epiphysis is fragmented. Because of this, the femoral head becomes flattened and splayed (Fig. 3–21). The hallmark

Text continued on page 39

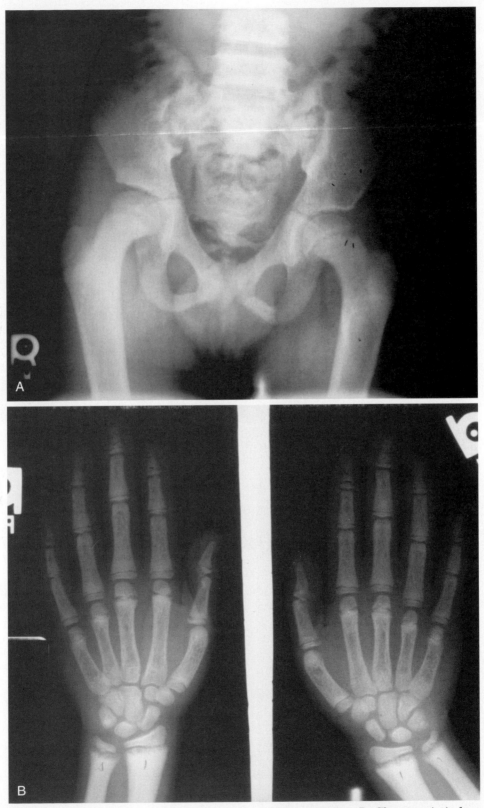

Figure 3–16. Osteodystrophy. *A,* Pelvis shows brown tumor. *B,* Characteristic lace-like pattern of the outer cortex of the digits.

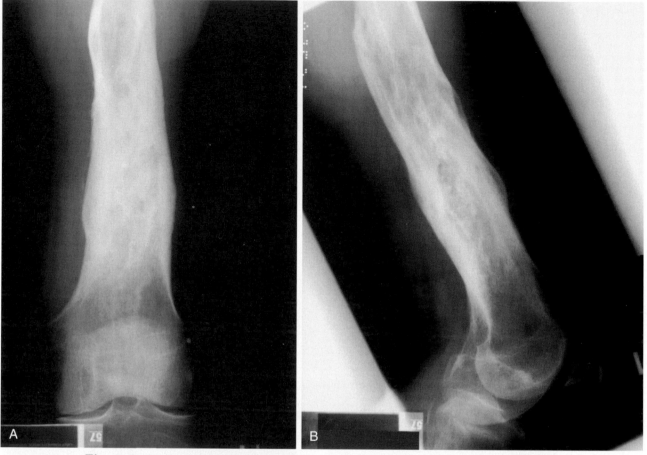

Figure 3–17. Anteroposterior *(A)* and lateral *(B)* views of the distal femur, demonstrating healed osteomyelitis. A Brodie abscess is seen on the anteroposterior view.

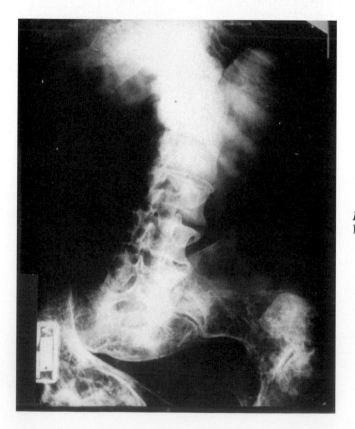

Figure 3–18. Generalized Paget disease of the pelvis and lumbar spine.

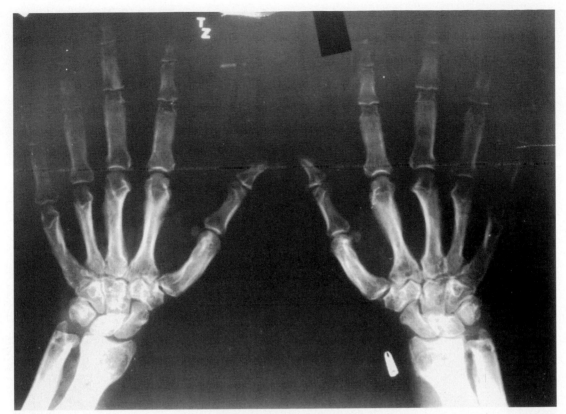

Figure 3–19. Acromegaly.

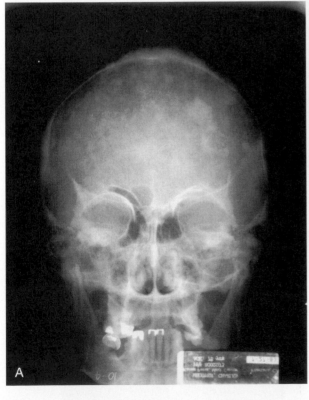

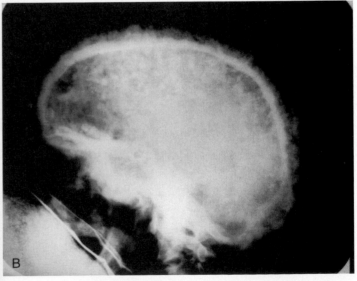

Figures 3–20. Anteroposterior *(A)* and lateral *(B)* view skull radiographs show the classic "cotton wool" appearance of Paget disease.

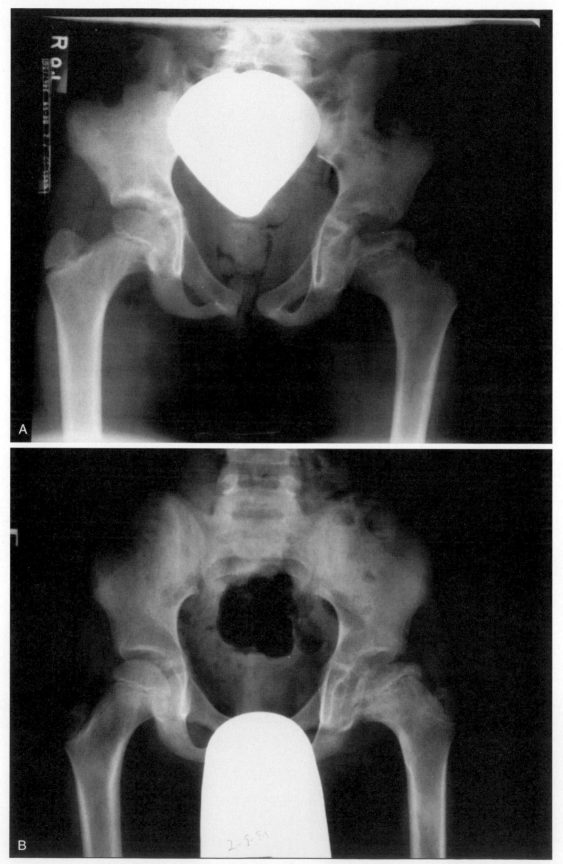

Figure 3–21. Legg-Calvé-Perthes disease: female *(A)* and male *(B)*.

of this disease is a flattened femoral head, which remains even after the lesion has healed and the bone regains some of its structure. The earliest clinical sign is a limp, but the radiograph will make the diagnosis, as early tuberculosis can cause the same clinical manifestations.

Neoplastic Bone Changes

Benign

Fibrous dysplasia is the fibrous displacement of osseous tissue. The bones that are involved are the long bones, ribs, and facial bones. Pathologic fractures are common because of expansion of the bone causing thin, eroded cortices. Angulation deformities result. The radiograph shows well-circumscribed expansile lesions in the shaft of a long bone containing bands of sclerosis causing a multilocular effect (Fig. 3–22).

A **bone cyst** is a wall of fibrous tissue filled with clear fluid, occurring in the proximal humerus and knee of children and adolescents. A bone cyst devel-

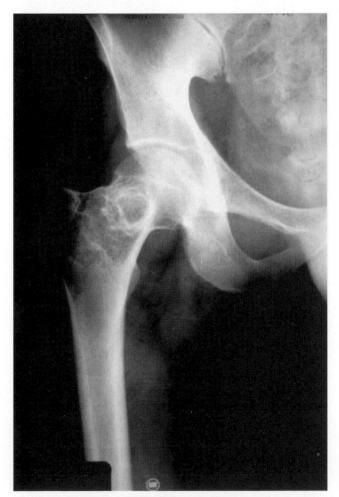

Figure 3–22. Fibrous dysplasia.

ops beneath the epiphyseal plate but migrates down the shaft with growth. The cysts are not usually noted on a radiograph but are detected only when pain due to cyst growth or a pathologic fracture occurs. When they do appear radiographically, they show as a lucent focus with a thin cortex and sharp boundary (Fig. 3–23).

A **chondroma** is a cartilaginous tumor that is sharply delineated with a thin inner cortex, as seen on the radiograph. It may be one of three types:

1. Exostosis
2. Enchondroma
3. Chondrosarcoma

The most common of the three is **exostosis,** also called **osteochondroma.** It is a common benign tumor arising from the cortex and growing parallel to the bone. The tumor points away from the adjacent joint and is capped by radiolucent cartilage. This cap may contain flake-like calcifications. Exostosis is caused by localized bone overgrowth at a joint, particularly the knee (Fig. 3–24). It enlarges during bone growth and then becomes static. Flat osteochondromas can occur in areas such as the pelvis and scapula. An **enchondroma** can occur anywhere that cartilage is present, but it is found most often in the bones of the hands and feet of adolescents and young adults. This benign tumor has little malignant potential when located in the hands or feet; however, the more centrally located the tumor, the greater the possibility of malignant transformation. Enchondromas are slow-growing tumors that are localized and small (Fig. 3–25). Chondrosarcoma will be discussed under the section on malignant neoplastic bone changes.

Giant cell tumors, or **osteoclastomas,** are benign tumors seen in young people in their early 20s. The most common location is in the long bones arising from the epiphysis after closure (Fig. 3–26). The joint space is not involved.

The tumor does extensive local damage to the bone, but does not metastasize. It is seen on a radiograph as large bubbles separated by thin strips of bone, likened to a mass of "soap" bubbles. This appearance is caused by the fact that it is a hemorrhagic mass.

Osteoid osteoma, a benign tumor usually found in the femur or tibia, is more likely to occur in adolescent males. This tumor is rare after the age of 30. Clinically, the classic symptom is pain that is markedly worse at night but is relieved by the use of aspirin. The radiograph will show an area of dense bone (Fig. 3–27) surrounding a radiolucent area of cartilage known as a **nidus.** In some cases, this can only be seen by tomography.

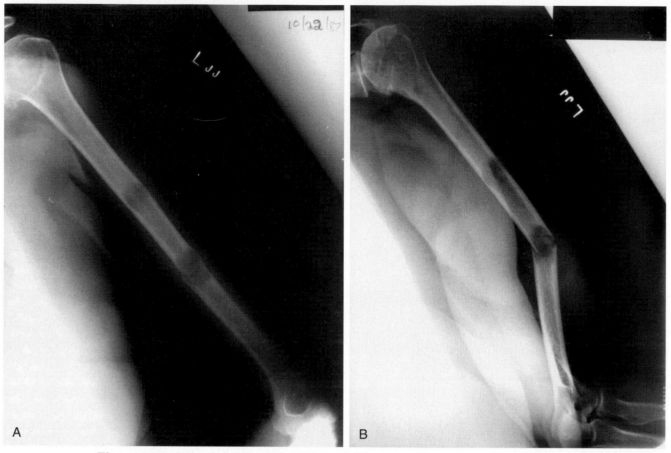

A

B

Figure 3–23. Anteroposterior *(A)* and lateral *(B)* views of bone cysts in the humerus. Radiographs made 3 days earlier showed no fracture. This pathologic fracture through the cyst occurred without trauma to the arm.

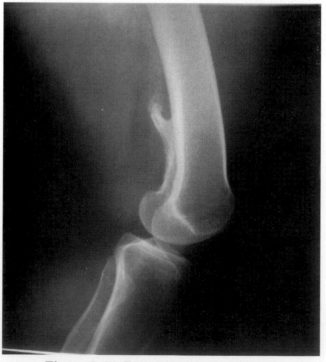

Figure 3–24. Exostosis (osteochondroma).

Malignant

The four chief primary malignant tumors of bone are chondrosarcoma, osteogenic sarcoma, Ewing sarcoma, and multiple myeloma.

A **chondrosarcoma** occurs three times more often in men over the age 45 than in women. The pelvis and long bones are the sites of a chondrosarcoma (Fig. 3–28).

As the name suggests, a chondrosarcoma is a malignant tumor of the cartilage. When the primary tumor is removed, there is often rapid growth or metastasis. However, the outlook for a chondrosarcoma is better than that for other malignant sarcomas.

Ewing sarcoma is the most common primary malignant bone tumor seen in a child of 5 to 15 years of age. It occurs in the diaphysis of long bones. This tumor is often misdiagnosed as osteomyelitis because of the constant low-grade pain, fever, and leukocytosis that are present. The bone has a stratified new bone formation, causing the "onion peel" appearance. By the time the tumor is seen on a radiograph, the prognosis is poor.

Of all the primary tumors of the bone, **multiple**

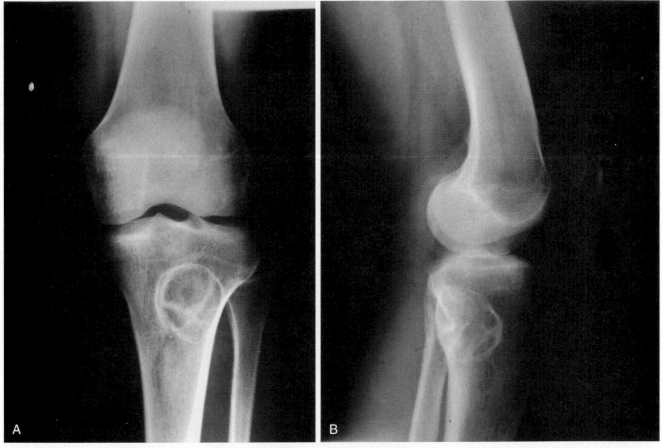

Figure 3–25. *A and B,* Endochondroma.

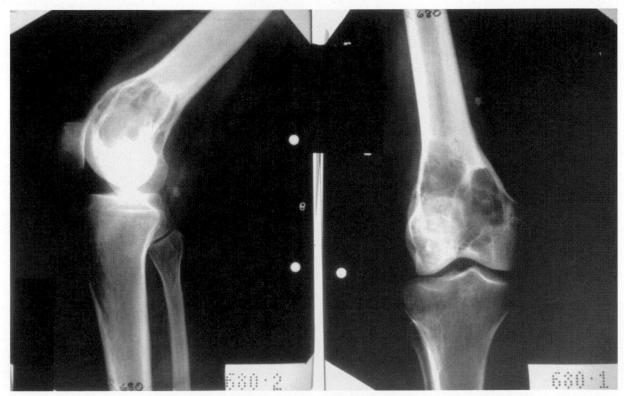

Figure 3–26. Osteoclastoma.

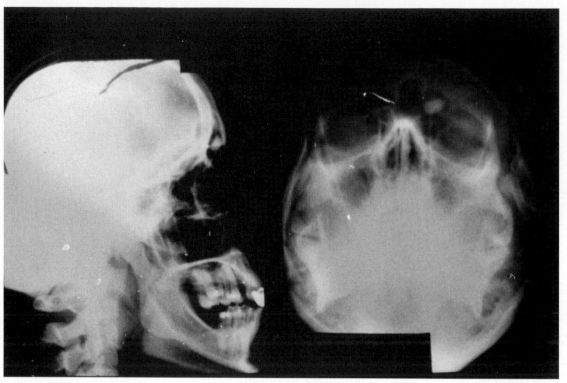

Figure 3–27. Osteoma. Lateral and Waters projections show a dense benign tumor in the frontal sinus.

myeloma is the most common. There may be only one tumor or, as the name suggests, multiple lesions in various areas of the body, particularly the flat bones. The disease is rare in persons younger than 40 years of age and is most often seen in persons over the age of 50. The tumor actually arises from the bone marrow plasma cells and occurs in bone marrow that is actively hemopoietic. Therefore, this is not a true osseous tumor.

The hallmark radiographic sign of multiple myelomas is punched out osteolytic lesions, not unlike a "Swiss cheese" (Fig. 3–29) effect. As the destruction of the bone continues, the chance of pathologic fractures increases. Also, the possibility of paraplegia increases as the bone marrow of the spinal column hypertrophies and exerts pressure on the spinal cord. This tumor is highly malignant and invariably fatal within a few years.

Osteogenic sarcoma, also known as **osteosarcoma** (Fig. 3–30A), is a highly malignant primary tumor occurring at 10 to 30 years of age, with the peak incidence rate at 20 years of age. A second peak incidence rate is found at age 60, if Paget disease is already manifested. This common neoplasm occurs most often in the long bones, particularly the lower ends of the femurs and upper ends of the humerus or radius. There is extensive destruction of bone, and metastasis occurs to the lungs at an early stage. The periosteum is lifted from the

bone by the tumor. Spicules of new bone are laid down, which radiate outward from the central mass. Radiographically, this presents as dense areas, radiolucent areas, or mixed areas to give it the characteristic "sunray" appearance (see Fig. 3–30B). A diagnosis of osteogenic sarcoma comes with a poor prognosis. Most patients die within 5 years. If osteogenic sarcoma is a complication of Paget disease and the patient is elderly, the 5-year prognosis changes to several months.

Metastatic bone tumors are much more common than primary bone tumors (Fig. 3–31). A metastatic tumor is the first sign that cancer is present somewhere else in the body; usually the breast, lung, prostate, and kidney are the primary sites. Metastatic tumors reach the skeleton through the circulatory system or lymph system or by invasion. Pathologic fractures occur as a result of the tumor weakening the bone. The bones that contain red bone marrow are the first to be affected by metastasis, including the spine, skull, ribs, pelvis, and femurs (Figs. 3–32 and 3–33).

Fractures

The most frequent injury to the skeletal system is a fracture. A **fracture** is a discontinuity of a bone caused by force applied either directly or indirectly to the bone. When a fracture occurs, there is a break

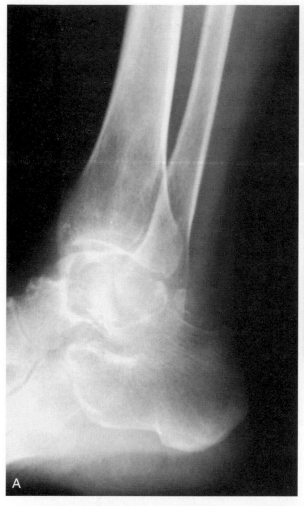

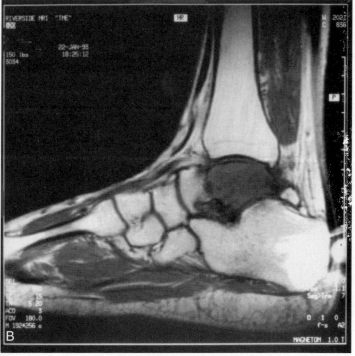

Figure 3–28. Chondrosarcoma. *A,* A radiolucent area is shown on the talus of the ankle. *B,* Magnetic resonance imaging confirms diagnosis.

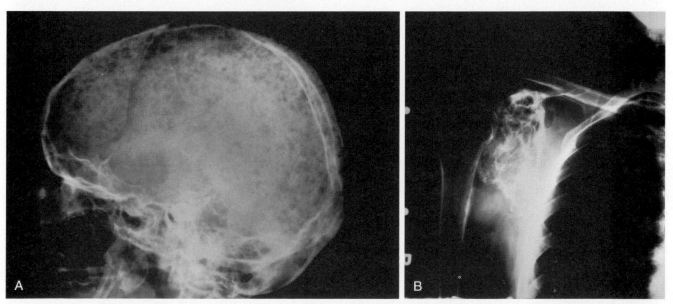

Figure 3–29. Multiple myeloma. *A,* Lateral skull shows the "swiss cheese" effect. *B,* Involvement of the scapula.

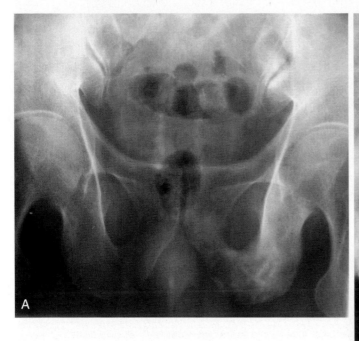

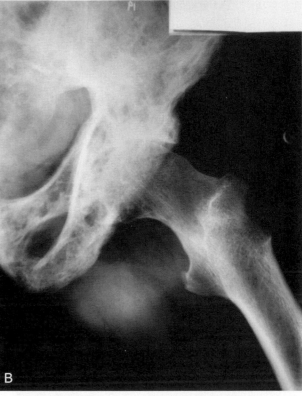

Figure 3–30. Osteosarcoma. *A,* Early stages. *B,* This lateral hip shows the "sunray" appearance near the head of the femur.

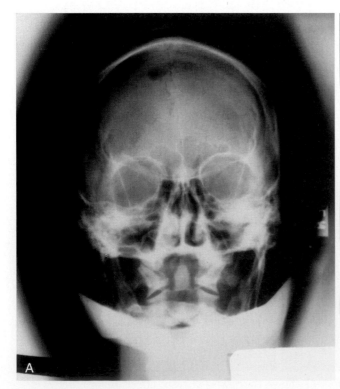

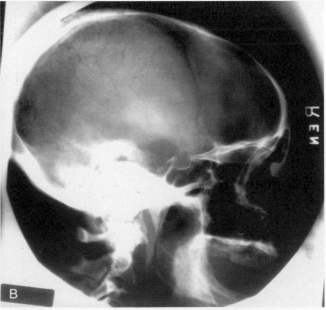

Figure 3–31. A and B, This single radiolucent area on the frontal bone turned out to be a primary bone carcinoma.

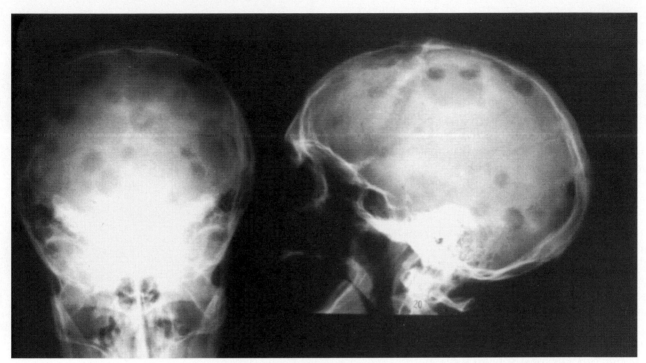

Figure 3–32. Towne and lateral projections of a 46-year-old male. Multiple small and large lytic areas are present throughout the skull, caused by metastases from a primary carcinoma of the lung.

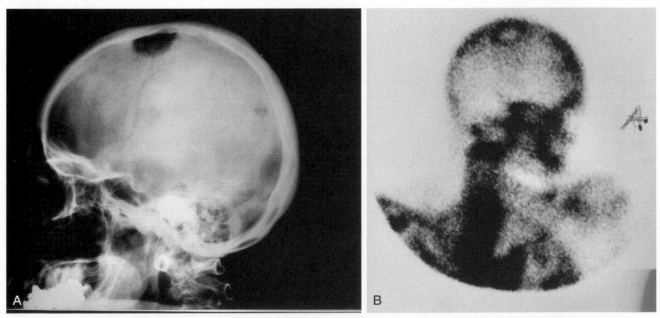

Figure 3–33. Metastatic bone carcinoma. *A,* Lateral skull radiograph shows large radiolucent area at the vertex. *B,* The nuclear medicine scan confirmed diagnosis of bone metastasis from a primary carcinoma of the prostate gland.

in the endosteum and damage to soft tissue and surrounding vessels. Fracture of long bones can lead to shock because as much as 1 liter of blood can be lost in the surrounding tissue.

Bleeding is necessary for the healing of fractures, however. The blood loss leads to inflammation and the formation of fibrous tissue. Blood, lymph, and tissue form a fibrin clot at the fracture site. Fibroblasts are then embedded in this clot, forming a stabilizing type of tissue called granulation tissue. This tissue in turn becomes a temporary callus (a fibrocartilaginous mass) that knits the fracture. Calcium is later deposited by osteoblasts to complete the healing process.

Since complication of a fracture is not unlikely, care must be taken to prevent this from occurring. Infection is likely with a compound fracture and delays union. Injuries to other organs, such as a lung punctured by a broken rib, with resulting pneumothorax, is another factor that must be watched for. There also may be ossification in surrounding muscles due to extensive soft-tissue damage or a fat embolism caused by the fat from the bone marrow entering the circulation.

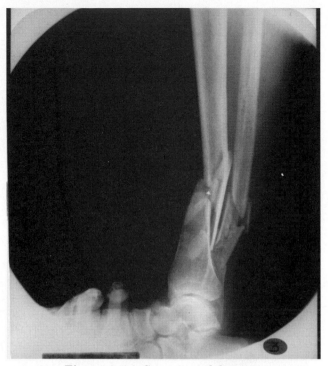

Figure 3–34. Comminuted fracture.

Types of Fractures

Most fractures are named or classified by the direction of the fracture line, whether the overlying skin is intact, and the shape, position, and number of the fragments of the fractured bone.

A **complete** fracture is one through the entire cross section of the bone, while an **incomplete,** or **fissure,** fracture breaks only one cortex. If broken skin is not involved, the fracture is known as a **closed** fracture. In order to be classified as a **compound (open)** fracture, the skin or mucosal surface must be pierced by at least one end of the fractured bone.

Simple fractures divide the bone into two complete pieces. Many technologists believe that **comminuted** fractures (Fig. 3–34) are those in which the bone is "shattered." Although this is also true, the bone must only be broken into three or more fragments for the fracture to be termed comminuted.

Terms such as **transverse, spiral, oblique,** and **longitudinal** simply describe the direction of the fracture in relation to the long axis of the bone (Fig. 3–35). A star-shaped fracture, particularly on the patella or the calvarium, is termed **stellate.** If the cortical shaft is driven into the cancellous bone by some force, the bone becomes **impacted** and the fracture is termed as such (Fig. 3–36). Figure 3–37 depicts several of these types of fractures.

The positioning of the fragments must be determined so that the fracture can be reduced (put back into place) prior to a cast being applied. **Displacement** refers to the lateral positioning of the fragments and **distraction** refers to the gap between the fragments.

When the tibia or fibula (or radius or ulna) is fractured, the other end of the paired bone should be checked for fractures. This is especially true in the case of spiral fractures, as the torquing force applied at one end of the bone is carried through to the other end and usually causes a second fracture.

Not all bones fracture when they are involved in trauma. They may become **dislocated,** which means the bones that form a joint no longer articulate (Fig. 3–38). If there is **subluxation** of the joint, it is only partially dislocated (Fig. 3–39).

Finally, there can be problems with healing of the fracture. When healing does not occur in the normal time it is referred to as **delayed union. Malunion** occurs when the bone ends have not been properly reduced and are misaligned, which impairs normal function. It is possible for the bone ends to never join at all, particularly in certain pathologies. This is known as **nonunion.**

Common Fractures

All fractures can be broken down into general categories, such as those just described, or can be labeled by terminology that refers to a specific type of fracture. There are many types and classifications

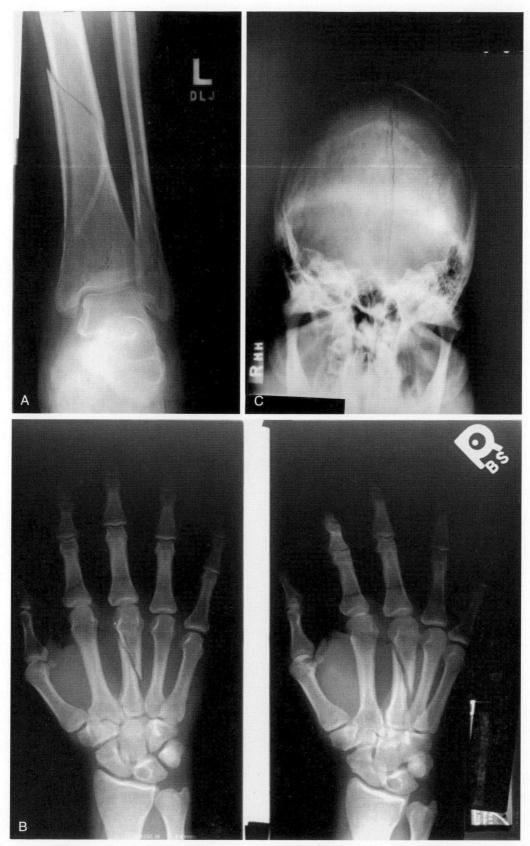

Figure 3–35. *A,* Spiral fracture; *B,* oblique fracture; *C,* longitudinal fracture.

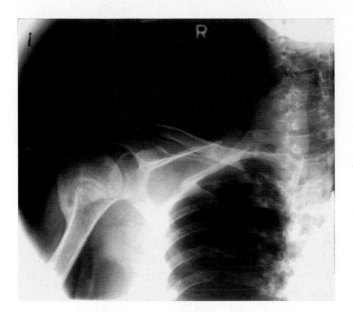

Figure 3–36. Impacted fracture.

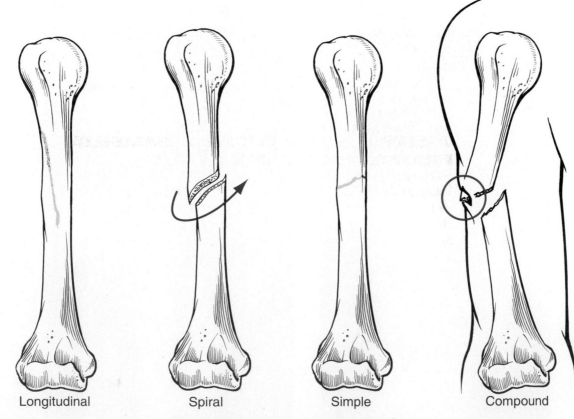

| Longitudinal | Spiral | Simple | Compound |

Figure 3–37. Common fractures of the bone.

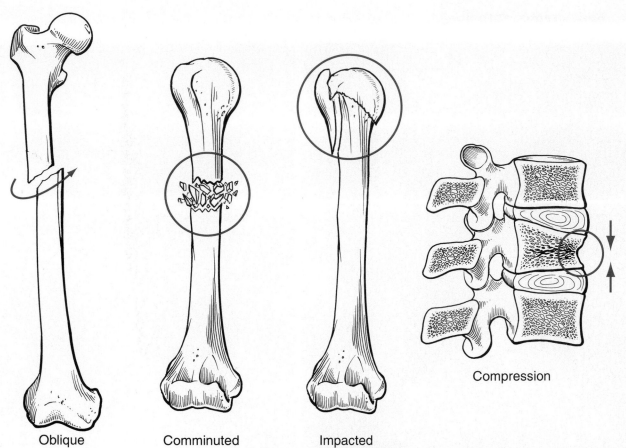

Oblique   Comminuted   Impacted   Compression

Figure 3–37 Continued.

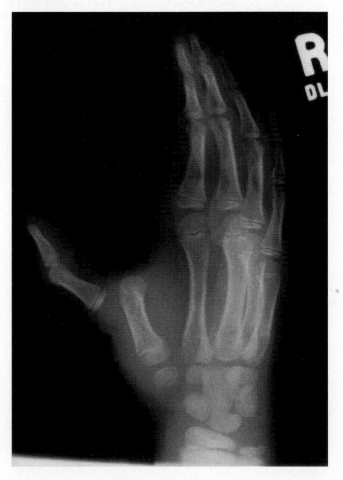

Figure 3–38. Dislocated thumb.

49

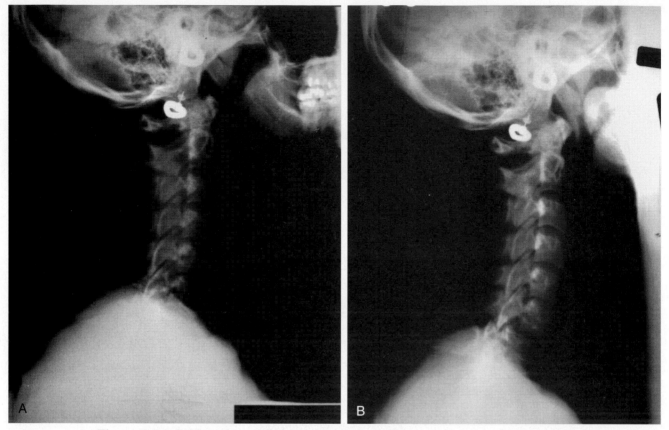

Figure 3–39. Subluxation. *A,* All seven cervical vertebrae are not seen. *B,* Shows the importance of seeing all seven cervical-spine vertebrae, as C-6 is subluxated over C-7.

of fractures that can occur; however, only the most common fractures that should be known by every radiographer will be discussed here.

Fractures that occur in children are usually not as serious as those that occur in adults because of the softness of children's bones. **Plastic** fractures occur when the soft young bone bends, but the cortex does not actually break (Fig. 3–40). A **greenstick** fracture (Fig. 3–41), on the other hand, is a break in the cortex but only on one side of the shaft. This is a type of fissure fracture. This angulated fracture produces a bowing of the bone. Another fracture that occurs in children is known as a **torus** fracture (Fig. 3–42). This is a type of greenstick fracture in which a driving force pushes down the shaft of bone, causing the cortex to fold back onto itself. A final fracture that involves children is the **epiphyseal** fracture that occurs through ununited areas of epiphyses (Fig. 3–43). There is no displacement, so a comparison view is needed. There are several classifications of epiphyseal fractures, but it is beyond the scope of an imaging radiographer to diagnose these types.

Fatigue (also known as a **march fracture** or a **stress fracture**) occurs at sites of maximum stress, usually the metatarsal bones. The fracture is the

result of repeated, relatively trivial trauma to an otherwise normal bone. Its name derives from the fact that these fractures are most commonly found in persons unaccustomed to vigorous physical activity in the form of marching or hiking. Often the fracture is not seen on an initial radiograph. It is usually seen after new bone formation has been completed. A fracture that occurs when normal stress is placed on diseased areas of bone is known as a **pathologic** fracture (see Fig. 3–23). The disease must be treated for healing of the fracture to take place.

Fractures can easily occur around joint articulations. When a small chip of bone breaks away when a joint has dislocated, an **avulsion** fracture (Fig. 3–44) has occurred. Compressing forces applied to both sides of the bone ends cause **compression** fractures (Fig. 3–45). These usually occur in the spine in postmenopausal women. As osteoporosis sets in, the bones become brittle. The spine, which normally holds the weight of the body upright, literally becomes bowed under the weight pushing down on the top of the vertebrae and the force of standing pushing up on the vertebrae. The anterior vertebral bodies collapse under the force.

Other fractures that will be encountered during

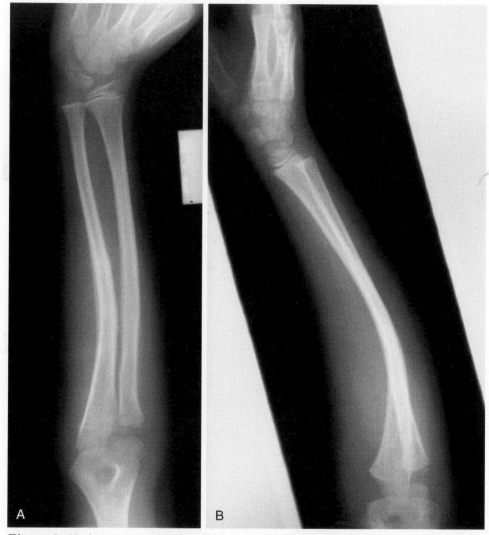

Figure 3–40. Anteroposterior *(A)* and lateral *(B)* views of the forearm of a young child showing bowing (plastic fracture) of bones but no actual fracture of the cortex.

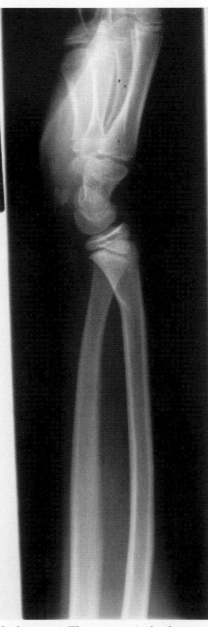

Figure 3–41. Greenstick fracture. The cortex is broken on one side, producing an angulated bowing of the bone.

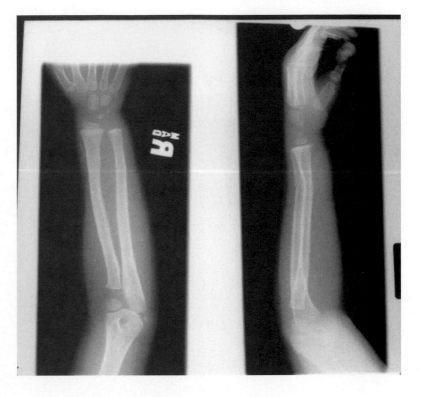

Figure 3–42. Torus fracture. The cortex can be seen to be pushed down or buckled on itself on the lateral projection.

the career of the radiographer have specific eponymic names to identify them. The **Galeazzi** fracture is of the radial shaft at the junction of the middle and distal thirds. It is associated with dislocation of the distal ulna. The **Monteggia** fracture (Fig. 3–46) involves the proximal third of the ulna with anterior dislocation of the radial head. Both fractures involve only one bone. It is essential in these instances to examine the elbow and wrist to determine whether any associated dislocations and possible avulsion fractures have taken place. The elbow itself may be fractured. A hallmark indication of a fracture here is the "fat pad" sign (Fig. 3–47). On lateral projections of a normal elbow, the anterior fat pad lies close to the distal end of the humerus and the posterior fat pad is not visible. When trauma occurs at this site, fluid effusion, either synovial or hemorrhagic in nature, displaces both fat pads. The anterior one separates from the bone surface. The normally hidden posterior fat pad becomes displaced posteriorly and shows up as a crescent-shaped lucency. Since this fat pad is normally not seen, its presence is an excellent indicator of effusion present within the joint.

Both Smith and Colles fractures occur at the wrist. A **Colles** fracture occurs when the distal radius fractures with the fragment being displaced posteriorly (Fig. 3–48). Conversely, a **Smith** fracture can be identified by the forward displacement of the fragments. Either of these fractures can be accompanied by an avulsion fracture of the ulnar styloid process. Fractures of the hand seen most often are the **Bennett** fracture, which is at the base of the first metacarpal (thumb) with proximal displacement, and the boxer's fracture, which occurs at the neck of the fifth metacarpal (Fig. 3–49). A boxer's fracture is so named because it usually occurs when the person hits a solid object with a tightly closed fist, causing the metacarpal of the little finger to snap.

The last fractures to be identified are of the ankle. A **bimalleolar** fracture (Fig. 3–50) is of the lateral and medial malleoli, and a **trimalleolar** fracture (Fig. 3–51) is of the lateral, medial and posterior malleoli of the ankle. These serious fractures require surgery to screw the fragments into place. A less drastic fracture of the ankle is the **Pott** fracture, which involves injury to the distal tibial articulation. This was originally described as a fracture of the fibula with dislocation of the tibia. Today, a Pott fracture refers to a bimalleolar fracture, wherein there is also an avulsion fracture of the medial malleolus caused by abduction and external rotation of the ankle.

Joint Pathology

Arthritis is the most common joint disease. It is an inflammation of the joint, but there can be degenerative changes without infection. Following are descriptions of six types of arthritis that are important radiographically.

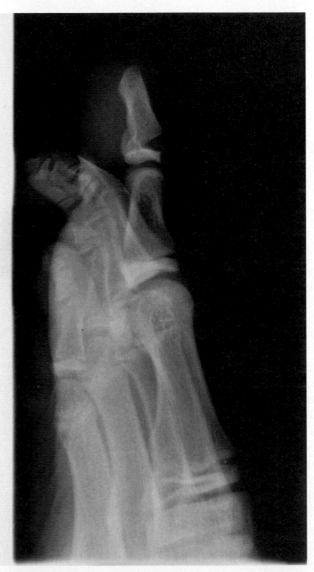

Figure 3–43. Epiphyseal fracture of the great toe.

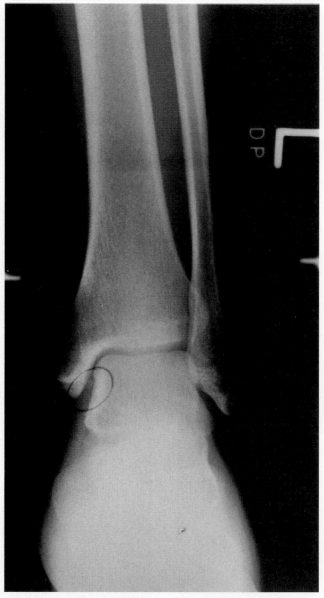

Figure 3–44. Avulsion fracture.

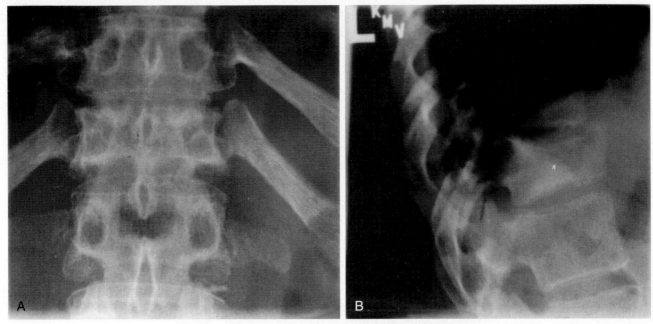

Figure 3–45. *A and B,* Compression fracture of T-12.

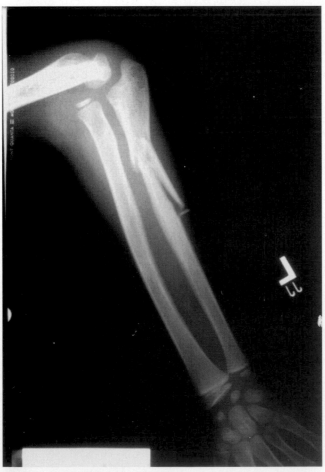

Figure 3–46. Monteggia fracture shows classic displacement of the radial head.

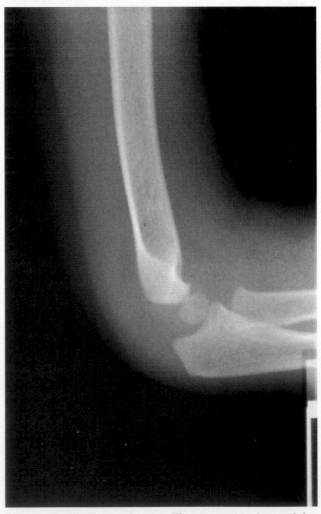

Figure 3–47. Fat pad sign. The posterior fat pad has been displaced and can be seen posterior to the humerus.

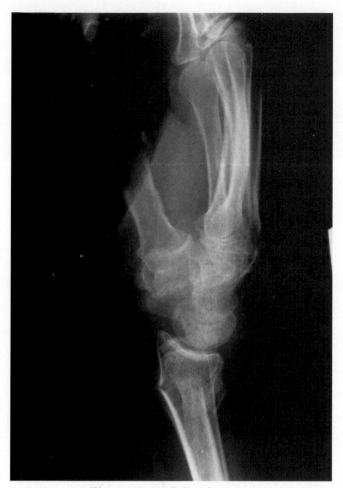

Figure 3–48. Colles fracture.

Gouty arthritis is an inherited type of arthritis that is more common in men and affects the joints of the foot, particularly the big toe (Fig 3–52). Because of a metabolic problem with nitrogen, increased levels of sodium uric acid are produced and deposited at the first metatarsophalangeal joint. Acute gout is characterized by inflamed synovium, whereas in chronic gout, the articular cartilage is damaged by deposited urates and inflammation.

The radiographer should look for uric acid crystal deposits, known as tophi, at the joint space, as well as calcified deposits in the soft tissues. In severe forms, tophi cause asymmetrical lumps that are readily noticeable. Complications such as kidney stones because of the excessive urates may also be noted on an abdominal radiograph. Loss of joint space and erosion of articular surfaces, signs of so many types of arthritis, are *not* seen in gouty arthritis.

Osteoarthritis, also known as **degenerative joint disease** and **hypertrophic arthritis,** is the most common of all types and occurs in older patients who have put a lot of "wear and tear" on the large weight-bearing joints of the body, such as the knees, or in obese patients who have extra weight that the joints have to carry. Joint changes in this disease are found to some degree in all persons older than 50 years of age.

Osteoarthritis is a noninflammatory deterioration of the articular cartilage with new bone forming at the surface of the joint. Radiographs of the joint show the hallmark sign, "spurring" (Fig. 3–53), or, in severe cases, mild subluxation or loose bodies within the joint space. Narrow joint spaces and some erosion may occur (see Fig. 3–53C).

Rheumatoid arthritis is the oldest of all known diseases. It affects the small joints of women in their 30s and 40s. It is a systemic disease characterized by chronic and progressive inflammatory involvement of the joints and atrophy of the muscles. The cause of rheumatoid arthritis is not known.

Widespread inflammation in the synovial membrane takes place, causing pain and stiffness and

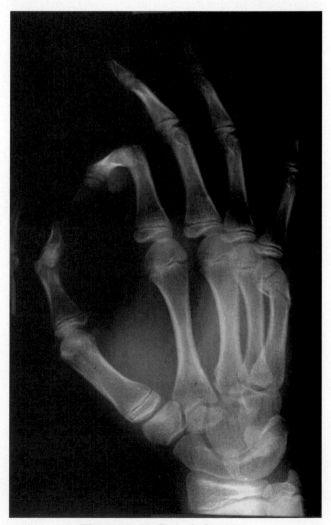

Figure 3–49. Boxer's fracture.

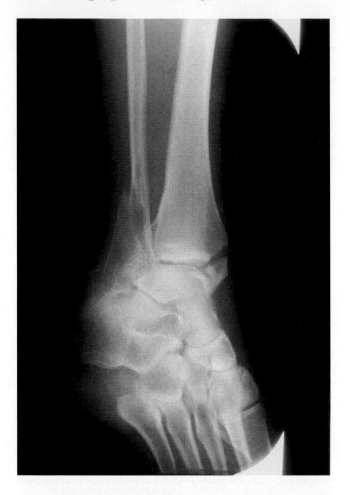

Figure 3–50. Bimalleolar fracture of the ankle.

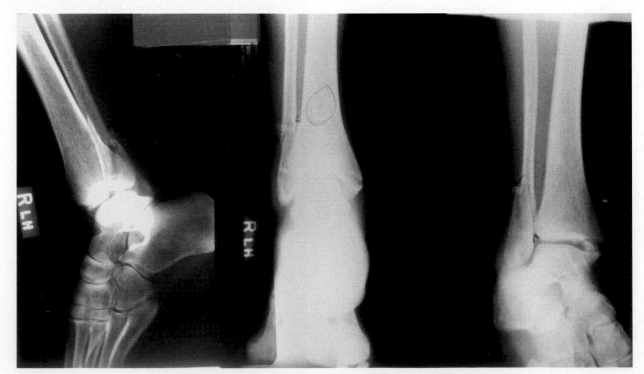

Figure 3–51. Trimalleolar fracture of the ankle.

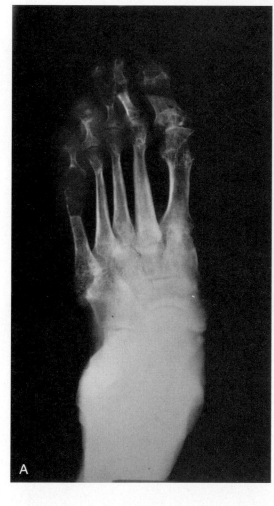

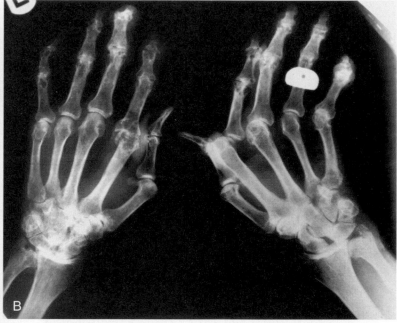

Figure 3–52. Gout not only affects the feet *(A)* but also can affect the hands *(B)*.

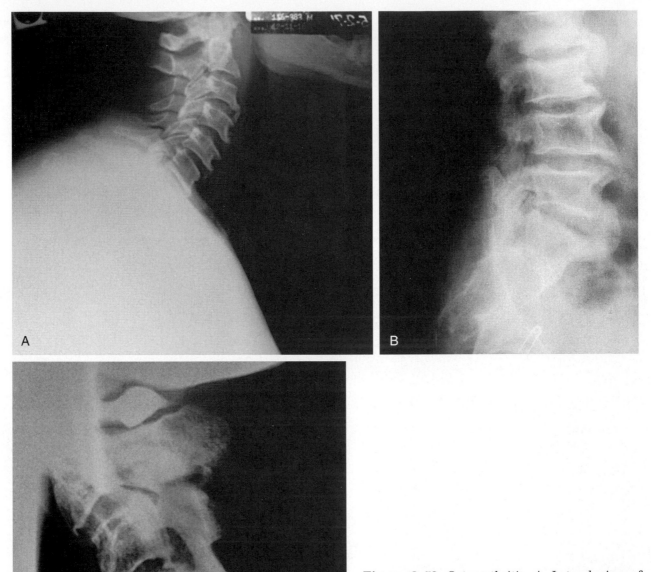

Figure 3–53. Osteoarthritis. *A,* Lateral view of the cervical spine shows spurring of the vertebral bodies. *B,* Note the blurring of the vertebrae as well as the lipping along the anterior borders of all the lumbar vertebrae. *C,* Lateral view of the cervical spine demonstrating subluxation and erosion.

thickening of the tissue. This thickened tissue grows inward and damages the cartilage. Later, the tissue becomes fibrous, which prevents motion of the joint (fibrous ankylosis). As the disease progresses, the fibrous tissue becomes calcified and becomes osseous tissue (bony ankylosis).

In the early stage of the disease, the radiograph shows soft-tissue swelling around the joints. Later, the films show a decrease in the joint space, with eroded bone ends and subluxation (Figs. 3–54 and 3–55). This leads to the gross deformities often encountered with rheumatoid arthritis. Ulnar deviation of the wrist with either "boutonniere deformity" (flexion) (Fig. 3–56) or "swan neck deformity" (hyperextension) of the proximal interphalangeal joint occurs. The distal interphalangeal joint is rarely affected.

Tuberculous arthritis is found in the patient who has pulmonary tuberculosis. The most common location for tuberculous arthritis is in the spine, where it is known as **Pott disease.** When it occurs in joints, usually only one joint is involved. It destroys the articular cartilage and disks but seldom shows any periosteal changes.

Ankylosing spondylitis, or **rheumatoid spon-** dylitis, affects the sacroiliac joints by fusing them. It also causes extensive calcifications of the anterior longitudinal ligament. This creates the characteristic "bamboo-spine" appearance on a radiograph (Fig. 3–57). Ankylosing spondylitis starts in the lumbar spine and works up. As it reaches the thoracic area, breathing becomes difficult and kyphosis develops. Ninety percent of the patients who have ankylosing spondylitis are male.

Reiter syndrome is common in young men between the ages of 20 and 40 and affects the lower extremities. Radiographs show eroded joint spaces with narrowing. Other complications include conjunctivitis, urethritis, and, occasionally, ulcerations on the palms of the hands and the soles of the feet. There are two forms of this disease. One, called dysenteric, results from infection by shigella or salmonella germs. The other is sexually transmitted, probably by chlamydia bacteria. The radiographic hallmark of Reiter syndrome is a "calcaneal spur," which is rather wide and fuzzy.

Table 3–1 summarizes all the pathologic conditions, causes, manifestations, and radiographic appearances that have been described.

Not all joint disease is arthritis. Many other

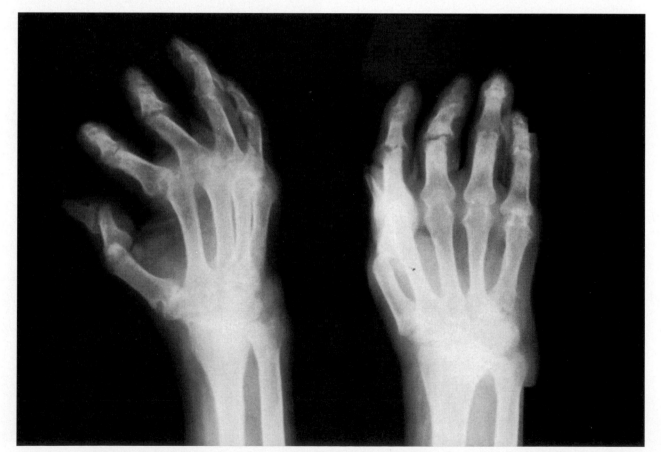

Figure 3–54. Rheumatoid arthritis in advanced stages. Note the subluxation of the finger joints and the loss of joint space.

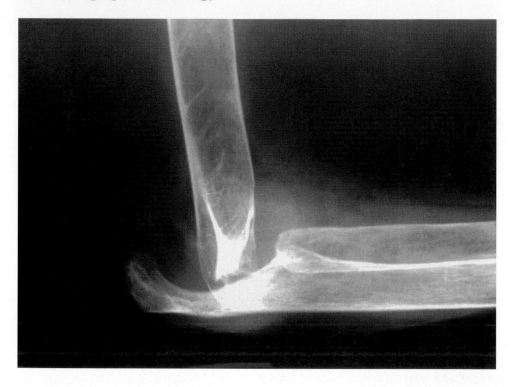

Figure 3–55. Severe bone-end erosion and subluxation due to rheumatoid arthritis.

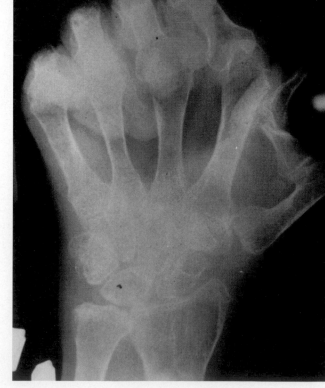

Figure 3–56. Boutonniere deformity of rheumatoid arthritis.

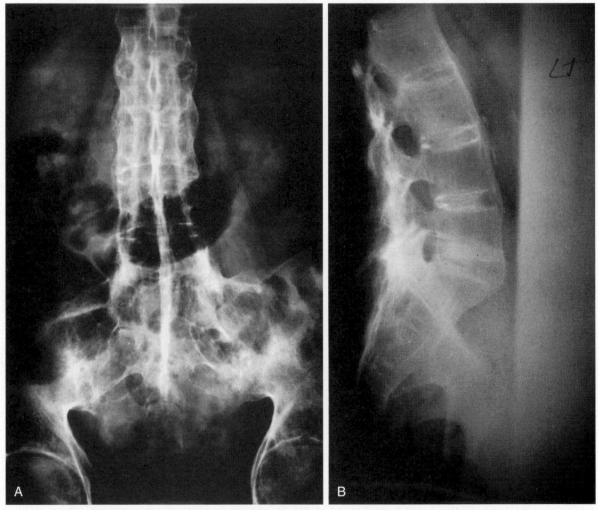

Figure 3–57. Rheumatoid spondylitis. Anteroposterior *(A)* and lateral *(B)* views of the lumbar spine shows classic "bamboo" spine. Note extensive calcifications of anterior longitudinal ligament on the lateral projection.

Table 3–1.
Clinical and Radiographic Characteristics of Common Pathologies

Pathologic Condition	Causal Factors*	Manifestations	Radiographic Appearance
Osteogenesis imperfecta, "brittle bone" disease	Congenital, autosomal dominant gene	Hypoplastic teeth, limb deformities, deafness	Multiple fractures, both old and new
Osteopetrosis, "marble bone" disease	Congenital, deficiency of osteoclast	Obliteration of marrow cavity, osteomyelitis, deformed skull	Extreme density of bones
Achondroplasia	Congenital, autosomal dominant gene	Failure of bone growth, dwarfism, bowed legs, bulky forehead, saddle nose	Scalloped posterior margins of lumbar vertebra; borders
Osteoporosis	Adulthood, aging, disuse of bone, hormonal changes, Cushing syndrome, prolonged steroid use	Back pain, fractures, normal calcium, lack of osteoid, kidney stones	Thin cortices and radiolucent bones due to decrease in density
Osteomalacia, rickets	Lack of calcium, vitamin deficiency, pregnancy	Normal osteoid, lack of calcium and phosphorus, skeletal deformities, bowing of lower limbs	Loss of density
Renal osteodystrophy	Renal failure	Brown tumor, heightened subperiosteal bone resorption, trabecular bone resorption	Salt and pepper skull, rugger jersey spine, lace-like pattern of digits, femur, and humerus
Osteomyelitis	Bacterial infection (Staphylococcus)	Inflammation, Brodie abscess	Poorly defined radiolucency
Osteitis deformans, Paget disease	Idiopathic	Overproduction of bone, soft, bowed tibias, acromegaly	"Cotton wool" mixed areas of radiolucent and radiopaque densities
Legg-Calvé-Perthes	Ischemic necrosis, osteochondritis	Femoral head fragments, limp, muscle spasm, muscle atrophy of thigh	Flattened femoral head
Osteochondroma	Localized bone overgrowth at a joint	Benign cortical tumor capped by radiolucent cartilage which may contain calcifications	Growth parallel to bone, pointing away from joint
Osteoclastoma, "giant cell tumor"	20 to 40 years, after epiphyseal closure	Extensive local bone damage, joint space not involved	"Soap bubbles," large radiolucencies separated by thin strips of bone
Osteoid osteoma		Pain at night relieved by aspirin	Radiolucent center (nidus) surrounded by dense bone
Ewing sarcoma	5 to 15 years	Low-grade fever, leukocytosis, misdiagnosed as osteomyelitis, located in diaphysis of long bone	"Onion peel" lesion, shows stratified layers of new bone formation
Multiple myeloma	40 to 60 years, unknown	Possible paraplegia, pathologic fractures, multiple lesions	"Swiss cheese," punched-out osteolytic lesions
Osteosarcoma	10 to 25 years, after 60 if Paget disease is present, unknown	Mass in bone, pathologic fractures	"Sunray," radiolucent areas mixed with dense areas
Gout	Adulthood, genetic	Uric acid deposits (tophi), sudden joint pain, deformed joints with masses, kidney stones	Uric acid deposits in joint space, great toe classically involved
Osteoarthritis	Late adulthood, wear and tear on joints, age, obesity	Pain, decreased mobility, enlarged joints, knees and hips involved	"Spurring" at joint space, mild subluxation
Rheumatoid arthritis	Adulthood, possible autoallergic	Pain, stiffness, deformity, soft tissue swelling	Decreased joint space, swan neck and boutonniere deformities
Rheumatoid spondylitis	Late teens, early adulthood	Fused sacroiliac joints, kyphosis, difficult breathing	"Bamboo spine" squared-off vertebrae
Reiter syndrome	Young male	Conjunctivitis, urethritis, ulcerations	Eroded joint space, "calcaneal spur"

*Includes age, if relevant.

types of disease processes, as well as trauma or infection, can destroy a joint. Probably the most common nonarthritic ailment of joints is **bursitis.** This is an inflammation of the synovial bursa caused by excess stress on the joint. Bursitis is generally found in the shoulder, and the radiographs may show calcified deposits in the tendon above the greater tuberosity of the humerus (Fig. 3–58).

Low back pain is the most common complaint of radiologic technologists. This is usually caused by improper body position when moving heavy objects. Diseases of the renal prostate area, or disk problems may be the cause of the pain in patients.

Spondylolisthesis is the forward displacement of one vertebra on top of another, usually occurring at the L-5/S-1 juncture (Figs. 3–59 and 3–60). This is usually caused by a defect of some kind of the pedicle. **Spondylitis** is inflammation of the spinal vertebrae, and **spondylosis** is a condition of the spine characterized by fixation and stiffness.

Disk herniations are common in the lumbar spine area. The fibrous ring of the disk degenerates to the point that the pulpy nucleus is forced out. Posterior herniation results in pressure on the spinal cord and nerve roots. This can cause neurologic symptoms. Radiographs show narrowing of the disk. Myelography or discography is used to demonstrate the extent of the damage.

No section on joint pathology would be complete without a mention of dislocations. Radiographers must be aware of the direction of dislocations of the shoulder and hip to avoid further injury to a patient. The shoulder dislocates anteriorly, with the head slipping into the subglenoid fossa (Fig. 3–61).

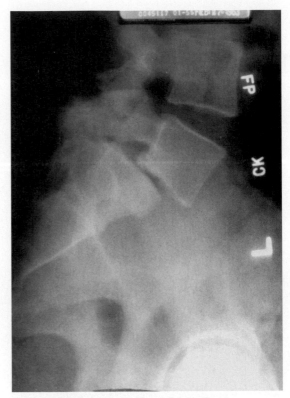

Figure 3–59. Spondylolisthesis.

A chip fracture is common with a shoulder dislocation. The hip dislocates posteriorly against the sciatic notch. Both dislocations are easily detected simply by viewing the patient. A patient whose shoulder is dislocated will carry the affected arm across the chest or abdomen while the shoulder droops noticeably below the ipsilateral shoulder. A patient with a dislocated hip will usually have the knee of the affected side bent while the lower extremity is rotated outwardly, similar to a fractured hip. The patient is most comfortable if the knee is supported slightly. The alert radiographer will avoid further injury to a patient if the situation is assessed prior to any movement of the body part.

Review Questions

1. Name the two classifications of the skeleton. List the five functions of the skeleton.
2. Name the five types of bones and give an example of each.
3. Describe the structure of a long bone.
4. Describe how bones heal following fractures. What complications can arise from fractures? Describe the following fractures: greenstick, fatigue, compression, pathologic, Colles, boxer's, Pott.
5. Name the 3 classifications of joints and describe.

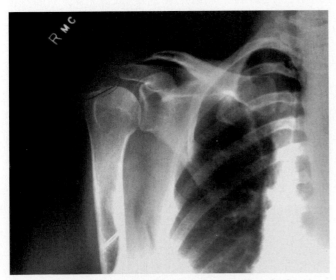

Figure 3–58. Bursitis. There are small calcifications above the humeral head.

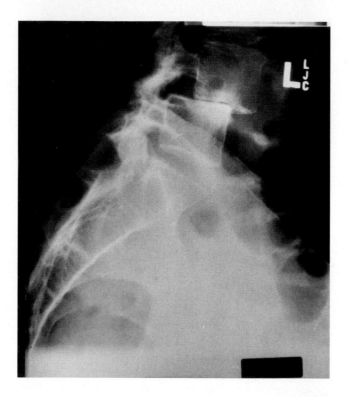

Figure 3–60. Lateral view of the lumbar region revealing an unusual spondylolisthesis of the fourth lumbar vertebra over the fifth.

Figure 3–61. Anterior shoulder dislocation.

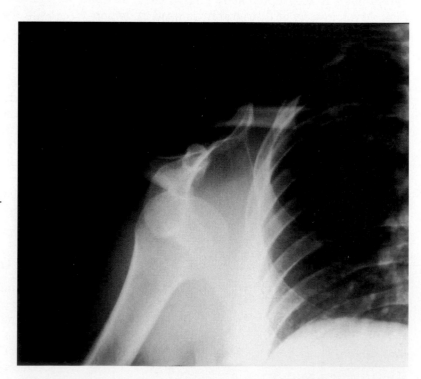

6. List and describe the six types of synovial joints and give an example of each.
7. Define and describe the process of ossification.
8. Explain how bones grow in length as well as in diameter.
9. Define each of the following as it relates to the skeletal system:

Tomography   Nuclear medicine
Angiography   Arthrography—
Computed tomography/   describe this
    magnetic resonance   procedure.
    imaging

10. Define achondroplasia and describe its effects.
11. Define osteomalacia and osteoporosis. Describe the difference between the two. What do the radiographs of each look like?
12. Define osteomyelitis. What happens to the bone in the acute stages? Why? Is radiography a good diagnostic tool? Explain.
13. Define osteitis deformans. Where does it occur? How does acromegaly relate to this disease? What do the radiographs demonstrate?
14. Define multiple myeloma. Describe its appearance on the radiograph. What causes this appearance? What is a complication of this disease? How does it occur?
15. Define arthritis. Describe each of the following types including the radiographic appearance: gouty, osteoarthritis, rheumatoid, ankylosing spondylitis.
16. Define the difference between spondylolisthesis, spondylitis, and spondylosis.
17. List and describe the radiographic hallmark sign for each of the following diseases. State which are neoplastic and which are non neoplastic bone changes.

Renal osteodystrophy   Ewing sarcoma
Osteoid osteoma   Osteogenic sarcoma
Osteoclastomas   Reiter syndrome

18. Define bursitis. Where is it usually located and what does the radiograph show? What technical factors should the radiographer use to demonstrate this?

CHAPTER IV

Hepatobiliary System

Goals

1. To review the anatomy and physiology of the liver, gallbladder, bile ducts, and pancreas.
2. To learn the special modalities and procedures that are used to image the liver, gallbladder, bile ducts, and pancreas.
3. To become acquainted with the pathophysiology and radiographic manifestations of all of the common disorders of the biliary system.

Objectives

At the completion of the chapter, the radiographer will be able to:

1. Identify the anatomy of the liver, gallbladder, bile ducts, and pancreas.
2. Explain the physiology and function of the liver, gallbladder, and pancreas.
3. Explain the impact that the function of each organ has on the other organs.
4. Describe the impact that the physiology and function of each organ has on pathologies.
5. List the various special imaging procedures for the liver, gallbladder, bile ducts, and pancreas.
6. List and describe the various forms of hepatitis.
7. Define the four forms of jaundice.
8. Explain acute and chronic cholecystitis.
9. Describe the difference between the different types of cholelithiasis.
10. List and describe the three pathologies of the pancreas discussed.

I. Anatomy
   A. Liver
      1. Lobes
         a. Right Lobe
            1. Right Lobe Proper
            2. Caudate Lobe
            3. Quadrate Lobe
            4. Riedel Lobe
         b. Left Lobe
      2. Falciform Ligament
         a. Ligamentum Teres
      3. Portal Vein
         a. Superior Mesenteric
            Vein
         b. Splenic Vein
   B. Gallbladder
      1. Fundus
      2. Body
      3. Neck
         a. Hartmann Pouch
   C. Bile Ducts
      1. Right Hepatic Duct
      2. Left Hepatic Duct
      3. Common Hepatic Duct
      4. Cystic Duct
         a. Spiral Heister Valve
      5. Common Bile Duct
         (Choledochus)
      6. Pancreatic Duct (Duct of
         Wirsung)
         a. Hepatopancreatic
            Ampulla (Ampulla of
            Vater)
      7. Hepatopancreatic
         Sphincter (Oddi
         Sphincter)
      8. Minor Pancreatic Duct
         (Duct of Santorini)
   D. Pancreas
      1. Head
         a. Uncinate Process
      2. Neck
      3. Body
      4. Tail
II. Physiology and Function
   A. Liver
      1. Digestion and Absorption
      2. Hematopoiesis
      3. Laboratory Tests
         a. Aspartate
            Aminotransferase
            (AST)
         b. Alkaline Aphosphaste
            (ALT)
         c. Alkaline Phosphatase

         d. Serum Bilirubin
   B. Gallbladder
      1. Concentrate Bile
      2. Store Bile
   C. Pancreas
      1. Endocrine
         a. Insulin
         b. Glucagon
      2. Exocrine
         a. Amylase
         b. Lipase
         c. Trypsin
III. Special Radiographic
     Procedures
   A. Liver
      1. Computed Tomography
         and Magnetic Resonance
         Imaging
      2. Ultrasonography
      3. Nuclear Medicine
   B. Gallbladder and Bile Ducts
      1. Computed Tomography
      2. Ultrasonography
      3. Nuclear Medicine
         a. Dimethyl Iminodiacetic
            Acid (HIDA)
         b. Paraisopropyl
            Iminodiacetic Acid
            (PIPIDA)
      4. Diagnostic Radiography
         a. Intravenous
            Cholangiography
         b. Operative
            Cholangiography
         c. T-Tube
            Cholangiography
         d. Percutaneous
            Transhepatic
            Cholangiography
         e. Oral Cholecystography
         f. Fatty Meal
   C. Pancreas
      1. Computed Tomography
      2. Ultrasonography
      3. Endoscopic Retrograde
         Cholangiographic
         Pancreatography
      4. Barium Studies
IV. Pathology
   A. Liver
      1. Inflammatory Processes
         a. Cirrhosis
         b. Hepatitis
            1. Deficiency
            2. Toxic

            3. Viral
         c. Jaundice (Icterus)
            1. Medical
               (Nonobstructive)
               a. Hemolytic
               b. Hepatic
            2. Surgical
               (Obstructive)
      2. Neoplasms
         a. Hepatoma
         b. Cholangiocarcinoma
         c. Metastatic Carcinoma
   B. Gallbladder and Bile Ducts
      1. Congenital Anomalies
         a. Duplication
         b. Variation of Shape
            1. Bilobed
            2. Hourglass
            3. Phrygian Cap
         c. Choledochal cyst
      2. Inflammatory Processes
         a. Nonfunctioning
            Gallbladder
            1. Hydrops
         b. Cholangitis
         c. Cholecystitis
            1. Acute
            2. Chronic
               a. Porcelain
                  Gallbladder
         d. Cholelithiasis
            1. Radiopaque
            2. Radiolucent
            3. Complications
               a. Gangrenous
                  Gallbladder
               b. Fistula
               c. Ileus
      3. Neoplasms
         a. Carcinoma
   C. Pancreas
      1. Congenital Processes
         a. Cystic Fibrosis
      2. Inflammatory Processes
         a. Pancreatitis
            1. Acute
            2. Chronic
            3. Enzymatic Necrosis
         b. Pseudocyst
      3. Neoplasms
         a. Islet Cell Tumors
            (Adenoma)
         b. Carcinoma
            1. Adenocarcinoma

The hepatobiliary system includes the liver, the gallbladder, and the bile ducts. The pancreas is an accessory organ in the digestive tract, as are the other three, but it is not a part of the biliary system. However, because the pancreas shares a portion of the biliary ductal system, discussion of it is included in this chapter.

ANATOMY

Liver

The liver is the largest organ in the body, weighing about 3½ pounds. It is roughly triangular in shape and is located immediately below the diaphragm in the right upper quadrant, but a portion of it does extend to the left of the midline.

The liver is divided into four lobes. The two main lobes are the right and left lobes, which are separated by the falciform ligament. The inferior portion of the falciform ligament has a free border which contains the ligamentum teres, a remnant of the fetal umbilical vein. As shown by Figure 4–1A, only the main right and left lobes can be identified anteriorly. Figure 4–1B demonstrates the posterior surface of the liver. As seen here, the right lobe is divided into three segments called the right lobe proper, the caudate lobe, and the quadrate lobe, which brings the total number of lobes in the liver up to four. In some women, a normal variant of the

right lobe is sometimes seen as an extra lobe. This is known as the Riedel lobe.

Each lobe is composed of numerous lobules. It is beyond the purpose of this text to provide an in-depth description of lobule structure. It should be known that the liver is able to send the bile out to the body by means of the minute bile ducts that lie in each lobule. These ducts unite to form the large bile ducts that enable bile to pass to other organs.

An important vessel to remember is the portal vein. Seen on the posterior surface of the liver, the portal vein is formed when the splenic vein and the superior mesenteric vein unite. Venous blood from the spleen and the gastrointestinal tract are sent to the liver for processing through this vital vessel.

Gallbladder

The gallbladder is a pear-shaped sac that lies in a shallow fossa on the posterior surface of the right lobe of the liver. It consists of three parts: fundus, body, and neck. In the posterior neck of the gallbladder, a small pouch is occasionally found that is known as a Hartmann pouch. This is a prime site for gallstones to collect, as it is the most dependent portion of the gallbladder. The neck merges with the cystic duct.

The wall of the gallbladder is composed of an outer serous, a muscular, and an inner mucous coat. The mucosal lining has rugae (folds) that help pro-

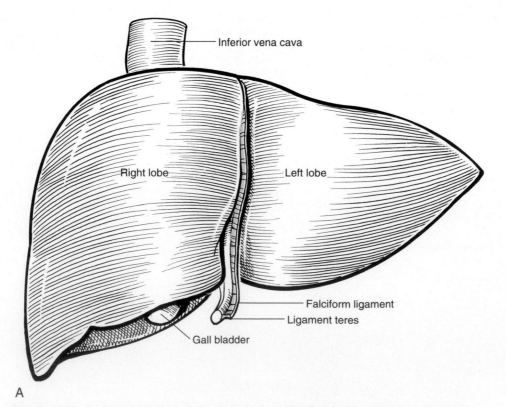

A

Figure 4–1. A, Anterior view of the liver as it is divided by the falciform ligament.

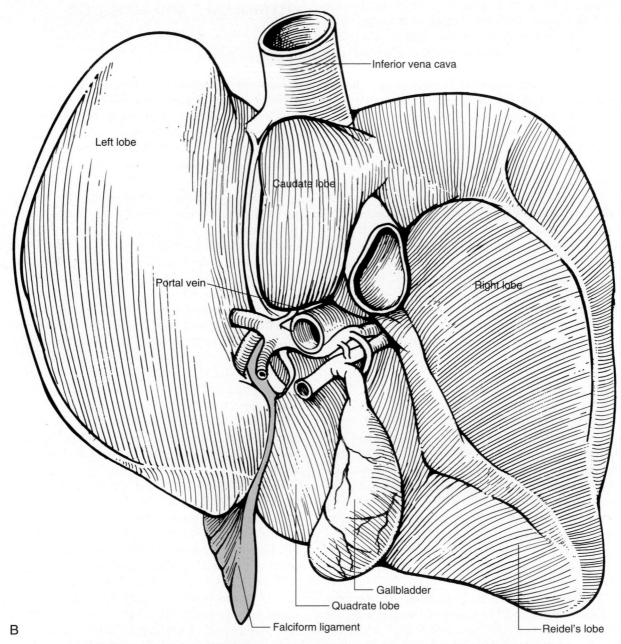

Figure 4–1 Continued. B, Posterior view of the liver, demonstrating the divisions of all lobes and the position of the gallbladder.

mote the passage of bile when the gallbladder contracts.

Bile Ducts

The minute bile ducts that are located in the lobules of the liver unite to form larger and larger bile ducts, which eventually form the right and left hepatic ducts that are located in the right and left lobes of the liver. The right and left hepatic ducts converge to form the common hepatic duct. Coming off the neck of the gallbladder is a small duct called the cystic duct. The lumen of the cystic duct contains membranous folds called the spiral Heister valve. This valve prevents the collapse or distention of the cystic duct. The common hepatic duct merges with the cystic duct and forms the common bile duct. The common bile duct, also known as the choledochus, descends posterior to the head of the pancreas. It joins the pancreatic duct near the duodenum and becomes the hepatopancreatic ampulla, better known as the ampulla of Vater. The hepatopancreatic sphincter, or Oddi sphincter, is located at the opening of the ampulla into the C-loop of the duodenum. The minor pancreatic duct, also known as the duct of Santorini, is an accessory duct that is sometimes present and may or may not empty into the duodenum.

Pancreas

The pancreas is divided into four areas: head, neck, body, and tail. The head sits in the C-loop of the duodenum. An inferior extension of the head that courses toward the midline is known as the uncinate process. The head constricts slightly to form the neck, then widens again to form the body. The body courses from the inferior vena cava toward the left across the midline. Part of the body is posterior to the stomach. The tail sits in the splenic hilum anterior to the left kidney. The entire organ is retroperitoneal.

The pancreas contains several types of cells. Beta cells, acinar cells, and the islets of Langerhans are all important, as tumors may arise from these cells.

The main pancreatic duct, also known as the duct of Wirsung, runs the entire length of the pancreas. It unites with the common bile duct after it enters the head of the pancreas. It is at this point that the ampulla of Vater is formed. A minor accessory duct is sometimes found branching off the superior aspect of the duct of Wirsung. This duct is called the duct of Santorini and enters the duodenum superior to the ampulla of Vater.

Figure 4–2 shows the biliary ductal system beginning with the left and right hepatic ducts. The anatomic locations of the ducts within the pancreas are important to remember, as special diagnostic radiographic examinations are done specifically for the areas.

PHYSIOLOGY AND FUNCTION

Liver

The liver plays an important part in digestion and absorption as well as in hematopoiesis. It is literally a chemical factory, responsible for manufacturing hundreds of enzymes necessary for bodily functions and for detoxifying many poisons and drugs, including alcohol, that enter the bloodstream. As the functions of the liver number more than 100, only a few will be noted here.

The most important function of the liver in regards to digestion and absorption is the production of bile, containing bile salts and bile pigments. The liver has an important part in the metabolism of carbohydrates, fats, and proteins by performing glycogenesis, glycogenolysis, and gluconeogenesis. The liver synthesizes fibrogen, albumin, and other blood proteins. It converts excessive amino acids to carbohydrates and urea to rid the body of these toxins through the renal system. The Kupffer cells of the liver destroy worn-out red blood cells and remove foreign substances from the blood. The liver stores some vitamins, such as A, D, E, K, and B_{12}. It inactivates the toxic products that pass from the spleen and the large intestine to the liver via the portal vein. The liver makes reticuloendothelial cells. It helps to maintain water balance and blood viscosity.

With all these processes taking place, it is easy to understand how disease can interfere with the body's functions by damaging one organ. There are several ways to detect liver damage. One is by liver function tests. Another is by special diagnostic procedures that will be discussed later in the chapter.

There are so many liver functions that one test cannot provide the total answer about disease. Measurement of serum bilirubin levels, the amount of bile pigment in the urine, and liver enzyme levels and sulfobromophthalein sodium and turbidity tests are valuable for the nonjaundice patient. In the jaundice patient, tests such as aspartate aminotransferase (AST), formerly known as **serum glutamic oxaloacetic transaminase** (SGOT), alanine aminotransferase (ALT), or **serum glutamic pyruvic transaminase** (SGPT), alkaline phosphatase, and serum bilirubin can help the clinician diagnose the correct type of jaundice.

The enzyme AST is released into the blood stream in abnormally high levels when death or

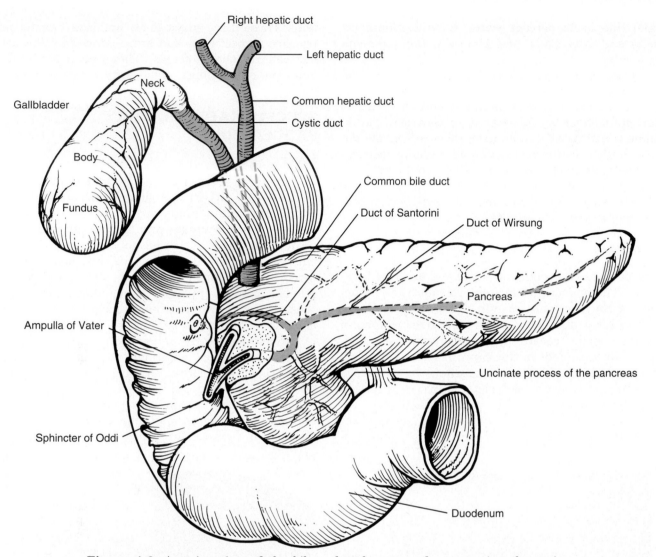

Figure 4-2. Anterior view of the bilary ductal system, demonstrating the main divisions and the course of the bile ducts.

injury occurs to the cells that produce it (for instance, cirrhosis causes the AST value to be anywhere from 10 to 100 times higher than normal).

The ALT test is more specific than the AST test in that the level of elevation differs with the pathology. The amount of ALT is mildly elevated in cirrhosis, moderately elevated in obstructive jaundice, and very high in toxic hepatitis.

Alkaline phosphatase is an enzyme that is produced by the liver and bone. Disease processes raise the levels of this enzyme.

Serum bilirubin is the product from the breakdown of hemoglobin in worn-out red blood cells. The liver converts bilirubin to bile. If bilirubin shows up in elevated levels, one of several pathologic processes is present. Either more red blood cells are dying than can be converted to bile, the Kupffer cells have failed to remove and excrete bilirubin, or

there is a blockage in the ducts leading from the cells that is causing a backup of bilirubin in the liver.

Gallbladder

Bile is manufactured in the liver, not in the gallbladder. It is secreted through the bile ducts to the right and left hepatic ducts. These ducts then convey bile to the common hepatic duct, where it passes through the cystic duct into the gallbladder. Bile is expelled by the gallbladder only when food has been ingested.

The liver produces 20 times more bile than the gallbladder can hold, so the gallbladder must concentrate the bile in order to store large amounts. The capillaries in the gallbladder wall extract the large amount of water that is a major component of bile. Bile is 97 percent water, 2 percent mineral salts and fatty acids, and 1 percent bile pigments and salts.

When food, particularly fat, is present in the duodenum, a hormone known as cholecystokinin is released into the bloodstream. The hormone reaches the gallbladder and causes it to contract. At the same time, the Oddi sphincter relaxes to allow the bile that the contracted gallbladder has pushed out to flow down the bile duct, into the ampulla of Vater, through the sphincter, and into the duodenum. The elapsed time between eating and gallbladder contraction is about 30 minutes.

Pancreas

The pancreas has both endocrine and exocrine functions. The endocrine functions include the production of the hormones insulin and glucagon. These are secreted directly into the bloodstream. Insulin exerts a major control over carbohydrate metabolism. Glucagon aids in this control. These hormones are made in the islets of Langerhans by two types of cells that comprise the islets: alpha$_2$ cells secrete the glucagon, and beta cells produce insulin.

The exocrine functions include the secretion of enzymes that digest carbohydrates, fat, and pro-teins. These three enzymes are amylase, lipase, and trypsin, respectively, and are produced by the acinar cells of the pancreas. They travel along the main pancreatic duct and empty into the duodenum.

SPECIAL RADIOGRAPHIC PROCEDURES

Liver

In abdominal radiography, the kidney, ureter, and bladder view (KUB) will show organ size, ascites, calcifications, and biliary air.

Computed tomography and **magnetic resonance imaging** are used to screen for hepatic masses. Both are the most sensitive modalities to detect small density changes. Computed tomographic scanning provides more information in an obese patient than does ultrasonography, which is more accurate in thin patients.

Ultrasonography relies on the technologist's ability to recognize abnormal echo patterns and to record them with normal settings. There are several "pit falls" in sonography, which must be guarded against, as they can present a confusing picture. For example, masses may appear twice their true size due to the specular reflector ability of the dia-

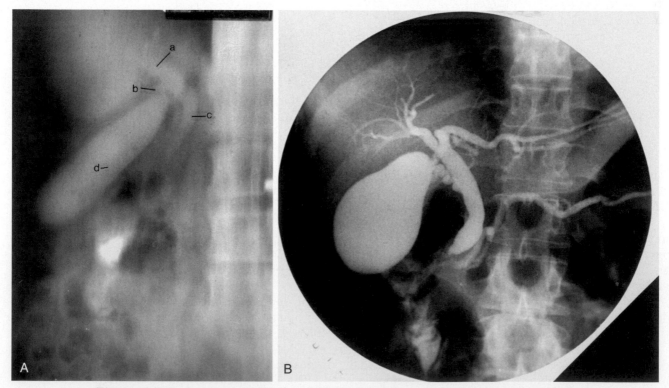

Figure 4–3. Intravenous cholangiography showing the main bile ducts and gallbladder. *A,* Anatomy demonstrated includes the common hepatic duct *(a),* the cystic duct *(b),* the common bile duct *(c),* and the gallbladder *(d). B,* All normal anatomy. Note the spiral valves located in the cystic duct and duct of Santorini immediately inferior to the common bile duct.

phragm, and gas in the loops of bowel may be mistaken for pathology. Ultrasonography is, however, an excellent noninvasive method to determine whether masses are cystic or solid and whether vital vessels have been invaded by tumors.

Although computed tomography, magnetic resonance imaging, and ultrasonography offer better anatomic display of the architecture of the liver, **nuclear medicine** provides an excellent assessment of space-occupying lesions. Unlike the other special modalities, nuclear medicine displays the liver in its entirety and not in cross section.

Gallbladder and Bile Ducts

Computed tomography is able to demonstrate dilated bile ducts. It usually cannot visualize stones in the gallbladder or ducts.

Ultrasonography is now the most widely used method to image a gallbladder. In most institutions, ultrasonography has replaced the routine oral cholecystogram. In a few facilities, it is utilized for a nonvisualized gallbladder or as a compliment study to the oral cholecystogram. Because the gallbladder normally appears as a cystic structure with no internal echoes, stones and sludge are easily demonstrated with ultrasonography. Dilated bile ducts are detected very easily within the liver, and many times the cause of the dilation is easily seen.

Nuclear medicine examinations of the hepatobiliary system are performed for functions that cannot be demonstrated by computed tomography, magnetic resonance imaging, or ultrasonography. Two such examinations involve the injection of technetium (^{99m}Tc) mixed with dimethyl iminodiacetic acid (HIDA) or technetium mixed with paraisopropyl iminodiacetic acid (PIPIDA). ^{99m}Tc-PIPIDA demonstrates the major bile ducts and gallbladder. Initial secretion into the duodenum is seen 30 minutes after injection on normal patients.

The radiographer should be familiar with special examinations, even though they may no longer be performed at certain institutions. One such examination is **intravenous cholangiography (IVC).** This examination involves the slow intravenous injection of a contrast medium, usually Cholografin, to demonstrate the extrahepatic biliary ducts and the gallbladder. It used to be the procedure of choice for determining acute cholecystitis.

The patient was placed in a right posterior oblique position for the entire examination, which could take as long as 2 hours or more. After a slow-drip infusion was begun, radiographs were taken approximately every 20 minutes until the biliary tree and gallbladder were well visualized (Figs. 4–3 and 4–4). Optimal visualization of the bile ducts

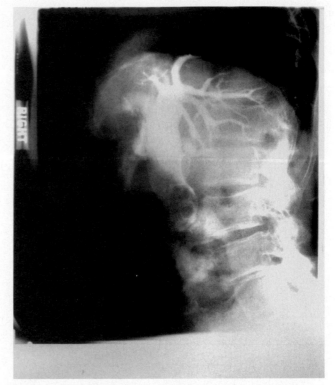

Figure 4–4. Intravenous cholangiography. Lateral position, showing an extremely dilated common bile duct.

took as long as 40 minutes to 1 hour after injection. If the gallbladder was present, it may not have been visualized until 80 minutes after injection. Tomography was helpful in obtaining optimum quality radiographs. Intravenous cholangiography is not as commonly used today because of the availability of other diagnostic modalities that take far less time and have a higher success rate.

Operative cholangiography is performed in the operating room while the patient is undergoing a cholecystectomy. It involves injecting the contrast medium directly into the common bile duct to ascertain if any stones are present in the duct. It also shows patency of the ducts and tests the Oddi sphincter. The radiographer is required to take overhead films with the portable equipment (Fig. 4–5). Usually, nothing more than fluoroscopy with the C-arm is required; however images of the right upper quadrant may be necessary. The left side of the patient should be elevated 15 degrees to eliminate superimposition of the biliary tract and the spine. Strict surgical technique must be adhered to in order to prevent contamination of the open wound. The C-arm is used for visualizing the entire procedure periodically, and replaces the radiographer's taking one to three overhead films with portable radiographic equipment (Fig. 4–6).

T-tube cholangiography is performed in the

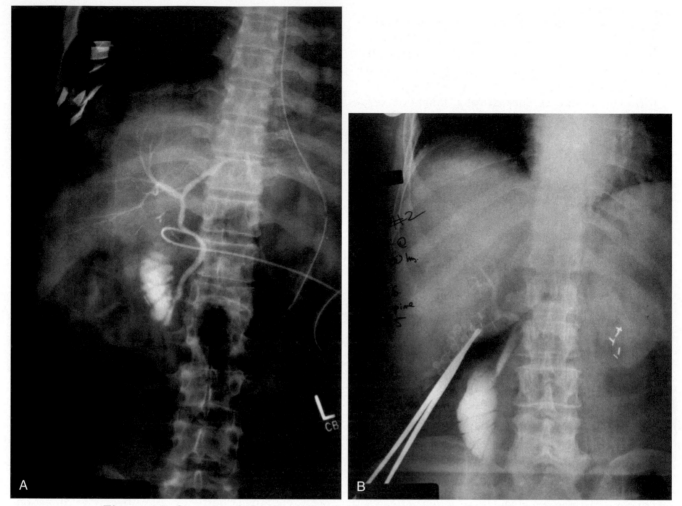

Figure 4–5. Operative cholangiography. *A,* Normal anatomy. *B,* Stone-filled gallbladder about to be removed in the operating room.

radiology department about 1 week after surgery. During surgery, a rubber tube that resembles a "T" is inserted into the common bile duct. The cross bar of the "T" runs vertically inside the duct, and the stem runs horizontally, to be brought outside of the skin. This allows bile to drain to the outside if the duct is still obstructed in some way. Biliary patency, residual stones, or strictures can be evaluated with this procedure. One day prior to the scheduled T-tube examination, the T-tube should be clamped. This concentrates bile in the tube and prevents the accumulation of air in the tube, which can be mistaken for stones in the biliary ducts. Under fluoroscopy, a positive contrast agent such as Conray, Renografin, or Isovue is injected through the stem of the tube and spot films are taken (Fig. 4–7).

A less common procedure for the bile ducts is **percutaneous transhepatic cholangiography (PTC).** This examination has been called a "skinny needle" examination because of the size and shape of the needle that is used to perform the procedure (Fig. 4–8).

Percutaneous transhepatic cholangiography is performed in the radiology department under sterile conditions. As this procedure is usually performed just prior to the patient being sent to surgery, the patient will be mildly sedated. A local anesthetic is then administered so that the radiologist can insert a long, thin-walled needle intercostally through the liver into a bile duct (Fig. 4–9). Contrast material is then injected directly into the duct, and spot films are obtained. This examination demonstrates the site of obstruction, particularly if it is in the common bile duct.

Percutaneous transhepatic cholangiography is not without risk. There is the possibility the liver may be damaged or that bile will spill into the peritoneum. However, the success rate of this examination many times outweighs the risks involved.

A successful **oral cholecystogram (OCG)** depends on the ability of the liver to remove contrast material from the portal bloodstream and excrete it with bile. The gallbladder should be opacified within 10 to 12 hours after the patient has ingested

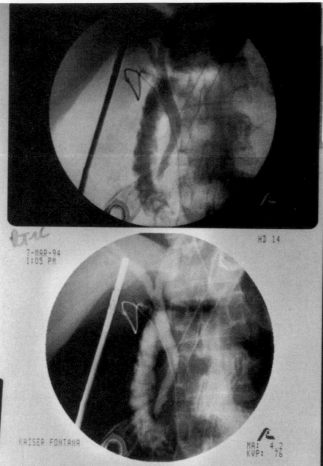

Figure 4–6. Cholecystography in the operating room using the C-arm fluoroscopic unit.

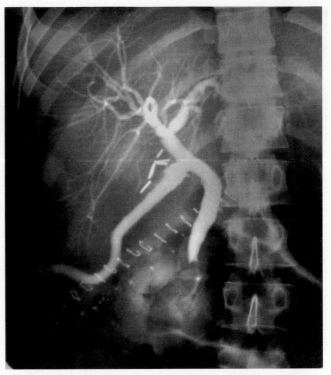

Figure 4–7. T-tube cholangiogram. Normal study.

of contrast medium is used or how much of it is given.

To determine whether the gallbladder is able to empty, a **fatty meal** is administered in the depart-

a contrast medium such as Telepaque tablets (Fig. 4–10). If the gallbladder cannot be visualized the morning after the ingestion of the contrast medium, there may be several explanations. The liver may be diseased and unable to send the contrast material to the gallbladder. There may be a blockage of the cystic duct or of the hepatic ducts leading to the cystic duct. Some patients forget over the years that the gallbladder was removed during surgery. The most common cause of nonvisualization of the gallbladder is poor patient preparation. If this is not the cause, the patient can be instructed to return the following morning with directions for a double dose of contrast agent, or a granulous contrast medium such as Oragrafin can be administered in the department. Depending on the solution, the gallbladder should be visualized in about 20 minutes (Fig. 4–11). If it is not, then the patient will be sent for ultrasonography. A patient who has a bilirubin level of 2 mg per 100 mL of serum is within normal range and the gallbladder should opacify. However, a bilirubin level of more than 4 mg per 100 mL is indicative of liver dysfunction and the gallbladder will probably not be visualized no matter what type

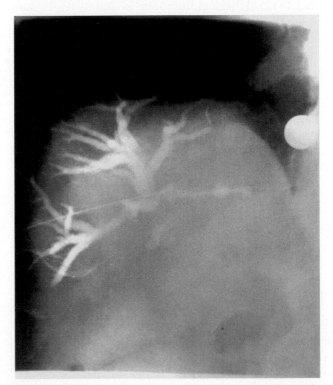

Figure 4–8. Percutaneous transhepatic cholangiography. Note the "skinny needle" to the left on the radiograph.

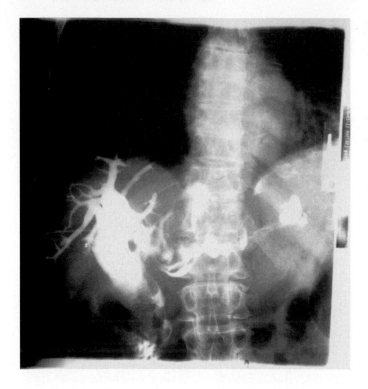

Figure 4–9. Percutaneous transhepatic cholangiography. Needle inserted into the common bile duct. The duct is obstructed and dilated.

ment. Approximately 20 to 30 minutes after the patient has ingested a cholecystagogue preparation, such as Bile-Evac or Neo-Cholex, the gallbladder contracts just as it would if the patient had eaten a meal. Radiographically, the gallbladder is quite small; however, the cystic duct and, occasionally, the outline of the spiral Heister valve can be seen (Fig. 4–12). If the gallbladder is inflamed, it does not contract to push out the bile and contrast material, regardless of how much time is allowed to pass.

Pancreas

Computed tomography plays a vital part in pancreatic imaging. It has an accuracy rate of almost 100 percent in the detection of pancreatic carcinoma and a 96 percent accuracy rate in the detection of pancreatitis.

Ultrasonography is used extensively to determine various pathologic conditions, such as the nature of a mass or the extent of disease. Along with computed tomography, ultrasonography can determine the degree of pancreatic inflammation. However, because of the pancreas' position posterior to the stomach, ultrasonography is not always the best modality for the entire organ.

Endoscopic retrograde cholangiographic pancreatography (ERCP) is a means of directly viewing the ampulla of Vater and portions of the common bile duct and duct of Wirsung (Fig. 4–13). It has a 95 percent detection rate for cancer of the pancreas.

A fiberoptic endoscope is passed through the patient's mouth into the duodenum under fluoroscopy. The fiberoptic feature allows the gastroenterologist to view the area of the Oddi sphincter. Once this area has been located, a cannula is passed through the endoscope and directly into the ampulla

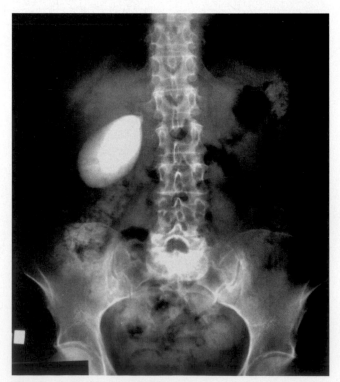

Figure 4–10. Normal findings on an oral cholecystogram.

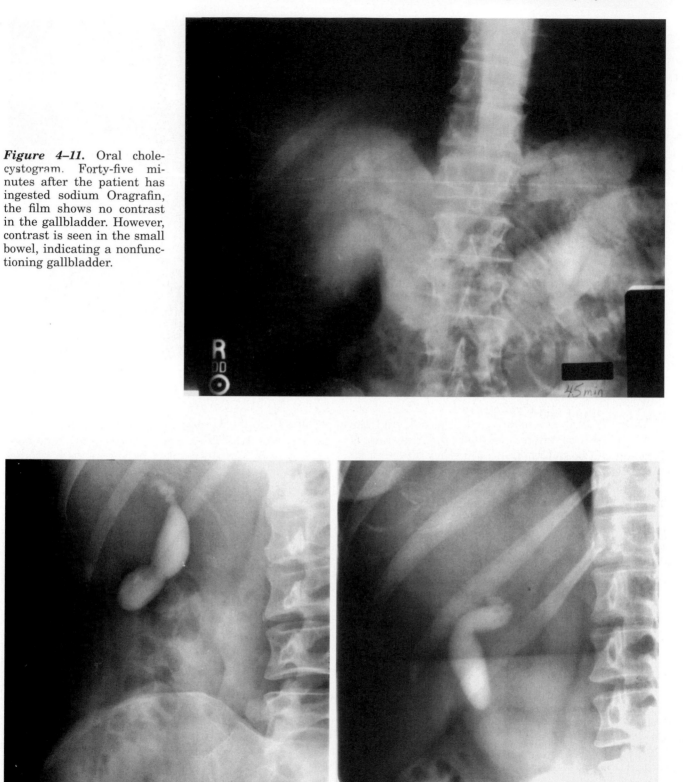

Figure 4–11. Oral chole-cystogram. Forty-five minutes after the patient has ingested sodium Oragrafin, the film shows no contrast in the gallbladder. However, contrast is seen in the small bowel, indicating a nonfunctioning gallbladder.

Figure 4–12. Oral cholecystogram after the patient has eaten a fatty meal. *A,* Note the smaller size of the gallbladder after ingestion of the cholecystogue. Also seen well is the cystic duct and the spiral Heister valves. *B,* Residual radiolucent stones in the neck of the gallbladder.

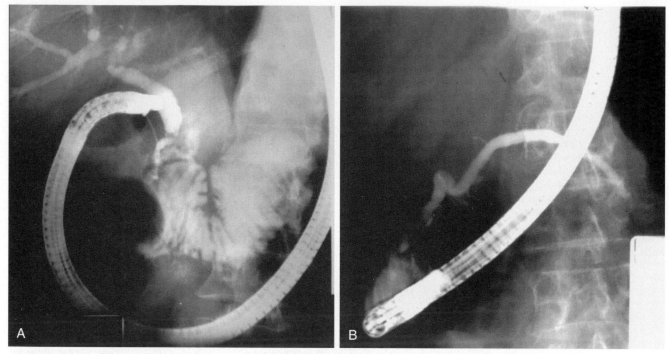

Figure 4–13. Endoscopic retrograde cholangiographic pancreatography visualizes all the bile ducts and small bowel *(A)* and shows the duct of Wirsung *(B)*.

of Vater. A contrast medium is injected, and the course of the common bile duct and the duct of Wirsung can be followed.

The patient is placed prone, and spot films and overhead radiographs are obtained. The contrast material leaves the normal ducts in about 5 minutes, so the films must be taken correctly and rapidly, as an opportunity to do repeat films is not available. The patient must take nothing orally (NPO) for approximately 10 hours following this examination, as the throat is temporarily paralyzed to allow passage of the endoscope down it.

Indications for ERCP include both clinical and radiographic findings that show abnormalities of the biliary system or pancreas (Fig. 4–14). An oral cholecystogram, ultrasonogram, and computed tomographic scan are all done prior to an ERCP to rule out conditions such as a pseudocyst, which would cause infection if contrast material were to be injected into it. Therefore, ERCP is contraindicated in acute pancreatitis.

Barium studies are not done routinely to visualize the pancreas, but rather masses in the head of the pancreas are detected on upper gastrointestinal films because of a displaced or distended C-loop of the duodenum (Fig. 4–15).

PATHOLOGY

Liver

Inflammatory Processes

Cirrhosis is one of humankind's most common serious diseases. It represents the fourth leading cause of death in the United States among people 25 to 65 years of age. This disease process may take anywhere from several months to several years to develop.

The term cirrhosis is used when changes occur in the structure of the liver as the result of any one of a number of chronic diseases. Normal tissue is destroyed and replaced by scar tissue, which diminishes the ability of the organ to function properly, hindering the circulation of the blood through the liver and reducing its power to remove toxins from the body.

Cirrhosis is usually the result of alcoholism, but may be caused by a viral hepatitis. It is the end stage of most serious chronic liver diseases.

The liver takes on a characteristic appearance in the early stages of the disease known as a "fatty liver." This appearance is caused by the engorgement of the liver by fat. At this stage, the damage is reversible. As the fat deposits continue, they interfere with normal function, and cell death occurs. Hepatitis is triggered by necrosis. The liver and the spleen are enlarged. Death can occur at this stage. The last stage of cirrhosis is characterized by fibrous scars, which disrupt the makeup of the liver cells. This interferes with blood flow to and from the liver because of obstruction of the portal vein. Portal hypertension causes ascites, jaundice, and esophageal varices. At this point, the liver is in failure and unable to detoxify ammonia, which can cause the patient to go into hepatic coma and die. If the diagnosis is made in the late stages of cirrho-

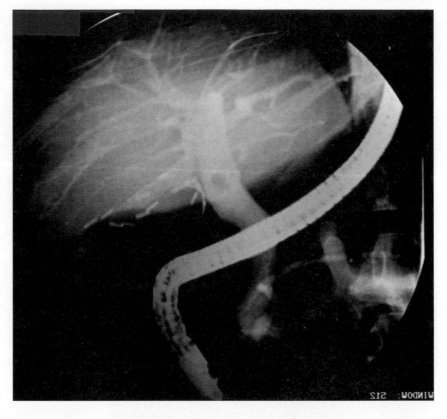

Figure 4–14. Endoscopic retrograde cholangiographic pancreatography shows a radiolucent stone in the common bile duct just superior to the endoscope.

sis, the patient will die within 1 to 2 years. If the disease is treated in the early stages and the patient is able to discontinue the activity that brought the cirrhosis on, the prognosis is only slightly better, with death occurring at a later date. Death by cirrhosis usually results from liver failure or internal hemorrhaging.

The radiographer should look for hepatomegaly, ascites, and air-fluid levels on the abdominal films. A computed tomographic scan will show hepatic nodules and lesions.

Hepatitis signifies inflammation of the liver cells. The cells die and are quickly replaced by new ones if the injury to the liver is slight. When the injury is more severe, cirrhosis results. There are three types of hepatitis, any of which may result in cirrhosis.

1. **Deficiency hepatitis:** Chronic alcoholism is generally associated with malnutrition, or a deficient diet, which causes the liver to suffer damage.
2. **Toxic hepatitis:** One of the functions of the liver is to detoxify poisons that enter the system. However, certain drugs, taken illicitly or for medical purposes, can result in necrosis of the liver.
3. **Viral hepatitis:** This can be subdivided into five groups: hepatitis A, formally known as infectious hepatitis; hepatitis B, previously called se-

rum hepatitis; hepatitis C; delta hepatitis, sometimes referred to as hepatitis D; and hepatitis E.

Hepatitis A, caused by an RNA virus, is the most benign form of viral hepatitis. It is rarely fatal and does not lead to chronic hepatitis. The virus is spread by fecal contamination. Another source is direct contact with infected food, such as raw clams, oysters, or mussels. Contaminated drinking sources or contaminated dishes from which food is eaten can spread the disease quickly.

In contrast, hepatitis B is much more serious. Caused by a DNA virus found in all body fluids of an infected individual, it is transmitted from one human to another by use of contaminated syringes and needles for such things as tattooing, ear piercing, or intravenous injection. Hepatitis B is a major health problem in that 1 in every 1000 people is a carrier. Chronic persistent hepatitis B is a mild illness that causes no permanent liver damage, and the patient can expect to eventually recover. Chronic active hepatitis causes the liver to undergo fibrosis and eventual progression to cirrhosis. This is the most severe form of hepatitis B, as it kills most liver cells and is eventually fatal.

The form of hepatitis previously known as nonA nonB is now referred to as hepatitis C. Caused by an RNA virus, this form of hepatitis is spread in a fashion similar to the way hepatitis B is spread. Hepatitis C has been found to be the cause of most

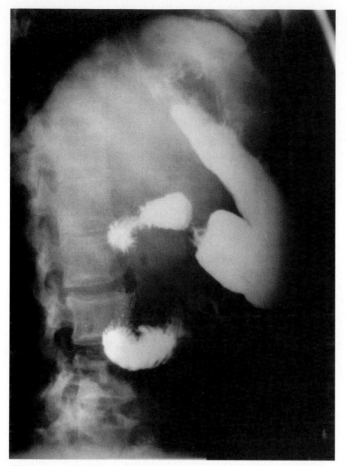

Figure 4–15. Upper gastrointestinal tract. The C-loop of the duodenum is distended. The patient was found to have a pancreatic pseudocyst.

cases of posttransfusion hepatitis, which was previously believed to be caused by hepatitis B. Unfortunately, hepatitis C has a greater probability than B of becoming chronic active hepatitis, leading to cirrhosis of the liver.

A rare cause of hepatitis is a delta agent. In order to contract hepatitis D, the patient must already be infected with hepatitis B. Another form of hepatitis not yet found in the United States, except in extremely rare instances, is hepatitis E. It is most frequently seen in India, South Central Asia, and the Middle East. A recent small outbreak in Mexico signals the arrival of the virus to the Western Hemisphere. The virus is transmitted by the fecal-oral route. Although there is no proven therapy or prevention for hepatitis E, it does not become chronic and the patient can fully recover.

Hepatitis shows as hepatomegaly and possibly jaundice. The alert radiographer is able to identify an enlarged liver shadow on the abdominal radiograph.

Jaundice, or **icterus,** denotes a yellowish cast to the skin and sclera of the eyes that is the result of excess bilirubin in the blood. It is an obvious sign of liver disease. There are several ways in which bilirubin can excessively accumulate in the blood and thereby give rise to jaundice.

1. **Medical jaundice** (also known as **nonobstructive jaundice**): Two forms of jaundice fall under the category of nonobstructive jaundice. **Hemolytic jaundice** occurs if an excessive amount of blood is broken down, causing more bilirubin to be formed than can be excreted by the liver. The excess remains in the blood. **Hepatic jaundice** occurs when the liver is extensively diseased so that it is unable to excrete the normal amount of bilirubin, causing an accumulation in the blood.

2. **Surgical jaundice** (also known as **obstructive jaundice**): The liver can excrete the normal amount of bile but because of an obstruction, usually a gallstone, it is unable to drain either into the gallbladder or to the duodenum. Under these conditions, bile backs up in the liver and is reabsorbed in the blood.

Neoplasms

Hepatomas are any tumor of the liver, but most often refer to malignant tumors of the liver originating in the parenchymal cells. Primary carcinoma of the liver is either massive, nodular, or diffuse. The right lobe is more often affected in the massive and nodular types of hepatomas. The incidence of hepatomas is on the rise; currently they are seen in 20 percent of cases of cirrhosis. This highly vascular neoplasm is best demonstrated by computed tomography and angiography. Clinically, there is an enlarging abdominal mass, pain in the right upper quadrant, and ascites. The changes in liver function result in an elevation of serum alkaline phosphatase levels.

Another primary carcinoma of the liver is known as **cholangiocarcinoma.** This neoplasm arises from the biliary ductule cells of the liver and is not nearly as common as the hepatoma.

Metastatic carcinomas of the liver are far more common than the primary tumors. These tumors arise, as a rule, from primary sources in the lung, gastrointestinal tract, and breast. Metastatic carcinoma usually involves both lobes of the liver, which becomes enlarged and easily palpable. Ultrasonography, computed tomography, and angiography all can be used to make the diagnosis.

Gallbladder and Bile Ducts

Congenital Anomalies

Congenital anomalies should be considered under pathology, even though they may not cause damage or are rare. **Duplication** of the gallbladder (Fig. 4–16) is a rare anomaly, whereas varying shapes of the gallbladder are more common. A gallbladder may have an internal septum dividing it into two chambers. This is termed a **bilobed** gallbladder. Another shape deviation occurs when the body is narrowed in the middle, creating an **hourglass** gallbladder. The most common anomaly of the gallbladder occurs when the fundus folds over the body. This creates the **phrygian cap** gallbladder (Fig. 4–17).

A rare congenital lesion that occurs in the common bile duct of young girls is called a **choledochal cyst.** It is caused by a weakness in the wall of the duct, allowing the formation of the cystic structure. This dilation of the duct causes jaundice and pain.

Inflammatory Processes

Failure of the gallbladder to become opaque can indicate several things. The contrast medium may not have been in the bowel long enough to have been absorbed, or the patient may not have been properly prepared for the examination. Liver disease may have caused decreased secretion of bile, which will not allow the medium to make the gallbladder opaque. A very common cause of nonvisualization is obstruction of the cystic duct. This obstruction may be caused by stones, a tumor, or

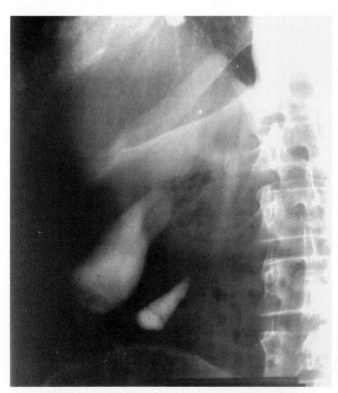

Figure 4–16. Duplication of the gallbladder.

disease of the gallbladder wall. If the cystic duct is blocked, the gallbladder can increase in size. This condition is known as **hydrops** and is best visualized via ultrasonography (Fig. 4–18). Hydrops means an abnormal accumulation of serous fluid in an organ. If this condition is not relieved, the gallbladder may perforate, spilling bile into the peritoneum.

Cholangitis is inflammation of the bile ducts. It is most often associated with gallstones of the common bile duct. This inflammatory process may spread into the intrahepatic biliary system, causing an abscess. **Cholecystitis** is inflammation of the gallbladder and is characterized by intermittent attacks of severe pain and belching. **Acute cholecystitis** is uncommon. The inability to visualize the gallbladder by any modality usually indicates a cystic duct obstruction, which is almost universally present in acute cholecystitis. The patient experiences a very sharp, painful attack in the right upper quadrant, usually after eating a large fatty meal. This pain is accompanied by fever, nausea, and vomiting. **Chronic cholecystitis** is very common, with the vast majority of patients having gallstones. Symptoms of chronic cholecystitis are vague but include an intolerance to fatty food, belching, and pain after eating. As a result of chronic cholecystitis, the gallbladder wall may completely calcify. This is known as a **porcelain** gallbladder (Fig. 4–19).

Cholelithiasis (gallstones) is reported to afflict a large number of the adult population in the United States. Although anyone in the general population can develop gallstones, there are several groups who are at a higher risk to do so. Those people who appear to be more prone to gallstones are women who are over 40 years of age and overweight. Also, pregnant women or women on oral contraceptives or estrogen therapy are more prone to develop stones. Any person who has lost a large amount of weight is also susceptible. Native Americans are at a higher risk than others to develop cholelithiasis.

Gallstones are composed of constituents of bile (cholesterol) that have formed into crystals. Some are pure cholesterol while others are pure bile pigment. These are radiolucent stones (Fig. 4–20). Other stones contain calcium carbonate and are radiopaque (Fig. 4–21). Of course a combination of any two, or all three, of these substances may comprise a stone (Fig. 4–22). Radiolucent stones are the most common type. About 80 percent of all stones are of mixed combinations of cholesterol, bile pigments, and small amounts of calcium. Only 10 percent of patients have enough calcium in their stones to make the stones radiopaque. Stones may not

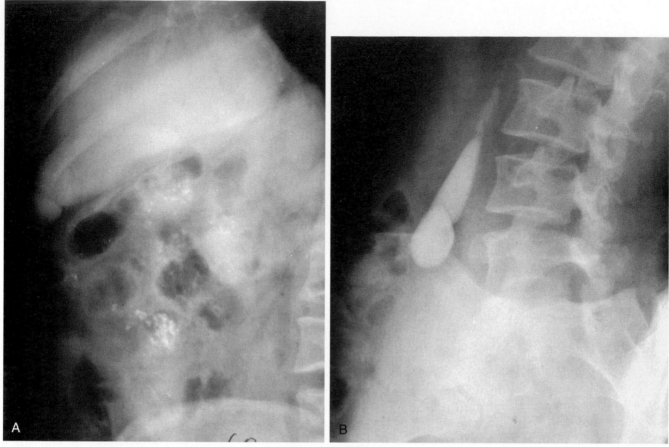

Figure 4–17. Phrygian cap. *A,* The fundus of the gallbladder has folded over the body. Contrast can also be seen in the small bowel. *B,* Image taken after a fatty meal shows a phrygian cap.

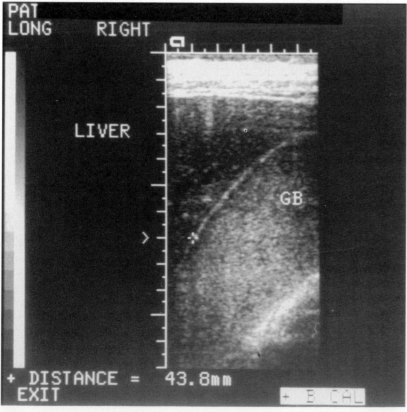

Figure 4–18. Hydrops: increased size of the gallbladder due to obstruction of the duct.

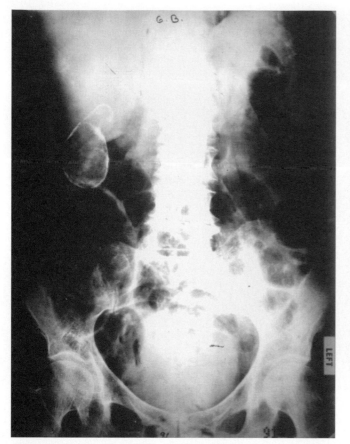

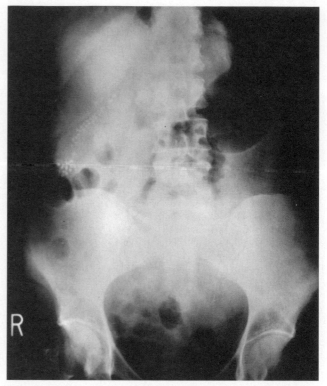

Figure 4–21. Radiopaque stones seen on a film taken with patient in supine position.

Figure 4–19. Porcelain gallbladder: the walls are calcified.

readily visualize and the radiographs with patient in various positions should be made to ensure adequate demonstration of gallstones. Erect (Fig. 4–23) or right lateral decubitis (Fig. 4–24) positions dem-

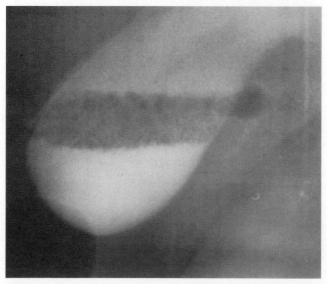

Figure 4–20. Lucent stones layered on a sludge-filled fundus. Many small stones have piled into a thick layer.

onstrate stratification of gallstones. Stones that may be too small to be seen on a flat abdominal film may float on the heavier constituents of bile. If the stones are heavier, they may layer out along the bottommost aspect of the gallbladder. Gallstones may be single (Fig. 4–25) or multiple, round or irregular, and range in color from yellow to brown to green.

Although no cause is known for sure, it is believed that stones are associated with the inability of the gallbladder to absorb properly. In 90 percent of patients with gallstones, the patient has more cholesterol in the bile and a lower amount of chenodeoxycholic acid than normal.

More and more patients are being treated with an oral medication known as ursodiol, which dissolves cholesterol gallstones. Ursodiol is a naturally occurring bile acid that lowers cholesterol levels in bile and slowly dissolves stones within 6 to 24 months, depending on the size of the stone. Chenodiol is another medication that is used to dissolve stones and may be used in conjunction with ursodiol.

Another alternative to cholecystectomy is shock wave lithotripsy, which uses external sound waves to fragment the stones into small pieces. The pieces are then dissolved by ursodiol or chenodiol. Some fragments of stones are so small after lithotripsy that they pass through the system naturally.

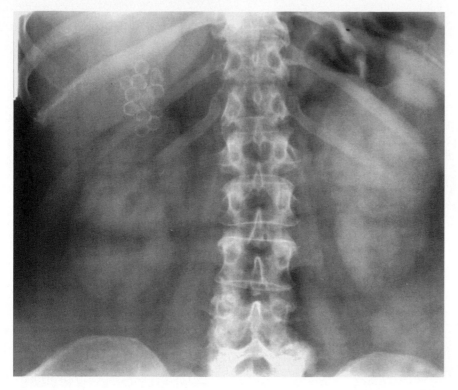

Figure 4–22. Mixed stones with both radiopaque borders and radiolucent centers.

Figure 4–23. Lucent stones fall to the most dependent portion of the gallbladder when the patient is in the erect position.

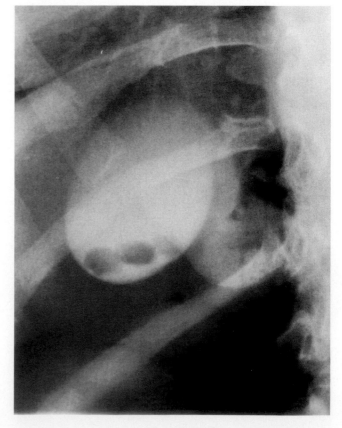

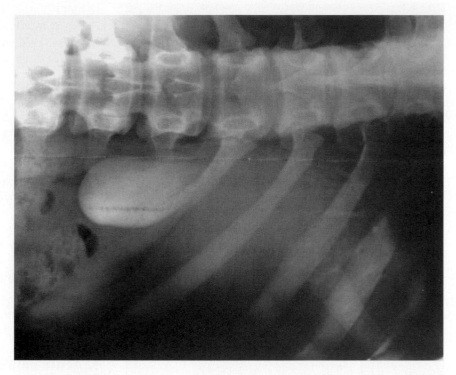

Figure 4–24. When the patient is in the decubitus position, the stones layer out in the most dependent portion of the gallbladder.

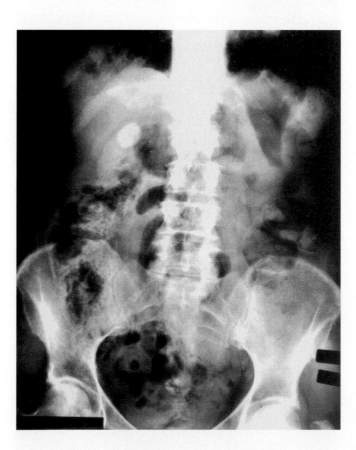

Figure 4–25. A single large radiopaque stone.

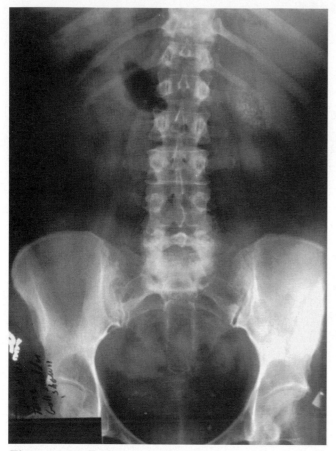

Figure 4–26. Radiopaque stones in the middle of a gallbladder on a film taken with patient in upright position. Note the thick wall around the stones, which indicates edema of the gallbladder. Situs inversus viscerum is also present.

Complications of gallstones are somewhat rare but include edema of the wall (Fig. 4–26) or inflammation caused by an impaction of a stone in either the cystic duct or the common bile duct. This can lead to a **gangrenous gallbladder.** A gallstone can erode through the wall into the bowel, creating a **fistula** between the gallbladder and bowel (Figs. 4–27 and 4–28). Another complication that is even less common is when the stone becomes impacted in the small bowel. If the stone is large enough to block passage through the bowel, an ileus will occur.

Neoplasms

Carcinoma of the gallbladder is the most common tumor of the biliary system. It occurs more often in elderly women. An association with gallstones is believed to be a factor because of the chronic irritation from the stones and any ensuing infection. If the tumor is in the fundus of the gallbladder, it will frequently invade the liver and peritoneum. Carcinomas found in the body and neck of the gall-

bladder often infiltrate the hepatic and biliary ducts, thus involving not only the liver but also the pancreas and the duodenum. Jaundice is associated as a late development of carcinoma that has spread to the ducts.

Pancreas

Congenital Processes

Cystic fibrosis of the pancreas is an inherited autosomal disorder. The pancreatic ducts fill with thick mucus, which leads to dilations of the ducts and fibrosis of the pancreas. Because the pancreas plays a vital role in digestion, malabsorption and weight loss are associated with cystic fibrosis of the pancreas. Pancreatic deficiencies eventually lead to death of the child.

Inflammatory Processes

There are two types of pancreatitis:

1. **Acute pancreatitis:** 40 percent of all cases are

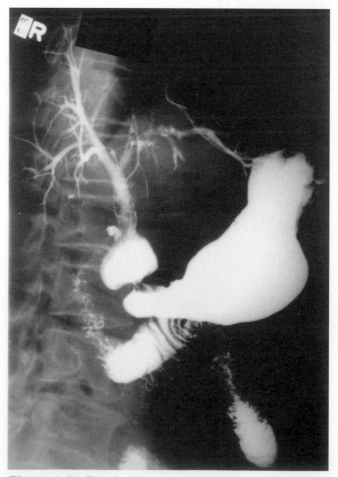

Figure 4–27. Fistula between the duodenal bulb and the bile ducts.

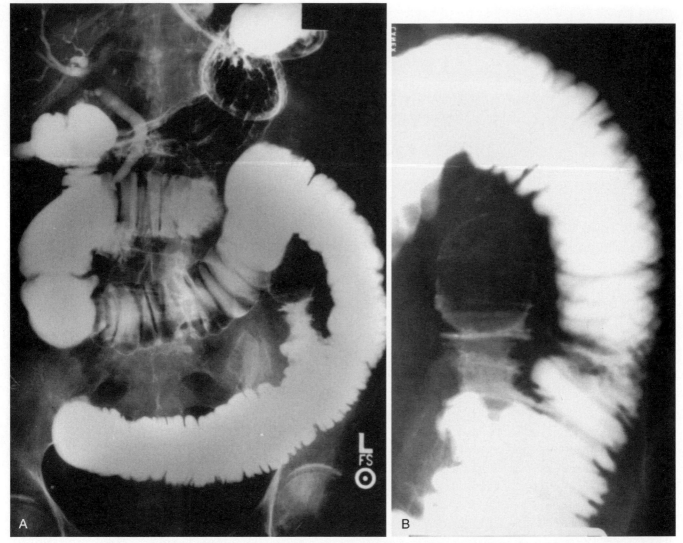

Figure 4–28. *A,* Film taken 90 minutes after ingestion of a contrast medium shows an obstruction of the small bowel. There is a fistula between the small bowel and the bile ducts. A large stone can be seen to have eroded through the bowel wall. *B,* Collimated radiograph of the stone.

caused by alcohol abuse and 40 percent are caused by gallstones. The other 20 percent are caused by either trauma (child abuse) or drug abuse. The symptoms include nausea and vomiting, fever, abrupt epigastric pain, and an increase in amylase and white blood cell count. A pseudocyst may be associated with acute pancreatitis (Fig. 4–29).

2. **Chronic pancreatitis** is a relapsing pancreatitis that causes progressive fibrosis and destruction of pancreatic cells. The pancreas increases in size. Late stages cause calcifications to form in the ductal system. Causes of chronic pancreatitis are a long history of alcoholism and recurring attacks of acute pancreatitis. Gallstones are rarely a cause of chronic pancreatitis.

Only 20 percent of people show radiographic signs of pancreatitis, which are a displaced stomach and effacement of bowel loops (Fig. 4–30). The difference between pancreatitis and another organ inflammation is that the powerful digestive enzymes secreted by the acinar cells may escape from the cells and start to digest the pancreas itself as well as the adipose tissue around it. This process is called **enzymatic necrosis.**

Pseudocysts are the most common cysts of the pancreas. These usually result from inflammation, but they have been known to develop following necrosis, hemorrhage, or trauma. Most often only one occurs at a time. Pseudocysts are commonly found in the subhepatic region. They contain enzymes and are capable of dissecting tissue, which allows them

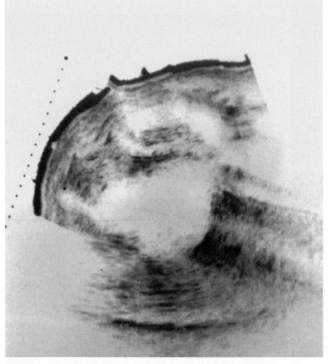

Figure 4–29. Static ultrasonographic scan, showing a large pancreatic pseudocyst below the left kidney.

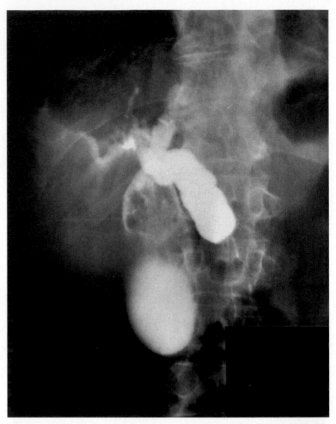

Figure 4–31. Complete obstruction of the common bile duct, causing dilation. No demonstration of the stone. Further testing revealed an adenocarcinoma of the head of the pancreas. Note the large gallbladder.

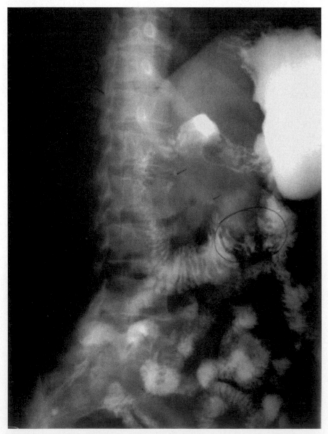

Figure 4–30. Classic signs of chronic pancreatitis: displaced stomach, effaced bowel loops, and calcification.

to travel anywhere in the body. Approximately 20 percent regress spontaneously and the remaining 80 percent are drained or left alone until they become so large that they begin to displace other organs.

Neoplasms

Benign neoplasms of the pancreas are called **islet cell tumors,** or adenomas. These occur in the beta cells and therefore contain high levels of insulin.

Carcinoma of the pancreas is not a common neoplasm; however, it ranks high among fatalities from malignancies in the United States. It is rare before the age of 40 and is more prevalent in men. **Adenocarcinoma** is the most common cancer; 90 percent of them arise from the ductal system and 10 percent from the acinar cells. The head of the pancreas is involved in 75 percent of all cases of carcinoma. Cancer of the head of the pancreas is an infiltrative process and frequently occludes the common bile duct, causing jaundice (Fig. 4–31). As bile backs up through the ductal system, the gallbladder can become massively distended. This is

Table 4–1.
Clinical and Radiographic Characteristics of Common Pathologies

Pathologic Condition	Causal Factors*	Manifestations	Radiographic Appearance
Cirrhosis	25 to 65 years, usually alcoholism, viral hepatitis	Ascites, jaundice, esophageal varices	Hepatomegaly ascites, air-fluid levels
Hepatitis			
Deficiency	Alcoholism	All types lead to jaundice	Hepatomegaly
Toxic	Drug use		
Viral			
A	Fecal contamination		
B	Blood and body fluid		
C	RNA virus		
Jaundice			
Medical	Hepatic or hemolytic	All types lead to yellow skin and sclera of eyes	
Surgical	Obstruction		
Chronic cholecystitis	Common with stones	Belching and pain after eating	May calcify gallbladder
Cholelithiasis	Women over 40 are more prone, no positive known cause	Asymptomatic or pain	Radiolucent, radiopaque, or mixed areas in right upper quadrant
Pancreatitis			
Acute	Alcoholism or gallstones	Nausea, vomiting, fever, abrupt epigastric pain	May have a pseudocyst
Chronic	Long history of alcoholism, recurring acute pancreatitis	Nausea and vomiting	Calcifications, displaced stomach and effaced bowel loop

*Includes age, if relevant.

known as Courvoisier gallbladder. The duct of Wirsung becomes dilated, as does the common bile duct. Causes of cancer are smoking and asbestosis but not alcoholism. Pancreatic carcinoma metastasizes to the liver in over 80 percent of the cases.

Radiographic examinations of the gastrointestinal tract can reveal abnormalities of the duodenum caused by the tumor. Percutaneous transhepatic cholangiography is an aid to diagnosis in obstructive jaundice, a complication of the tumor. Nuclear medicine and angiography are also quite helpful in differentiating the tumor.

Table 4–1 summarizes the common pathologies of the hepatobiliary system.

Review Questions

1. List and describe four tests that are used to detect liver disease. How do abnormalities of the tests correlate with changes in the liver?
2. Describe the anatomic relationship of the pancreas to the duodenum, inferior vena cava, stomach, splenic hilum, and left kidney. Where is the entire organ located?
3. Explain the composition of bile. Where is it made? How is the gallbladder able to hold the amount that is produced? Describe this process.
4. Describe the action of food on cholecystokinin and the relationship of cholecystokinin to the function of the gallbladder.
5. List the functions of the pancreas. Define each.
6. Describe a T-tube cholangiography procedure.
7. What is PTC? Describe the procedure. What risks are involved with this procedure?
8. What is ERCP? Describe the procedure. What are the indications for it? What care must the patient be made aware of following the examination? Why?
9. Describe the procedure known as a "fatty meal" for the gallbladder. What anatomy will a radiograph demonstrate? Why?

10. List and define the three types of hepatitis. Be sure to explain any subgroups.
11. Name and describe the pathologic conditions of the liver and the pancreas that result from alcohol abuse.
12. Define enzymatic necrosis. When does this occur? How does it occur?
13. Describe the composition of gallstones. Which are more common? What population of people is prone to gallstones?
14. List and describe three complications associated with gallstones.
15. List and describe the two types of pancreatitis. What causes them and what will radiographs of each demonstrate?
16. Define jaundice. List the two types and explain each.

CHAPTER V

Gastrointestinal System

Goals

1. To review the basic anatomy of the esophagus, stomach, small bowel, and large bowel.
2. To review the physiology and function of the esophagus, stomach, small bowel, and large bowel.
3. To learn the special imaging modalities and procedures that are performed on the esophagus, stomach, small bowel, and large bowel.
4. To understand the pathophysiology and radiographic manifestations of all of the common pathologic conditions of the gastrointestinal system.

Objectives

At the completion of the chapter, the radiographer will be able to:

1. Identify all anatomic components of the esophagus, stomach, small bowel, and large bowel and explain their relationship to each other as well as to other organs.
2. Explain the physiology and function of these four areas of the digestive tract.
3. Describe how each organ functionally affects the others.
4. List and describe the various special imaging procedures performed for each area.
5. Identify the radiographic manifestations of the listed pathologies of the gastrointestinal tract.
6. Describe the various pathologic conditions affecting the gastrointestinal system.

I. Anatomy
  A. Esophagus (Gullet)
    1. Esophageal Hiatus
    2. Cardiac orifice
  B. Stomach
    1. Fundus
    2. Body (Corpus)
    3. Curvatures
      a. Greater
      b. Lesser
    4. Incisura Angularis
      (Angular Notch)
    5. Cardiac Orifice (Cardia)
    6. Pylorus
    7. Rugae
    8. Muscular Coats
      a. Oblique
      b. Circular
      c. Longitudinal
  C. Small Bowel
    1. Duodenum
      a. Superior
      b. Descending
      c. Horizontal
      d. Ascending
    2. Jejunum
      a. Ligament of Treitz
    3. Ileum
      a. Ileocecal Valve
  D. Large Bowel
    1. Cecum
      a. Appendix (Vermiform
      Process)
    2. Colon
      a. Ascending
      b. Transverse
      c. Flexures
        1. Hepatic
        2. Splenic
      d. Descending
      e. Sigmoid
    3. Rectum
      a. Houston Valves
      b. Rectal Columns
    4. Teniae (Taeniae) Coli
      a. Haustra
      b. Semilunar Folds
II. Physiology and Function
  A. Esophagus
    1. Passes Food and Liquid
    to Stomach
  B. Stomach
    1. Initiates Digestion
    2. Reservoir
    3. Absorption
      a. Water
      b. Alcohol
  C. Small Bowel
    1. Secretes Enzymes
    2. Completes Digestion
    3. Absorption of Digested
    Food

  D. Large Bowel
    1. Elimination of Waste
    2. Absorption of Water and
    Vitamins
III. Special Radiographic Procedures
  A. Endoscopy (Endoscopic
    retrograde cholangiographic
    pancreatography)
  B. Hypotonic Duodenography
  C. Computed Tomography and
    Magnetic Resonance Imaging
  D. Nuclear Medicine
  E. Interventional Radiography
    1. Percutaneous
      Transluminal Angioplasty
IV. Pathology
  A. Esophagus
    1. Congenital Anomalies
      a. Atresia
      b. Fistula
    2. Acquired Pathology
      a. Achalasia
        (Cardiospasm,
        Megaesophagus)
      b. Corkscrew
      c. Esophageal Web
      d. Foreign Bodies
      e. Hiatal Hernia
        1. Sliding
          a. Schatzki Ring
          b. Intrathoracic
          Stomach
        2. Paraesophageal
        (Rolling)
      f. Spasms
        1. Cricopharyngeal
        2. Esophageal
      g. Spontaneous Rupture
    3. Inflammatory Processes
      a. Diverticula
        1. Pulsion
          a. Zenker
          b. Epiphrenic
          c. Pharyngeal
          Pouch
        2. Traction
      b. Reflux Esophagitis
        1. Barrett Esophagus
      c. Strictures
        1. Peptic Esophagitis
      d. Varices
    4. Neoplasms
      a. Benign
        1. Leiomyoma
      b. Malignant
        1. Esophageal
        Carcinoma
  B. Stomach
    1. Congenital Anomalies
      a. Pyloric Stenosis
    2. Acquired Pathologies
      a. Bezoar

        1. Phytobezoar
        2. Trichobezoar
      b. Prolapse
    3. Inflammatory Processes
      a. Gastritis
      b. Ulcers
        1. Gastric
        2. Duodenal
      c. Zollinger-Ellison
        Syndrome
    4. Neoplasms
      a. Benign
      b. Malignant
        1. Papillary
        (Fungating)
        2. Ulcerating
        3. Infiltrating
          a. Leather Bottle
          Stomach
  C. Small Bowel
    1. Congenital Anomalies
      a. Meckel Diverticulum
    2. Acquired Pathologies
      a. Hernia
    3. Inflammatory Processes
      a. Diverticula
      b. Malabsorption
        Syndrome
        1. Sprue (Celiac
        Disease)
      c. Bowel Obstruction
        1. Mechanical
        2. Paralytic Ileus
        (Adynamic Ileus)
      d. Regional Enteritis
        (Crohn's Disease)
  D. Large Bowel
    1. Congenital Anomalies
      a. Hirschsprung disease
        (aganglionic
        megacolon)
      b. Imperforate Anus
      c. Rectal Atresia
    2. Acquired Pathologies
      a. Cathartic Colon
      b. Intussusception
        1. Adult
        2. Infantile
      c. Volvulus
    3. Inflammatory Processes
      a. Colitis
        1. Granulomatous
        2. Ulcerative
        3. Ischemic
      b. Diverticulosis
      c. Polyps
        1. Adenomatous
        2. Villous
    4. Neoplasms
      a. Adenocarcinoma
        1. Annular Lesions
        2. Polypoid Lesions

The gastrointestinal system is also called the digestive system by some authors. This system includes the mouth, pharynx, esophagus, stomach, and small and large intestines (bowel). As mentioned in the previous chapter, the liver, gallbladder, bile ducts, and pancreas are all accessory organs to the digestive tract. Other accessory organs are the teeth and salivary glands.

ANATOMY

Esophagus

The esophagus, also known as the gullet, is a vertical tube approximately 25 cm (10 inches) long. It extends from the level of C-6, inferior to the pharynx, to the stomach at the level of T-11. The esophagus lies posterior to the trachea and heart and anterior to the spine. The descending thoracic aorta lies posterior to the esophagus.

The esophagus lies in the thoracic cavity but pierces the diaphragm at an opening called the esophageal hiatus. It passes through this hiatus and opens into the medial side of the stomach. The opening of the esophagus into the stomach is termed the cardiac orifice (cardia).

The esophagus is not covered with peritoneum but rather has a covering of fibrous connective tissue. The esophagus is different from the trachea in that it is a completely collapsible tube, as it lacks the cartilage rings that the trachea contains.

Stomach

The stomach is a large collapsible sac that is located in the left upper quadrant of the abdomen. It is the most dilated portion of the digestive tract; it can hold almost 1.5 L (1½ quarts).

The fundus of the stomach is an enlarged, bulblike portion located to the left and above the opening from the esophagus. The central portion is called the body or corpus. The greater curvature is along the lower border of the stomach and the lesser curvature is along the upper medial border. The incisura angularis, better known as the angular notch, is a sharp indentation along the lesser curvature.

The cardiac sphincter is located at the cardiac orifice to prevent regurgitation of stomach contents into the esophagus. Located at the opening from the stomach into the duodenum, between the lesser curvature and the pyloric channel, is an area known as the pylorus (also known as the pyloric orifice). It is guarded by the pyloric sphincter.

When the stomach is empty, it collapses into many folds called rugae. These internal mucosal folds help to move the stomach contents into the duodenum. Rugae disappear when the stomach is full. Figure 5–1 shows the separate areas of the stomach.

The muscular coat of the stomach is actually three muscle layers. The most internal layer is known as the oblique layer. A circular layer of muscle is the middle section and a longitudinal layer of muscle is the outermost layer, which is visceral peritoneum.

Small Bowel

The small bowel (small intestine) extends from the pyloric sphincter to the cecum. It is called the small bowel not because it is short (it measures 5.5–7 m [18–23 feet] in length), but because its lumen is smaller than that of the large intestine.

There are three divisions of the small bowel: duodenum, jejunum, and ileum. The duodenum is the shortest, widest portion, being approximately 25 cm (10 inches) long. It is made up of four divisions to form a C shape.

The superior portion is immediately adjacent to the pyloric opening. It includes the duodenal bulb. The descending duodenum connects with the superior portion and passes to the right of the median plane. The ampulla of Vater opens into this portion of the duodenum. The horizontal portion of the duodenum crosses over the median plane to the left and connects with the ascending duodenum, which travels upward to connect with the jejunum just posterior to the stomach.

The jejunum is the second portion of the small bowel and is approximately 2.4 m (8 feet) long. The junction between the duodenum and jejunum is marked by the ligament of Treitz. The jejunum coils back and forth to fill the left upper quadrant of the abdomen. A loop is made in the right upper quadrant before the jejunum joins the third portion of the small intestine, the ileum.

The ileum extends about another 4 m (13 feet) before terminating at the ileocecal valve of the cecum. The ileum forms coils in the lower quadrants of the abdomen and in the pelvis.

Large Bowel

The large bowel averages 1.5 to 1.8 m (5–6 feet) in length. It extends from the cecum to the anus. Many people mistakenly believe the colon to be synonymous with the large bowel. The colon, along with the cecum and rectum, is a part of the large bowel. The portion known as the cecum is an area that

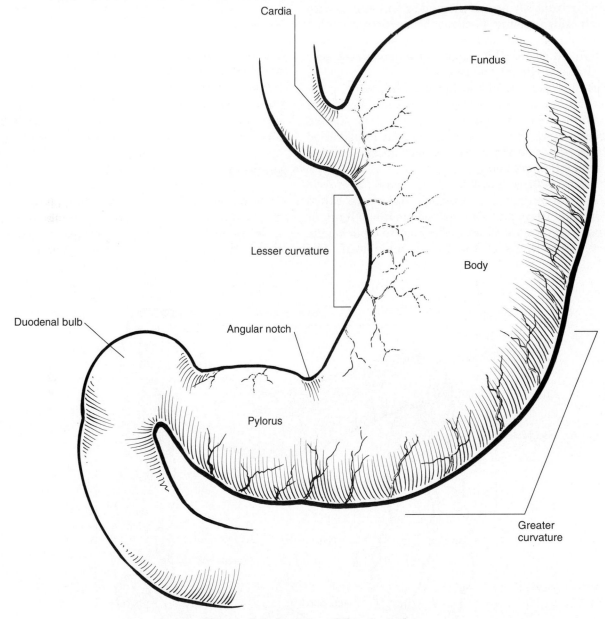

Figure 5–1. Anatomy of the stomach.

forms a sac-like structure inferior to the ileocecal opening in the right lower quadrant. The appendix (vermiform process) is a long, narrow tube attached to the base of the cecum.

The colon is divided into the ascending colon located on the right side of the abdomen and extending to the liver; the transverse colon, which begins at the right colic (hepatic) flexure and extends horizontally across the abdomen, ending with the left colic (splenic) flexure; the descending colon located on the left and continuing vertically; and the sigmoid colon, which is an S-shaped curved portion that attaches to the rectum.

The last portion of the large bowel, which contains the anus, is known as the rectum. There are transverse folds located within the rectum known as Houston valves, as well as vertical folds called rectal columns. It is these columns that can enlarge to become hemorrhoids.

The entire large bowel has three bands of muscle running its length. These muscle fibers are called teniae coli. (Teniae is also spelled taeniae. Tenia or taenia is the singular form.) They cause a puckering effect of the walls of the cecum and colon. The

pouches that are formed by the puckering of the teniae coli are called haustra. Semilunar folds are located between each haustrum and are helpful in differentiating the large bowel from the small bowel. Figure 5–2 clearly shows each area of the large bowel.

PHYSIOLOGY AND FUNCTION

Esophagus

The only function of the esophagus is to pass food and liquids from the mouth to the stomach. Since the esophagus is a fairly straight tube, liquids pass down mainly by gravity. Food passes by gravity also, but because it is a bolus of solid material, its passage must be facilitated by peristalsis.

Stomach

As food and liquid pass from the esophagus through the cardiac orifice and into the stomach, digestion is initiated. The stomach secretes a gastric juice that is the combination of pepsinogen, gastrin, and

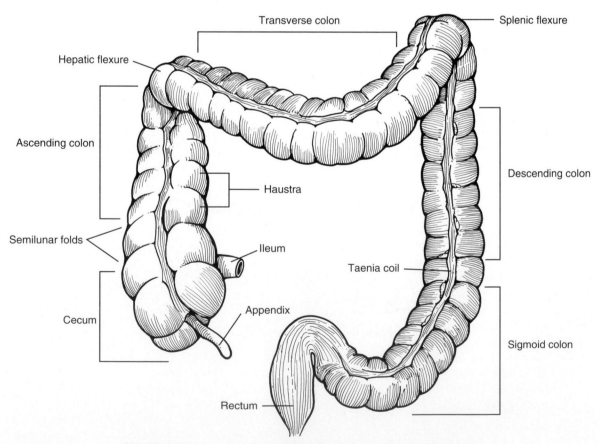

Figure 5–2. Large bowel showing the cecum, colon, and rectum.

hydrochloric acid. The pepsinogen is converted to pepsin, an enzyme that digests food. Mucus and alkaline fluid are also produced to keep the stomach from digesting itself. The stomach prepares the food so that it can be moved along the alimentary tract. By contracting the three muscular coats, the stomach breaks the food into small particles. Once the food is broken down, it is mixed with the gastric juices. If the pyloric sphincter is closed, the stomach acts as a reservoir to store food until it is sufficiently digested to be moved, a bit at a time, into the duodenum.

Not all of the digestion process takes place in the stomach. In fact, only a small amount of absorption of water and alcohol takes place there.

Small Bowel

The structure of the small bowel was designed to carry out the processes of digestion and absorption. The tiny tubes that are found inside the mucous membrane lining secrete an enzyme that acts on the food that is being passed through the bowel. When the food becomes liquefied by bile, digestive juices from the pancreas, enzymes from the stomach, and acid from the bowel, it is considered to be digested and is ready for absorption.

The finger-like projections, called villi, that are located in the bowel each have a blood vessel. When the liquid food passes these villi, nutrients are absorbed into the blood vessels of each villus. From there, the blood vessel transports the nutrients to the liver by way of the portal vein.

In summary, the small bowel has three functions: secretion of an enzyme to act on food; completion of the digestive process; and absorption of the digested food.

Large Bowel

The mucous membrane of the large bowel does not contain any villi but is lined with tubular glands that are packed closely together. These glands do not secrete any digestive juices, as all digestion is accomplished before material enters the large bowel. This leaves the large bowel with two major functions: elimination of waste and absorption of water. Bacteria produce some vitamins that the body needs, such as vitamins K and D. These, too, are absorbed by the large bowel.

SPECIAL RADIOGRAPHIC PROCEDURES

Special procedures for the esophagus, stomach, and large and small bowel are limited. Radiography that does not fall under the category of "special procedures" is usually all that is necessary to demonstrate the various pathologic conditions of the gastrointestinal system. However, a few procedures are covered here briefly.

When a special instrument that illuminates the internal aspect of an organ (endoscope) is inserted into the body for examination of the esophagus, stomach, duodenum, or colon, the procedure is called **endoscopy.** The endoscope allows cannulation and injection of a contrast medium into the ducts. **Endoscopic retrograde cholangiographic pancreatography,** described in Chapter IV, is an example of this type of opacification of the ampulla of Vater and bile ducts.

Hypotonic duodenography is the study of the duodenum with the use of barium and air. Probantheline bromide (Pro-Banthine), a drug that causes atonicity and dilation of the duodenum, is injected intramuscularly. Barium, followed by air, is then introduced into the duodenum through a tube. Lesions located both inside and outside the duodenum are then easily identified. Modern technology in the form of computed tomography and magnetic resonance imaging have replaced this once routine examination.

Computed tomography has a somewhat limited role in the evaluation of the gastrointestinal tract. It is useful in evaluating retroperitoneal and omental metastases from carcinoma of the digestive tract. Computed tomography can clearly reveal a gastric carcinoma diffusely infiltrating the wall of the stomach. **Magnetic resonance imaging** of the gastrointestinal tract is not as specific as computed tomography because the images are degraded by both respiratory motion and peristalsis. Artifacts from peristalsis can be decreased by intramuscular administration of glucagon just prior to the examination. In the colon, bowel preparation is necessary to avoid misinterpretation of the stool as an abnormally thickened bowel wall.

Nuclear medicine examinations provide a convenient, noninvasive, direct method of assessing gastrointestinal motility, including gastric emptying rate, esophageal transit, and gastroesophageal or enterogastric reflux. Nuclear medicine not only has the advantage of being noninvasive, but it has also proved more sensitive than angiography for the detection of lower gastrointestinal bleeding, particularly in the case of a Meckel diverticulum.

Interventional radiography is also utilized, as it offers an alternative to more invasive means of treatment. **Percutaneous transluminal angioplasty (PTA)** uses balloons to either occlude or dilate blood vessels and is performed in a specialized angiography suite. The catheters are placed under fluoroscopy.

PATHOLOGY

Esophagus

Congenital Anomalies

Atresia is a congenital anomaly of the esophagus manifested as a lack of development of the esophagus at any point. The most common type, occurring in about 90 percent of cases, is the ending of the upper segment of the esophagus in a blind pouch near the level of the bifurcation of the trachea, with a lower segment from the stomach connected to the trachea by a short fistulous tract (Fig. 5–3). In another, less common type, both upper and lower segments of the esophagus are connected by a common fistulous tract to the trachea. A barium swallow study with thin barium readily identifies the termination of the esophagus of the fistulous tract with the trachea.

A passageway between the trachea and the esophagus is known as a fistula. Although there are both congenital and acquired fistulas, the most common is the congenital type III, in which the lower end of the upper segment of the esophagus

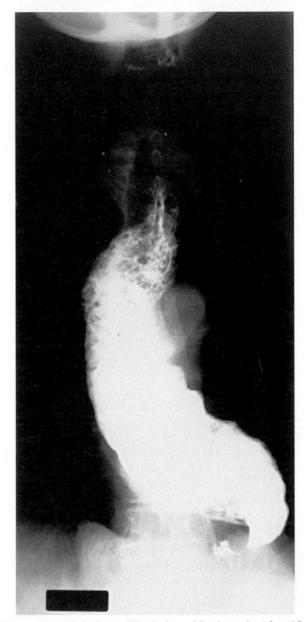

Figure 5–4. Achalasia. The bolus of food can be identified at the proximal end of the esophagus. The distal end of the esophagus is narrowed.

ends in a blind pouch. The upper end of the lower segment of the esophagus is attached to the trachea by a short fistulous tract. An upright abdomenal radiograph will demonstrate air in the bowel.

Acquired Pathology

Achalasia has two other names, **cardiospasm** and **megaesophagus,** and refers to the combined failure of peristalsis to pass food down the esophagus and relaxation of the cardia. The esophagus becomes dilated because of food that cannot pass into the stomach. Past the gastroesophageal junction

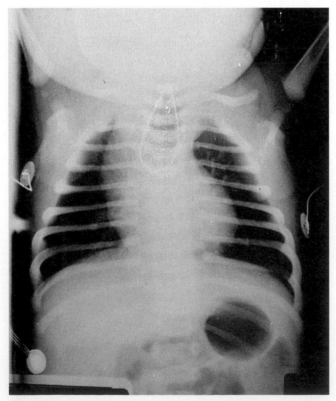

Figure 5–3. Esophageal atresia. Note the looped feeding catheter that was unable to pass to the stomach.

(where the cardia is located), the esophagus is normal in size. Symptoms include dysphagia (difficult or painful swallowing) and heart burn. Radiographically, the esophagus shows as a dilated area (Fig. 5–4) with a narrowing of the distal esophagus, producing the classic "rat tail" appearance. Normal esophageal motility is absent in the middle and lower esophagus. Often, the trapped food particles are readily identifiable.

A **corkscrew esophagus** is caused by asynchrony of peristalsis (tertiary contractions). This disorder is seen more often in elderly patients and sometimes in hiatal hernia cases. The radiographs show a curling or corkscrew appearance, hence its name (Fig. 5–5).

An **esophageal web** is seen on middle-aged women, most often those with anemia. A mucosal band of tissue lies across the lumen of the esophagus, causing difficulty in the passage of food down the esophagus. It is important that an esophageal web be demonstrated early, as it has a predisposition to malignancy. A barium swallow with thick paste or some material soaked in thin barium may identify the web, as the tissue may deter the barium and allow radiographs to be taken of the area.

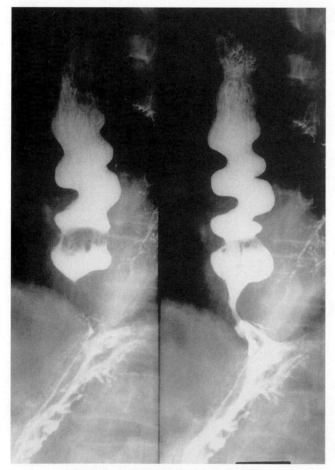

Figure 5–5. Corkscrew esophagus.

Foreign bodies in the esophagus can cause dysphagia or can be asymptomic. A radiopaque object (such as a coin) can be easily demonstrated without the use of a contrast agent (Fig. 5–6). Radiolucent objects, such as chicken bones, pose a problem. The object, especially if it is a small bone, can perforate the esophagus, and an infection or abscess can occur. It is important that these objects be demonstrated. A barium swallow with a thick paste may be all that is required to visualize the objects. Other times, some material soaked in thin barium and then swallowed by the patient is necessary to try to locate the foreign body.

When the abdominal viscera herniates through a defect in the diaphragm, it is known as a **hiatal hernia.** This condition can be found in approximately one half of the population.

The esophageal opening through the diaphragm can become weak, which allows a portion of the stomach and gastroesophageal junction to bulge up through the hiatus. Some authors state that the only true sign of this type of sliding hernia is the presence of the gastroesophageal junction (Schatzki ring) above the diaphragm (Fig. 5–7). After a time, the hiatus becomes so large that the patient acquires a gastric volvulus or **intrathoracic stomach** (Figs. 5–8 and 5–9). In this condition, almost the entire stomach has herniated through the esophageal hiatus into the chest and has assumed an inverted or upside-down configuration. This may be associated with a congenitally short esophagus if the condition exists at birth. Rarely, traction or torsion of the stomach at or near the level of the hiatus may lead to obstruction, infarction, or perforation of the intrathoracic stomach. Patients with this condition often undergo emergency surgery without preoperative barium studies because of their rapidly deteriorating clinical condition.

Another type of hernia occurs through an opening adjacent to the normal hiatus and is known as a **rolling,** or **paraesophageal hiatal hernia** (Fig. 5–10). In this type, only a portion of the stomach slides above the diaphragm, leaving the gastroesophageal junction in place.

A hiatal hernia can be demonstrated by placing the patient in a Trendelenburg position during a series of upper gastrointestinal radiographs. Symptoms of hiatal hernias are related to inflammatory changes of the esophageal mucosa caused by the action of gastric juices on it. These symptoms are heartburn and dysphagia.

Several types of spasms can occur in the esophagus that may be detected radiographically. A **cricopharyngeal spasm** occurs when the muscle around the proximal end of the esophagus does not completely relax to allow food to pass from the phar-

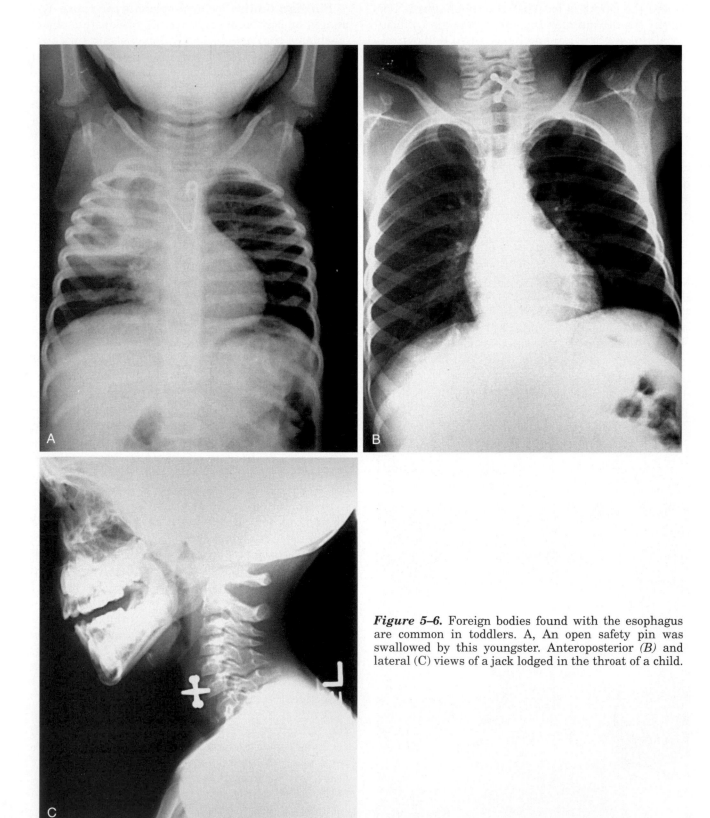

Figure 5–6. Foreign bodies found with the esophagus are common in toddlers. A, An open safety pin was swallowed by this youngster. Anteroposterior *(B)* and lateral (C) views of a jack lodged in the throat of a child.

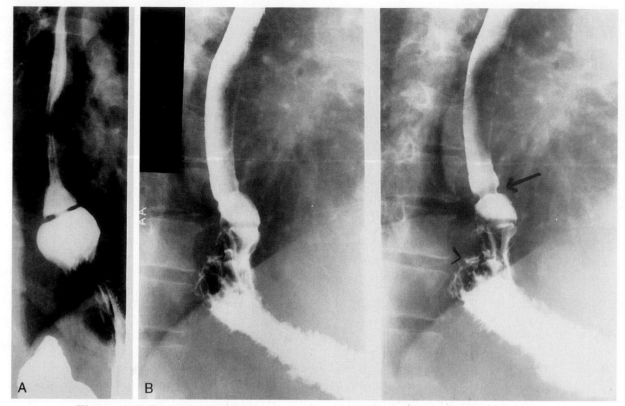

Figure 5–7. Hiatal hernia demonstrating Schatzki's ring. *A,* A very good demonstration of Schatzki's ring proximal to a fundus. *B,* Schatzki's ring can be seen on the right *(arrow).* The fundus of the stomach can be seen above the level of the diaphragm, demonstrating the sliding hiatal hernia *(arrowhead).*

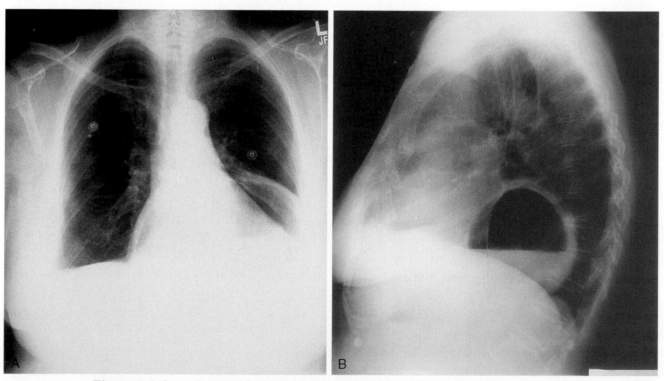

Figure 5–8. Intrathoracic stomach. Posteroanterior *(A)* and lateral *(B)* chest examinations demonstrate the air-fluid level behind the heart shadow.

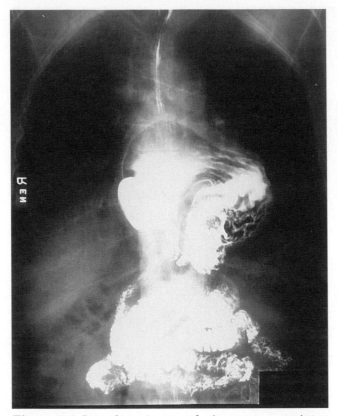

Figure 5–9. Intrathoracic stomach. An upper gastrointestinal study that shows the stomach in a horizontal position with the majority of it located within the thoracic cavity (different patient than the one shown in Figure 5–8).

ynx into the esophagus. A barium swallow study shows a marked indentation on the posterior aspect of the esophagus. An **esophageal spasm** is a transitory process that may cause substernal pain and difficulty in swallowing. A barium swallow study shows a normal esophagus, unless the examination is performed at the same instant that a spasm occurs. In this case, the esophagus will become constricted at the site of the spasm, allowing only a small trickle of barium to pass.

Spontaneous rupture is caused by violent vomiting. When the patient vomits, the distal portion of the esophagus is suddenly overdistended and splits. This leads to escape of gas and fluid, which causes pneumomediastinum and left pleural effusion.

Inflammatory Processes

There are two common types of diverticula of the esophagus, pulsion and traction. **Pulsion diverticula** are more common than traction ticks. Usually located at the esophageal-pharyngeal junction, they have a narrow neck with a round head protruding from the weakened esophageal wall. A **Zenker di-**

verticulum (Fig. 5–11) is located in the upper esophagus, and an **epiphrenic diverticulum** (Fig. 5–12) is located just above the hemidiaphragm. A **pharyngeal pouch** is another type of pulsion tick that occurs at the cricopharyngeal junction. Food has a tendency to go into this pouch instead of down the esophagus. Eventually, enough food collects to cause the diverticulum to be a noticeable mass on the outside of the neck.

Traction diverticula (Fig. 5–13) occur at the tracheal bifurcation, or middle one third of the esophagus. These ticks are caused by scarring of the esophagus from a disease such as tuberculosis. They are triangular in shape, with the apex of the triangle pointing toward the area of disease.

Diverticula go unnoticed until they have reached a size large enough to cause a mechanical obstruction. In addition, reoccurring pneumonitis may result from the contents of the diverticulum draining and being aspirated into the lungs while the patient is recumbent.

Reflux esophagitis is an inflammation of the mucosa and submucosa of the lower esophagus. Reflux of gastric acid from the stomach back up into the esophagus eventually causes erosion of the pro-

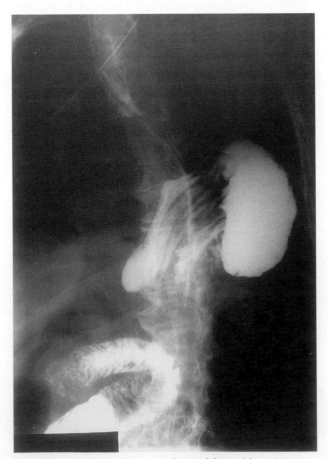

Figure 5–10. Paraesophageal hiatal hernia.

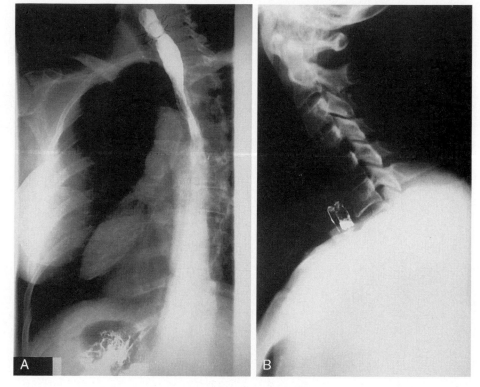

Figure 5–11. Zenker's diverticulum. *A,* Oblique view of the esophagus shows a coin-shaped object in the proximal area *(arrows)*. *B,* The lateral view shows the round object clearly outlined by barium. This 40-year-old female patient had taken a pill several hours before and had the feeling that something was caught in her throat. The pill had gone into a Zenker's diverticulum of the esophagus.

tective mucosa, resulting in heartburn and pain. This gastric reflux is caused by increased abdominal pressure and incompetence of the sphincter at the cardiac orifice. It is readily identifiable with a contrast study and a water siphonage test. The patient is placed in the left posterior oblique position so that the fundus of the stomach fills with barium. With the use of fluoroscopy, the radiologist observes the gastroesophageal junction while the patient drinks water from a straw. If barium flows from the stomach back into the esophagus, reflux has been demonstrated.

Reflux esophagitis may be a mild inflammation or it may become severe enough to cause ulcerations. The ulcerative areas of the esophagus are known as **Barrett esophagus** (Fig. 5–14). Adenocarcinoma may occur in these areas. If persistent, the ulcerations lead to scarring. Contraction of the scar tissue causes a stenosis and closure of the esophagus.

Strictures can occur secondary to inflammatory lesions, gastric reflux (Fig. 5–15), or a nasogastric tube that is left in the esophagus too long. **Peptic esophagitis** is the most common cause of esophageal stricture. A hiatal hernia and reflux are demonstrated in most cases. Symptoms develop slowly as first food and then liquid will not pass into the stomach. Long-standing esophagitis may lead to shortening of the esophagus. A benign stricture is demonstrated as a dilated esophagus above the stricture and normal below it, with a smooth mucosal contour. In contrast to a stricture caused by peptic esophagitis, a malignant stricture usually shows a sharply outlined "shelf" of tissue at the point where normal tissue meets diseased tissue (Fig. 5–16). A malignant stricture is often irregular, and the mucosal contour may be slightly or markedly ragged in appearance, as opposed to the usually smooth margins of a benign stricture.

Varices are very important to diagnose, as fatal hemorrhage may result if they rupture. These dilated tortuous veins are located in the wall at the end of the esophagus and the top of the stomach. They occur more frequently in alcoholic patients with portal venous hypertension and secondary to cirrhosis of the liver. The hardening of the liver restricts the blood flow and causes increased pressure in the portal venous system, which forces the veins to become enlarged and form a bypass. An enlarged spleen is associated with varices.

A barium swallow done with the patient in the recumbent position will show multiple filling defects that look similar to "rosary beads" or "worm tracings," which can be accentuated by the Valsalva maneuver (Fig. 5–17). Thin barium should be used, as thick paste may cover the varices.

Neoplasms

The esophagus can have both benign and malignant tumors. The most common benign esophageal neo-

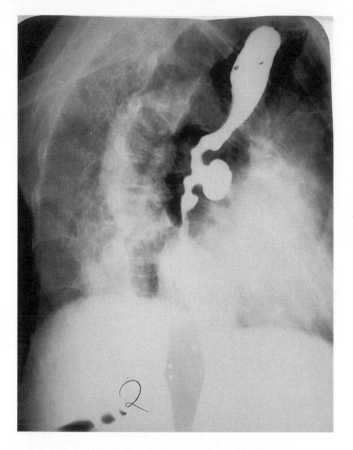

Figure 5–12. Excellent example of a pulsion diverticula of the esophagus. Because of its location above the hemidiaphragm, this is an epiphrenic diverticulum.

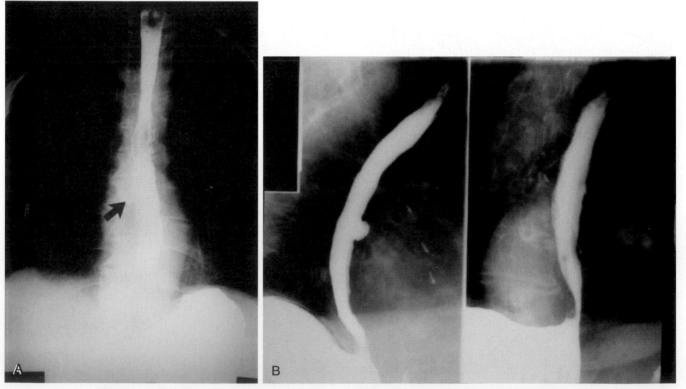

Figure 5–13. Traction diverticula of the esophagus occur at the tracheal bifurcation of the esophagus. *A,* The *arrow* points to a traction "tick." *B,* The radiograph on the *left* shows the broad base of this type of esophageal diverticula.

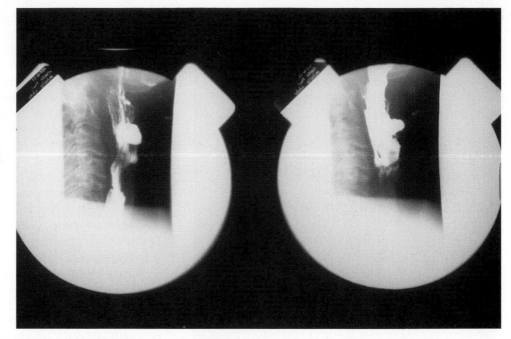

Figure 5–14. Barrett's esophagus caused by reflux esophagitis. The ragged edges of the esophagus denote the ulcerations.

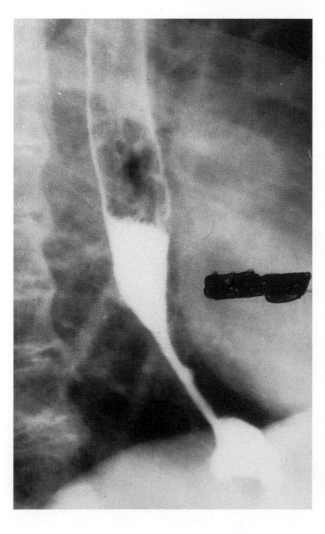

Figure 5–15. Stricture caused by gastric reflux. The distal esophagus has been narrowed considerably and presents as a stricture. There is shortening of the esophagus with resultant small hiatal hernia.

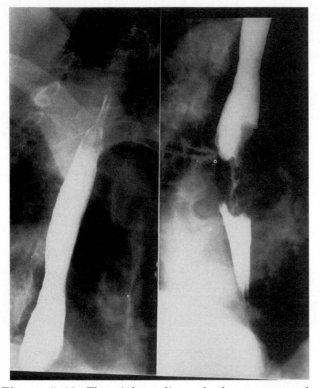

Figure 5–16. The *right* radiograph demonstrates the sharply demarcated "shelf" that the normal esophageal tissue makes when it meets the malignancy. There is a stricture and the mucosa contour is somewhat ragged, unlike in the case of a peptic esophagitis stricture.

plasm is a **leiomyoma** (Fig. 5–18). Radiographically, benign tumors within the esophagus characteristically produce an intraluminal polypoid defect with smooth narrowing of the lumen.

The most important tumors of the esophagus are malignant neoplasms. When a person 40 years of age or older experiences difficulty swallowing, **esophageal carcinoma** should be suspected until disproven. The incidence of squamous cell carcinoma is higher in men than in women, and there is a strong correlation between excessive alcohol intake, smoking, and esophageal carcinoma. Two sites of carcinomas are at the middle of the esophagus where it is crossed by the left bronchus, and in the lower third of the esophagus. These carcinomas usually stem from cancer of the stomach.

Malignant tumors demonstrate a definite division between normal tissue and tumor. This division is known as "shelving" (Fig. 5–19). The tumor grows into the lumen, causing narrowing and dysphagia.

About 50 percent of acquired fistulas between the trachea and esophagus are the result of malignancy in the mediastinum. The remaining 50 percent result from infectious processes or trauma. As in the congenital type, an upright abdominal radiograph shows air in the bowel.

Stomach

Congenital Anomalies

A narrowing of the lumen of the pylorus caused by hypertrophy of the muscle is called a **congenital pyloric stenosis.** This common anomaly occurs almost exclusively in males. Symptoms of projectile vomiting after feeding begin 2 to 4 weeks after birth. This condition will cause the stomach to become dilated, as the contents can not pass. If the

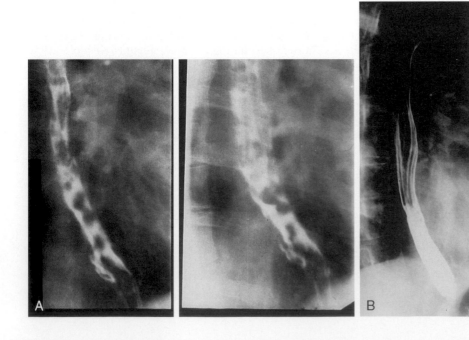

Figure 5–17. Varices. *A,* A 46-year-old man with hematemesis caused by portal cirrhosis. The film demonstrates both the "rosary bead" *(left)* and "worm tracing" *(right)* patterns common to esophageal varices. *B,* A different patient with the classic worm tracing pattern of the upper esophagus, indicating distended and elongated submucosal veins.

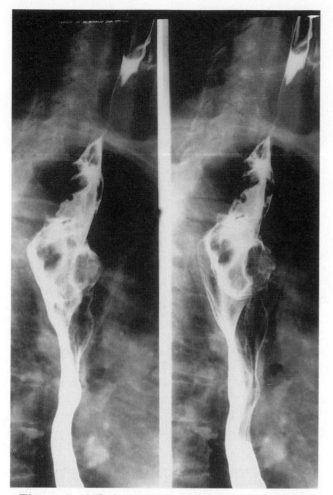

Figure 5–18. Leiomyomata of the upper esophagus.

stomach contents have not emptied after 7 hours, retention is present. As the stomach continues to fill, the patient becomes greatly distressed, and vomiting will result. A simple surgical incision to cut the thickened pyloric muscle remedies the situation.

The radiographic appearance of pyloric stenosis is that of a distended stomach filled with contrast medium. A "string sign" may appear as a very small amount of contrast trickles through the pylorus to the duodenum (Fig. 5–20).

Acquired Pathologies

Foreign bodies usually pass through the stomach without difficulty. There are several types of foreign bodies that persist in the stomach, however. **Bezoars** are just such a type. When the accumulation is of organic material such as vegetable matter, the bezoar is known as a **phytobezoar** (Fig. 5–21). These are most often found after a gastrectomy, when the remaining stomach portion does not break the food down and prepare it for digestion. The food

remains, collecting more material with each meal until it finally becomes a mass. When the mass is made of hair and fingernails, it is called a **trichobezoar** (Fig. 5–22). Such masses are usually found in patients suffering from mental or anxiety disorders, as these patients have a tendency to chew their nails or even eat their hair.

When the mucosa of the stomach is not well attached to the gastric musculature, peristalsis can push this mucosa through the pyloric channel into the duodenal bulb. This **prolapse** of gastric mucosa is a common finding (Fig. 5–23).

Inflammatory Processes

Gastritis is inflammation of the mucosa of the stomach. The most common cause is alcohol. Other causes are chemicals of a corresive nature and bacterial or viral infections. The mucous membrane of the stomach becomes red, swollen, and inflamed.

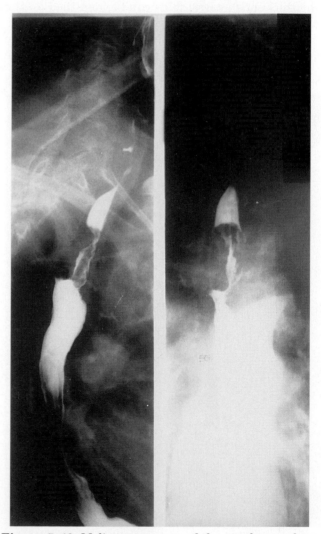

Figure 5–19. Malignant tumors of the esophagus showing the "shelf" sign.

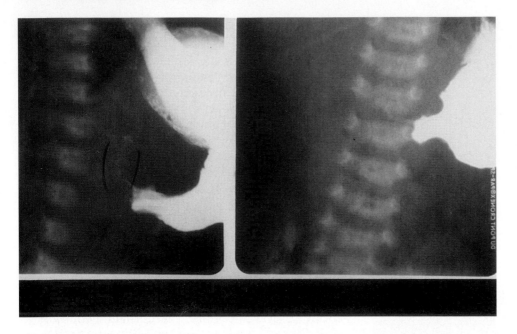

Figure 5–20. Congenital pyloric stenosis. The film on the left demonstrates the small string sign seen between the ( ).

The thickened gastric folds can be identified on the upper gastrointestinal series. After repeated bouts of gastritis, the condition becomes chronic. The early signs of inflammation are gone, and the rugae become thin and atrophy, even to the point of becoming absent in the fundus.

Any **ulcer** of the stomach is called a peptic ulcer because of the digestive acid in the stomach, pepsin. When necrosis of the stomach wall occurs, the acid gastric juice acts on this dead tissue as it would on

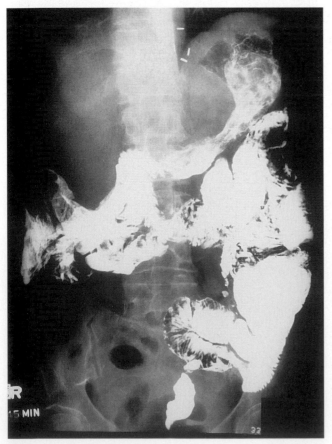

Figure 5–21. Phytobezoar that formed after gastric surgery.

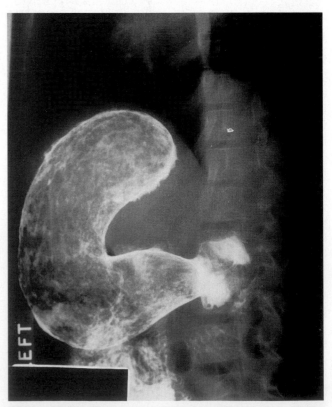

Figure 5–22. This posteroanterior oblique view of the abdomen of a 13-year-old boy shows a massive trichobezoar.

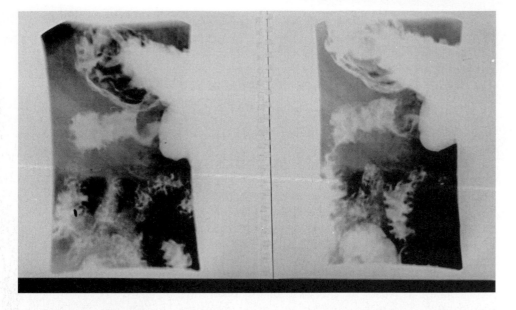

Figure 5–23. Prolapse of the mucosa into the duodenum.

any other object in the stomach to prepare it for digestion. The juice actually "eats away" and penetrates the muscle layer of the wall. The upper gastrointestinal study shows contrast material protruding outside the lumen of the organ.

The ulcers may occur in two places. **Gastric ulcers** are most common along the lesser curvature of the stomach (Fig. 5–24). As most gastric ulcers

heal, they leave behind little scar tissue, which allows normal peristalsis to resume. These ulcers are suspicious for malignancy. Radiographically, benign ulcers display radiolucent mucosal folds running to the edge of the ulcer. Seen on edge, the appearance of the crater is round and smooth. Malignant ulcers show obliterated mucosal folds with irregular borders that continue into the ulcer crater and merge with its edges.

Duodenal ulcers occur in the duodenal bulb or near the pylorus (Fig. 5–25). As this type of ulcer

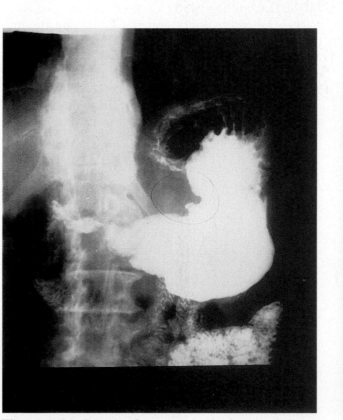

Figure 5–24. Gastric ulcer seen in the lesser curvature of the stomach.

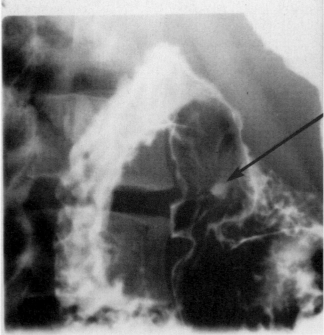

Figure 5–25. Duodenal ulcer seen in the bulb of the duodenum.

heals, scar tissue is produced, which narrows the lumen. As the ulcer becomes chronic, the lumen may actually close, causing obstruction. This scarring produces the classic radiographic appearance of a "clover-leaf" deformity. Duodenal ulcers are more common than gastric ulcers and occur more frequently in men in the 30 to 50 years age group. Duodenal ulcers are almost never cancerous, and most respond to medical treatment.

Complications of ulcers can develop. Perforation occurs if the erosion goes through the muscle layer and into the peritoneal cavity. As the contents from the stomach pour into the abdominal cavity, peritonitis occurs, which can prove fatal unless surgery is undertaken to close the opening. An upright abdominal film shows free air in the abdomen.

A frequent complication is hemorrhage. Bleeding occurs when a vessel at the base of the ulcer has been eroded. The blood may be passed by vomiting (hematemesis) or in the feces (melena).

A less common complication of ulcers is a benign stricture in the body of the stomach. As excessive scar tissue builds up, the stomach takes on the appearance of an hourglass.

Zollinger-Ellison syndrome is a disease caused by tumors in the pancreas, which causes hypersecretion of acids. It is the most common cause of thickening of the gastric folds in the fundus and body of the stomach. An overactive stomach produces excessive acid that overwhelms the natural mucosal barrier of the stomach, resulting in inflammation of the inner lining. This is a cause of ulcers. Zollinger-Ellison syndrome causes multiple ulcers in unusual places like the duodenum or jejunum.

Radiographically, increased gastric fluid content, thickened, tortuous gastric rugae, and ulceration in atypical locations suggest the presence of Zollinger-Ellison syndrome. Dilatation of the duodenum may be seen.

Neoplasms

Benign tumors of the stomach are uncommon and usually are a smooth muscle leiomyomata (Fig. 5–26). The majority of stomach tumors are adenocarcinomas, with three types being recognized. **Papillary (fungating)** tumors are polypoid masses that project into the lumen of the stomach near the cardioesophageal junction. Because these lesions are extremely difficult to demonstrate on conventional single-contrast barium studies, a double-contrast technique is essential for diagnosing them at the earliest possible stage. Papillary tumors are the least malignant type of the three. **Ulcerating** tumors show ragged mucosa and may be confused

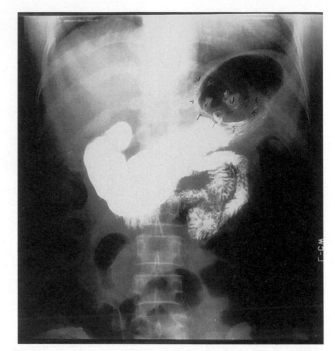

Figure 5–26. Leiomyomata of the fundus of the stomach.

with benign ulcers. They have a predilection for areas of the stomach near the greater curvature and the pylorus. **Infiltrating (linitis plastica)** is the third type of adenocarcinoma. These tumors spread within the walls of the stomach, causing thickening of the walls and fibrous tissue production. The tumor commonly begins near the pylorus and continues upward toward the fundus. Eventually, the thickening leads to an obstruction as the opening is closed off (Fig. 5–27A). The walls of the stomach become shrunken and rigid ("leather bottle stomach") in the region of the tumor (see Fig. 5–27B).

In the United States, the incidence of stomach carcinoma has been declining. The cause of stomach cancer is unknown, but dietary factors appear to be a determinant. Tumors present early symptoms of weight loss, loss of appetite, and vague abdominal discomfort. Later developments include weakness, anemia, and loss of blood through the stool or by vomiting. Metastasis to lymph nodes along the greater curvature is frequent.

Small Bowel

Congenital Anomalies

Meckel diverticulum is a congenital diverticulum found in the ileum. It is a rounded sac that represents the persistence of the yolk sac. In contrast to an acquired tick, a Meckel diverticulum always contains all the muscular layers of the bowel wall

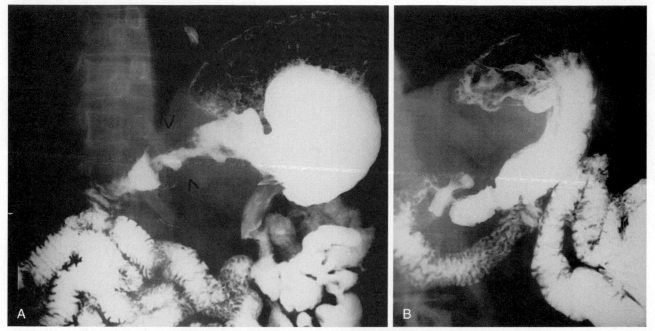

Figure 5–27. Infiltrating carcinoma of the stomach. *A,* The malignancy has caused narrowing of the pyloric channel. *B,* As the tumor advances toward the fundus, the walls of the stomach shrink. Note the decrease in the lesser curvature. This is known as the "leather bottle syndrome."

(Fig. 5–28). This allows for rapid emptying on a barium study which makes diagnosis of this type of diverticulum difficult. Nuclear medicine studies are best for demonstrating this anomaly (Fig. 5–29).

Acquired Pathologies

A **hernia** occurs when a loop of bowel pushes its way through a weak spot or opening in the abdominal wall. The common sites for hernias are the groin and umbilicus. A strangulated hernia is one in which so much bowel has been forced through the opening that the lumen of the bowel is closed off. The blood vessels that supply the herniated loop are also cut off. Unless the hernia is treated rapidly, gangrene develops and peritonitis sets in.

Inflammatory Processes

Diverticula in the duodenum are common. These "ticks" are usually singular and become quite large (Fig. 5–30). They hold no significance unless they perforate.

A group of diseases that cause food not to be digested and absorbed normally are lumped together under the general heading of **malabsorption syndrome.** The mucosal cells of the small bowel are defective in that they will not absorb fat, proteins, and carbohydrates. The best known malabsorption disorder is **sprue.** When the disease

occurs in children it is called **celiac disease.** It is characterized by poor food absorption and an intolerance of gluten, a protein of wheat and wheat products. The malabsorption in the bowel results from the atrophy of the villi and a decrease in the activity of the bowel. The patient exhibits weight loss, and stools are large and foul-smelling because of bacterial action on unabsorbed fat. The bowel shows as either diffusely or segmently dilated, depending on how much is affected. The mucosal folds are very thin or totally absent. Peristalsis slows or stops. The radiograph shows a dilated bowel without the appearance of mucosal folds. This is termed the "moulage" sign. Intermittent intussusception is associated with this disease.

Seventy-five percent of all **mechanical small bowel obstructions** are caused by fibrous adhesions. Other causes include volvulus, intussusception, and tumors. Distended loops of bowel can be demonstrated on a kidney, ureter, and bowel scan within hours of the obstruction. In a complete mechanical small bowel obstruction, little or no gas is found in the colon. The upright radiograph shows air-fluid levels at different heights in the bowel. This helps to differentiate it from adynamic ileus in which gas is seen within distended loops through the bowel.

Paralytic ileus (adynamic ileus) is a common problem in which fluid and gas do not progress normally because of inactivity of the bowel. The

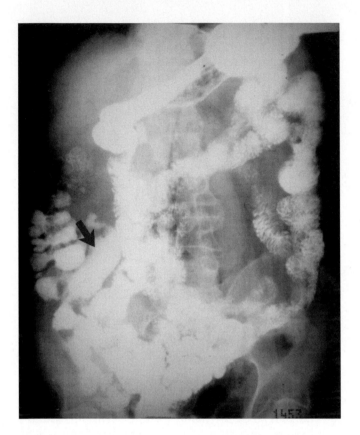

Figure 5–28. A Meckel's diverticulum *(arrow)* can be seen on this film of the small bowel.

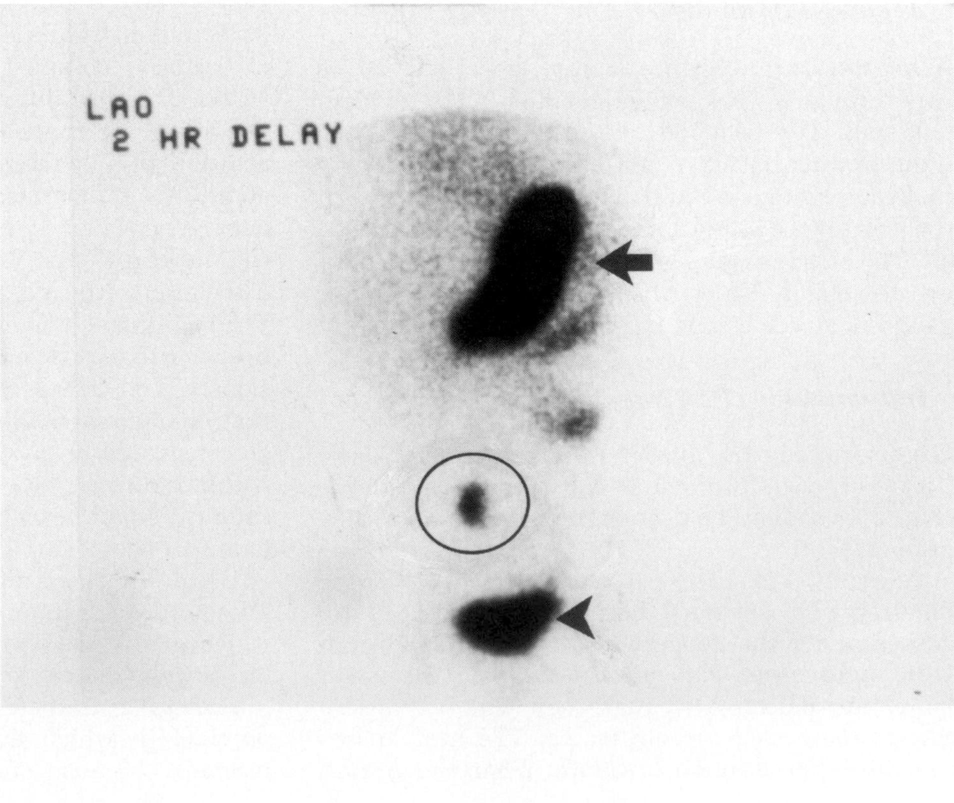

Figure 5–29. Nuclear medicine scan. The *arrow* points to the stomach, the *arrowhead* to the bladder. The *circled* area demonstrates the Meckel's diverticulum.

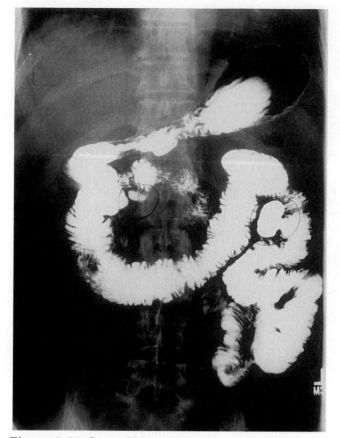

Figure 5–30. Several large duodenal and jejunal diverticula.

of the time in the terminal ileum. The condition may extend into the cecum and sometimes into the ascending colon (Fig. 5–34) (see granulomatous colitis). Early stages of the disease affect the bowel wall by causing it to become thickened. If the thickening continues, fibrosis can occur, which leads to an obstruction. As the wall thickens, the lumen must become narrowed. A segment of bowel with this narrow lumen is demonstrated as the "string sign" on radiographs. The combination of mucosal edema and ulcerations give the bowel a "cobblestone" appearance on the radiograph. Lesions affect only certain areas of the bowel, leaving unaffected areas in between. These normal areas of bowel are termed "skipped areas" and are characteristic of this disease. Treatment is medical, as the disease tends to become chronic.

Intussusception and **volvulus** can both occur in the small bowel. A description of each of these conditions can be found in the following section on colon pathology.

Large Bowel

Congenital Anomalies

Hirschsprung disease is also known as **aganglionic megacolon** because it is the congenital absence

bowel is not obstructed. It is usually seen in postoperative patients or those receiving medications that decrease bowel activity. Because of decreased motor activity, peristalsis cannot pass material from one portion of the bowel to the next. This causes a dilation of the whole bowel. Supine and erect views (Fig. 5–31) of the abdomen demonstrate large amounts of gas and fluid in the small and large bowel. There is uniform dilation with no obstruction demonstrated. This classic radiographic appearance is called the "step ladder" sign (Fig. 5–32).

If only a small isolated segment of bowel is dilated, it is a localized ileus (Fig. 5–33). It is important to differentiate between small and large bowel obstruction. This should not be too difficult if the radiographer recalls that the small bowel occupies the central portion of the abdomen. Colonic ileus refers to distention of the large bowel and can be identified along the lateral aspects of the abdomen.

Regional enteritis is more commonly known as **Crohn's disease.** An idiopathic disease, it tends to begin at an early age (teens and twenties), and males are affected more often than females. It is a chronic inflammatory disease that occurs 80 percent

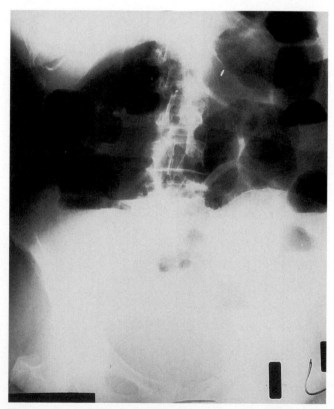

Figure 5–31. Film of a mechanical obstructic, taken with the patient in upright position.

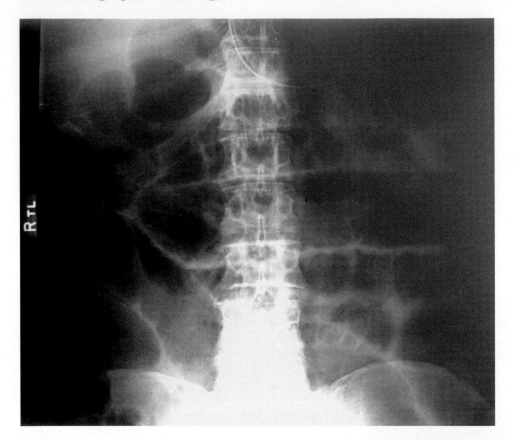

Figure 5–32. Classic stepladder sign of a paralytic ileus.

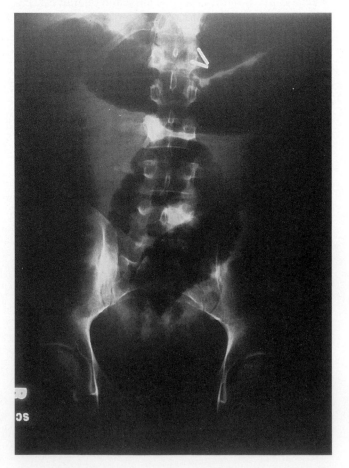

Figure 5–33. Loop of bowel with a localized ileus.

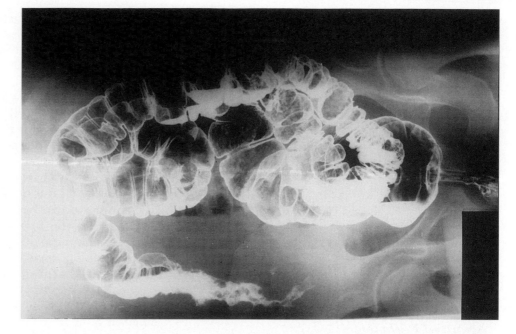

Figure 5–34. Crohn's disease. Radiograph taken with the patient in decubitus position, showing the inflamed ascending colon. Note the ragged edges and the narrowed string sign.

of neurons in the rectum and a small segment of the colon, which prevents peristalsis and passage of the colon contents. This causes a greatly enlarged colon proximal to the affected area. The rectum and sigmoid areas seem to be the areas that are affected most, but the entire bowel may also be involved (Fig. 5–35). Eighty percent of the patients with Hirschprung disease are male and almost all of them become symptomatic within the first week of life. Symptoms include failure to thrive, constipation, abdominal distention, and episodes of vomiting. The newborn may fail to pass meconium in the first 24 to 48 hours after birth. A high incidence of complications, such as enterocolitis or perforation of the transverse colon or the appendix, is found. The important plain film finding includes dilation of the entire small bowel, air-fluid levels on a decubitis view, and no evidence of air in the rectum.

The most significant finding on the barium enema is the transition zone, the boundary between the normal dilated portion and the aganglionic portion of the bowel. The aganglionic colon is spastic, narrowed, and empty of stool. The normal (ganglionic) colon is dilated, hypertrophied, and filled with

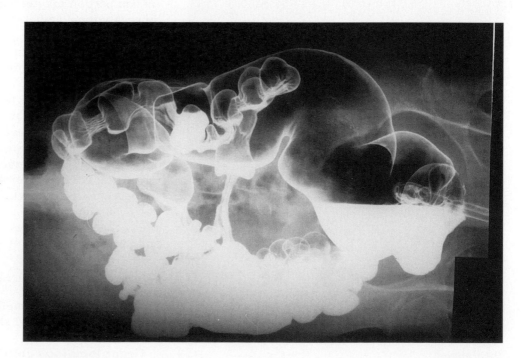

Figure 5–35. Megacolon with constriction.

feces. This transition is found 80 percent of the time in the rectosigmoid area. If barium is forced in too rapidly, the transition zone or the spastic portion of the colon may not be recognized. Barium is often retained in the colon for as long as 48 hours after the study.

Two other congenital abnormalities are an **imperforate anus** and **rectal atresia.** An imperforate anus is a condition that exists when there is no opening at the end of the anal canal (Fig. 5–36). Rectal atresia describes the failure of the distal rectum and anus to develop at all. Both of these abnormalities are causes of obstruction. Visual inspection will diagnose each of these conditions, but radiography is performed to determine the extent to which they exist. Also, a complication of imperforate anus or rectal atresia is a fistula into the genitourinary tract. These fistulas can be detected by contrast studies.

Acquired Pathologies

A **cathartic colon** is one that develops after the prolonged use of laxatives. As the patient becomes

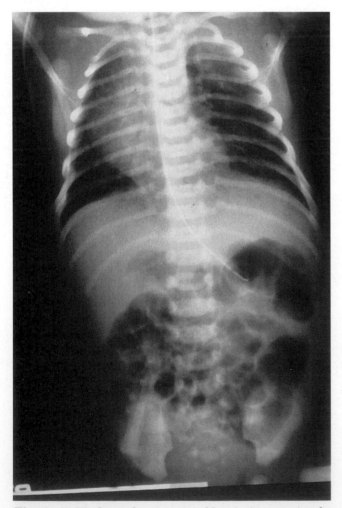

Figure 5–36. Imperforate anus. No air is seen in the distal bowel.

dependent on the laxatives, mucosal atrophy and neuromuscular changes take place in the colon. There is almost total loss of the haustral markings (Fig. 5–37); however, the walls of the colon remain distensible. The lack of rigidity, as well as the elongation of the colon, serves to differentiate this condition from ulcerative colitis.

Intussusception is the telescoping of a proximal part of the bowel into a distal part because of peristalsis. It causes bowel obstruction and compromises the vascular supply to the bowel wall. **Adult intussusception** is usually secondary to some type of mass located within the lumen of the bowel (Fig. 5–38). The presence of a mass is often obscured by the intussusception itself and is not shown until the intussusception is reduced. This is not as common as **infantile intussusception,** which occurs idiopathically in males under the age of 1 year (Fig. 5–39). The most common site for intussusception in children is near the cecum and ileum. Usually the ileum spontaneously invaginates into the colon. In many cases, the barium enema reduces the affected parts of the bowel if it does not totally correct the situation.

Classic signs are colicky abdominal pain leading to shock. Many times the condition temporarily corrects itself and the patient recovers and appears to be normal. Radiographically, the classic appearance is that of a "coiled-spring," not unlike a Slinky toy, which is caused by barium being caught between the layers of bowel wall encased within the surrounding bowel.

Intussusception must be corrected early, as the portion of the bowel that is encased within the outside portion may become strangulated, at which time gangrene may set in. Once the invaginated portion is pulled back into normal position, the intestine is properly secured with sutures.

A **volvulus** is a more commonly seen condition than intussusception. It generally occurs in the highly mobile sigmoid area and is the twisting of bowel onto itself, producing an obstruction which, like intussusception, can lead to gangrene if the blood supply from the vessels is shut off. The radiograph shows a large amount of air in the sigmoid colon because of the obstruction. The barium enema shows a classic hallmark sign called the "beak" sign. The beak sign refers to a tapered narrowing at the site of the volvulus caused by twisting of the bowel and narrowing of the lumen (Fig. 5–40).

Inflammatory Processes

Colitis, as its name implies, is an inflammation of the colon, but there are several types of colitis that should be recognized.

Granulomatous colitis (Crohn's colitis) is the

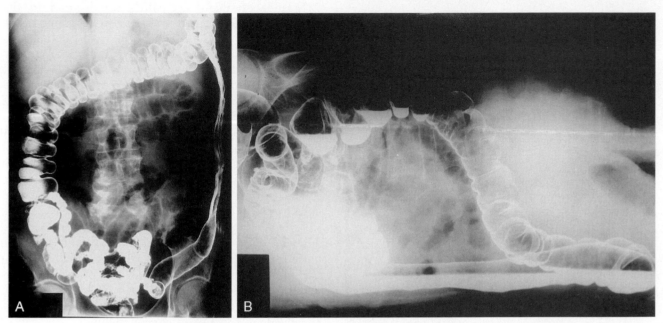

Figure 5–37. Cathartic colon. The descending colon has lost almost all of the haustral markings. Films taken with patient in supine *(A)* and decubitus *(B)* positions show the tubular appearance of the colon.

Figure 5–38. Adult intussusception. Note the cap-like defect of advancing barium-filled intussuscipiens pressing the invaginated intussusception.

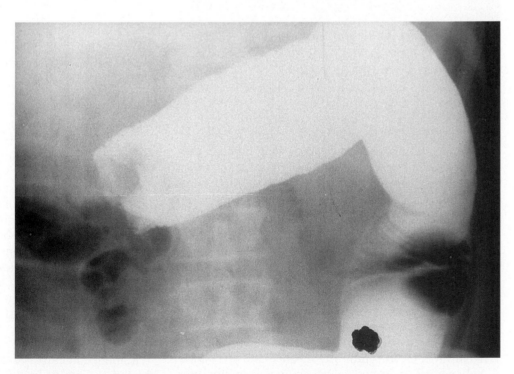

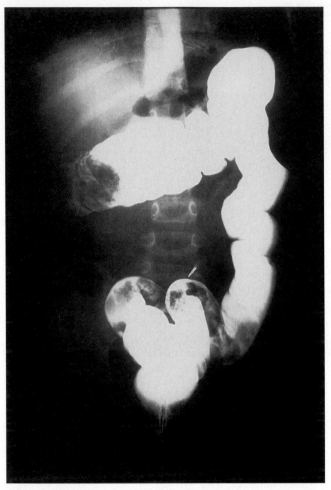

Figure 5–39. Infantile intussusception.

almost daily. Toxic megacolon is a complication of ulcerative colitis.

Lesions of ulcerative colitis are located in the mucosa. Unaffected areas of mucosa become edematous and may appear as pseudopolyps. Such a finding should not be confused with skipped areas, which are found in granulomatous colitis. The air contrast enema examination reveals these pseudopolyps as multiple, ring-shaped filling defects. As the disease advances, the ulcerations in the bowel wall heal because of fibrosis, which causes rigidity and creating the classic sign "leadpipe". In most cases, the disease becomes chronic even though there are periods of remission. Chronic ulcerative colitis causes haustral folds to be irregular and asymmetrical (Fig. 5–42).

Cancer of the colon is not an automatic consequence. The risk appears to be confined to those patients who have extensive ulcerative colitis for a period of 10 years or more. The risk of carcinoma is about 10 percent and increases with each decade of affliction. Again, this is unlike granulomatous colitis, in which the risk of cancer is low.

A final type of colitis that will be discussed is **ischemic colitis.** This usually occurs in patients over the age of 50 who have a history of cardiovascular disease. It is characterized by abrupt onset of lower abdomenal pain and rectal bleeding. The first sign seen radiographically is superficial ulcerations. As the disease progresses, the ulcerations become deeper and pseudopolyps, as seen in ulcerative colitis, are identified. The characteristic "thumbprint" sign is demonstrated (Fig. 5–43). Thumbprinting refers to well-defined indentations along the margins of the bowel wall that appear to have been made by a finger pressing in on it.

Diverticulosis of the large bowel is found in 25 percent of the population over 65 years of age, which makes it a common disorder of the bowel. Diverticulosis is a condition of having diverticula in the colon. If these diverticula become inflamed, the patient has the condition called diverticulitis.

Diverticula are outpouchings that occur through weakened areas of the bowel wall, especially along sites of vessel insertion in the sigmoid area. The usual size is that of a large pea. They rarely occur singularly. Rather, they are multiple protuberances found in clusters. These protruding points of mucosa contain fecal matter, which, if they become infected and perforate, may cause a pericolic abscess.

Radiographically, the diverticula are demonstrated as multiple barium-filled pouches off the outside of the bowel wall (Fig. 5–44). They are best demonstrated on the postevacuation film because of their poor emptying capabilities.

The most frequent benign neoplasms of the gas-

same process as regional enteritis in the small bowel and is similar to ulcerative colitis in its clinical manifestations. It begins near the terminal ileum, cecum, and ascending colon. Involvement of the rectum is rare. The etiology is unknown but psychosomatic causes are believed to be linked to it.

All radiographic appearances described under regional enteritis (cobblestone, string sign, and skip areas) are encountered in the large bowel (Fig. 5–41). As the disease becomes chronic, the inflexibility of the bowel wall has been compared to that of a "lead pipe." Carcinoma of the colon in association with this type of colitis is not often found.

Ulcerative colitis begins in the rectosigmoid region in about 75 percent of cases and involves the ileum in about 25 percent of cases. It is first noticed in persons between the ages of 15 and 30. Ulcerative colitis is an autoimmune disease and the cause is believed to be linked to stress; however, this has not been proven. It usually starts with a series of attacks of crampy abdominal pain and is characterized by the passage of bloody mucus with stools and a large number of discharges of watery diarrhea

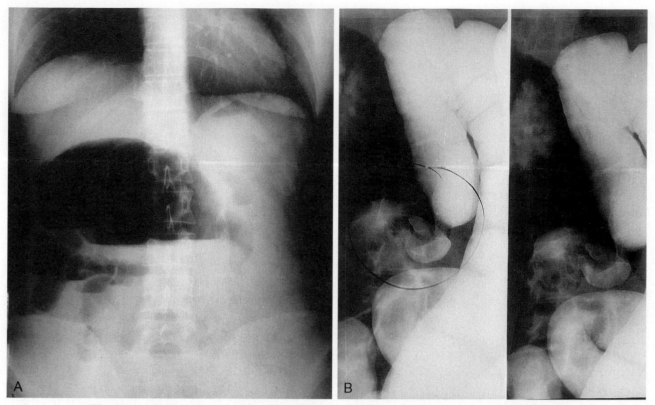

Figure 5–40. Volvulus. *A,* Upright abdomen shows obstruction in the right abdomen. *B,* Barium enema shows the twisting of the bowel.

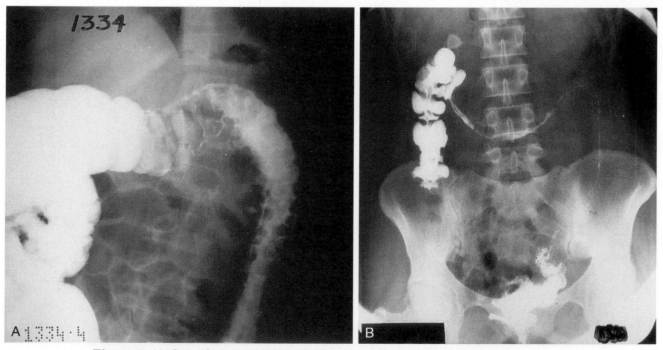

Figure 5–41. Granulomatous colitis. *A,* Note the difference between the left and right sides of the colon. There is an absence of haustral folds, with mucosal ulcerations and a cobblestone pattern because of longitudinal ulcerations. *B,* Large string sign.

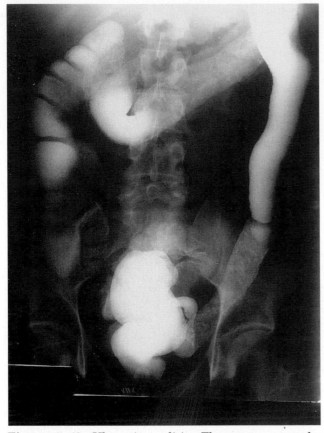

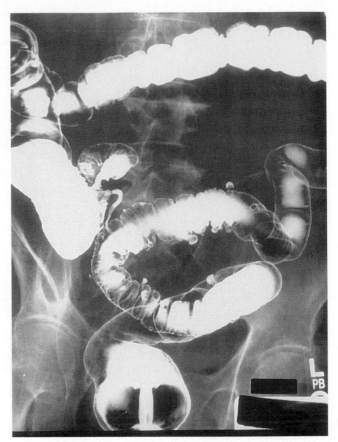

Figure 5–42. Ulcerative colitis. The transverse colon shows dense areas within the bowel, representing pseudopolyps. There is almost a complete loss of haustral markings ("stove pipe" appearance). These two signs are classic indicators of ulcerative colitis.

Figure 5–44. Diverticula of the large bowel.

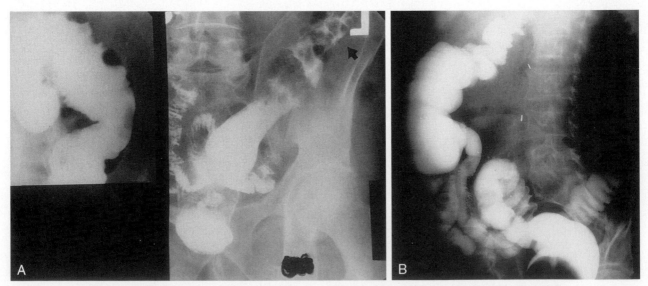

Figure 5–43. Ischemic colitis. Classic thumbprint sign is seen on both parts *A* and *B*.

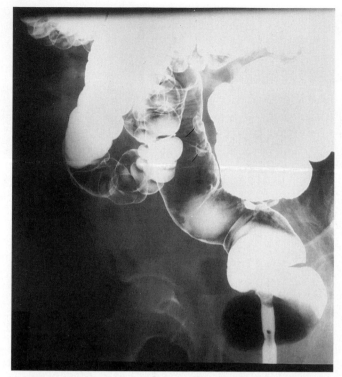

Figure 5–45. Adenomatous polyps of the large bowel.

trointestinal tract are **polyps.** Polyps differ from diverticula in that they project into the lumen of the bowel. **Adenomatous polyps** are sac-like projections that have a peduncle. They are small and rarely are cancerous (Fig. 5–45). Adenomatous polyps are more common than are the villous polyps. **Villous polyps** are usually over 2 cm in size, grow a broad base, and are not pedunculated (Fig. 5–46). About 20 percent contain cancer cells at the time of diagnosis. The likelihood that a polyp is malignant increases rapidly as the size increases.

Polyps are found in the descending colon and sigmoid and rectal areas. Any polyp that is larger than 2.5 cm or is thought to be a source of bleeding is surgically removed. The most serious potential complication of the polyp is that it can undergo a degenerative change and become malignant.

Neoplasms

Malignant neoplasms are almost exclusively in the form of **adenocarcinomas** (95%). They occur in the rectosigmoid area about 75 percent of the time. However, in severe cases, they spread to the entire colon. Colon cancer does not metastasize early, but if not diagnosed and treated in the first stages, it will metastasize to the liver and lungs.

There are different types of lesions that appear differently on the radiographs. **Annular lesions** slowly surround the bowel and cause gradual nar-

rowing of the lumen and chronic intestinal obstruction. Radiographically, the colon has the unmistakable appearance of a "napkin ring" or an "apple core" (Fig. 5–47). The edges of the lesion tend to overhang and form acute angles with the bowel wall. **Polypoid lesions** project into the lumen as does a benign polyp (Fig. 5–48). Large polypoid colonic masses destroy the mucosal pattern and are highly suspect of malignancy. Radiographic appearance is not a reliable means of differentiating benign from malignant polyps.

Table 5–1 summarizes the clinical and radiographic characteristics of common pathologies of the gastrointestinal system.

Review Questions

1. Describe where the cardiac orifice is located. What is the function of the stomach? What function do rugae serve? Describe the anatomy of the stomach and duodenum. Where does the duodenum begin?
2. List the three functions of the small bowel. Explain how the structure of the small bowel was designed to carry out the processes of digestion and absorption. How do the nutrients pass from the small bowel to the liver?
3. Name the three parts of the large bowel. What

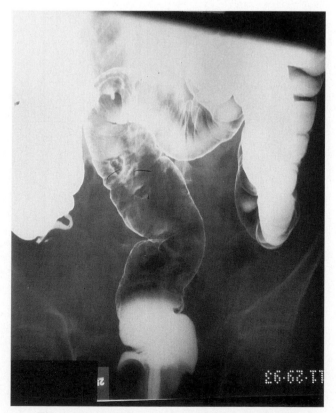

Figure 5–46. Villous polyps of the large bowel.

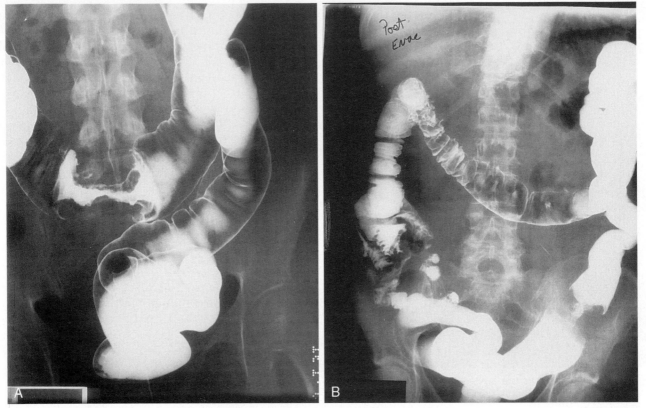

Figure 5–47. Annular carcinoma of the large bowel. Apple core sign of the transverse colon *(A)* and of the sigmoid colon *(B)*.

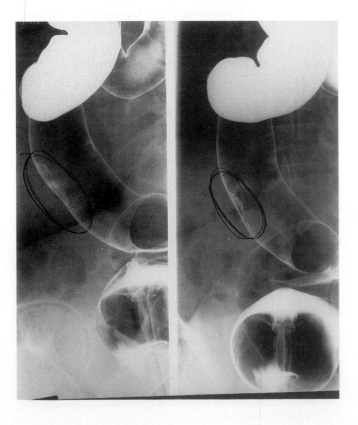

Figure 5–48. Polypoid malignancy of the large bowel.

Table 5–1.
Clinical and Radiographic Characteristics of Common Pathologies

Pathologic Condition	Causal Factors*	Manifestations	Radiographic Appearance
Achalasia	Esophageal stenosis	Dilated esophagus	"Rat tail" sign
Corkscrew esophagus	Elderly, tertiary contractions	Associated with hiatal hernia	Curling or "corkscrew" of the esophagus
Sliding hiatal hernia	Weakened gastroesophageal junction	Heartburn, feeling of fullness	Schatzki ring; in severe cases, an intrathoracic stomach
Pulsion diverticula	Weakened esophageal wall	Feeling of something caught in throat	Narrow neck with a round head
Esophageal varices	Dilated veins from portal hypertension	Vomiting with blood	"Rosary beads" and "worm tracings"
Esophageal carcinoma	Men over 40 years, excessive smoking and alcohol intake	Dysphagia	"Shelving"
Pyloric stenosis	Newborn males, hypertrophy of pyloric muscle	Projectile vomiting	"String sign"
Gastric ulcer	Excess gastric acid	Heartburn, pain	Radiolucent mucosal folds radiating out from center of ulcer
Duodenal ulcer	Males, 30 to 50 years, excessive gastric acid	Heartburn, pain	"Cloverleaf" deformity after healing due to scar tissue
Sprue or celiac disease	Nonabsorption of fat, proteins, and carbohydrates	Weight loss, foul-smelling stools	"Moulage" sign
Mechanical small bowel obstruction	Fibrous adhesions	Severe abdominal pain	Distended loops of small bowel
Paralytic ileus	Decreased bowel activity (postoperative)	Abdominal pain	"Step ladder"
Regional enteritis	Teens and 20s, idiopathic	Diarrhea, cramping	String sign, skip areas, "cobblestone"
Hirschsprung disease	Newborn males, absence of neurons in the rectum	Failure to thrive, constipation, abdominal distension	"Transition zone," spastic narrow rectum, dilated sigmoid
Intussusception	Children: idiopathic Adult: mass	Bowel obstruction	"Coiled spring" sign
Volvulus	Mobility of sigmoid	Bowel obstruction	"Beak" sign
Granulomatous colitis	See regional enteritis	—	Cobblestone, string sign, skipped areas, "lead pipe"
Ulcerative colitis	15 to 30 years, autoimmune	Crampy abdominal pain	"Pseudopolyps," "lead pipe"
Ischemic colitis	Over 50 years, history of cardiovascular disease	Lower abdominal pain, rectal bleeding	"Thumbprint" sign
Colonic diverticula	Over 60 years, weakened bowel wall	Asymptomatic	Barium-filled pouches
Polyps	—	May cause rectal bleeding	Filling defect in bowel lumen
Annular adenocarcinoma	—	Inhibits fecal passage	"Napkin ring" or "apple core"

*Includes age, if relevant.

is the transition from the small bowel to the large bowel? How do they differ anatomically? What function does the large bowel perform?

4. Describe how the hepatobiliary system and the gastrointestinal system work together to acomplish digestion.

5. Define achalasia. What causes it? What will the radiograph demonstrate above and below the gastroesophageal junction?

6. List and define the two common types of diverticula of the esophagus. What do they look like on a radiograph? Which is more common? Describe the three different types of pulsion ticks. Explain where all types of diverticula occur. What are the complications associated with diverticula of the esophagus?

7. Describe the procedure performed to demonstrate radiolucent foreign objects of the esophagus on a radiograph. What complications can occur from foreign objects lodged in the throat?

8. Fully describe a hiatal hernia. Include how such hernias occur, how common they are, and the difference between sliding and rolling types. What is an intrathoracic stomach and what causes it?

9. Describe where malignant tumors of the esophagus occur. What will they demonstrate on the radiograph?

10. Define varices and explain the cause. Who is more likely to acquire them? Why? Describe the radiographic procedure that will demonstrate them. What is the appearance on the radiograph?

11. Define bezoar. What are the two types and what are they composed of?

12. List and describe the three types of adenocarcinomas of the stomach.

13. Why is an ulcer called a peptic ulcer? How does one occur? Compare and contrast gastric and duodenal ulcers. Include where they occur, what happens as they heal, the radiographic appearance (if any), which is more common, who is more prone to acquiring them, and their predisposition to malignancy.

14. Describe three complications associated with ulcers. How does each of these occur?

15. Define Zollinger-Ellison syndrome. What does this disease process cause? What is seen on the radiograph?

16. Compare and contrast mechanical small bowel obstruction and paralytic ileus. List and describe the two variants of paralytic ileus.

17. Define regional enteritis. Where does it occur, what causes it, how does it affect the bowel wall, and what happens as the disease progresses? What are the classic signs on the radiograph? What causes them?

18. Define colitis. Describe the three types.

19. Compare and contrast features of ulcerative colitis and regional enteritis. Refer to question number 17 and contrast these features to ulcerative colitis.

20. Describe the two types of polyps.

21. Describe intussusception. What are the two types? How is intussusception different from volvulus?

22. Describe malignant neoplasms of the colon. What type are they, where do they occur, where will it metastasize, what are the different lesions and how do they appear on the radiograph?

CHAPTER VI

Urinary System

Goals

1. To review the anatomy and basic physiology of the urinary system.
2. To learn theories that will enhance understanding of the special procedures used to demonstrate the urinary system.
3. To learn pathologic conditions related to the urinary system.

Objectives

At the completion of the chapter, the radiographer will be able to:

1. Draw the structure and internal architecture of the kidney.
2. Describe the process of urine production and passage.
3. Describe cystography.
4. List and define the two types of intravenous pyelograms.
5. Define the difference between retrograde pyelography and retrograde urethrography.
6. Explain the use and advantage of ultrasonography in renal imaging.
7. List two types of nuclear medicine studies of the urinary system.
8. Describe extracorporeal shock wave lithotripsy.
9. Define the basic urinary pathology terminology.
10. Describe the different types of congenital anomalies found in the urinary system.
11. Recognize the various types of benign conditions on a radiograph and explain each condition.
12. Define the various types of malignant conditions.

I. Anatomy
  A. Kidneys
    1. Capsule
    2. Cortex
      a. Renal Columns
        (Columns of Bertin)
    3. Medulla
      a. Pyramids
        1. Collecting Tubules
        2. Papillae
    4. Minor Calyx
    5. Major Calyx
    6. Renal Pelvis
    7. Hilum
  B. Ureters
  C. Bladder
    1. Trigone
  D. Urethra
    1. Urinary Meatus
II. Physiology and Function
  A. Kidneys
    1. Urine Production and
      Secretion
      a. Glomerular Filtration
      b. Tubular Reabsorption
      c. Tubular Secretion
    2. Regulate Fluid Content of
      Blood
    3. Regulate Concentration of
      Electrolytes (Blood pH)
  B. Ureter
    1. Passage of Urine
  C. Bladder
    1. Reservoir
  D. Urethra
    1. Female
      a. Passage of Urine
    2. Male
      a. Passage of Urine
      b. Passage of Sperm

III. Special Radiographic
  Procedures
  A. Intravenous Pyelography
    1. Nephrography
    2. Hypertensive
    3. Drip Infusion
  B. Cystography
    1. Voiding Cystogram
    2. Bead-Chain Urethrogram
  C. Retrograde Urethrography
  D. Retrograde Pyelography
  E. Percutaneous Antegrade
    Pyelography
  F. Percutaneous Nephrostomy
  G. Angiography
  H. Computed Tomography
  I. Ultrasonography
  J. Nuclear Medicine
    1. Architectural Renal Scan
    2. Dynamic Renogram
  K. Extracorporeal Shock Wave
    Lithotripsy
IV. Pathology
  A. Terminology
    1. Oliguria
    2. Polyuria
    3. Anuria
    4. Retention
    5. Hematuria
    6. Uremia
    7. Cystitis
    8. Pyelitis
  B. Congenital Anomalies
    1. Double System
    2. Horseshoe
    3. Crossed Ectopy
    4. Nephroptosis
    5. Polycystic Kidneys
      a. Infantile

      1. Newborn
      2. Childhood
    b. Adult
    6. Renal Agenesis
    7. Hypoplasia and
      Hyperplasia
    8. Renal Ectopia
  C. Inflammatory Processes
    1. Bright Disease
      (Glomerulonephritis)
    2. Diverticula
      a. Ureteral
      b. Bladder
    3. Ureteroceles
    4. Prostatic Hypertrophy
    5. Hydronephrosis
    6. Hypertension
    7. Nephrosis
    8. Pyelonephritis
      a. Acute
      b. Chronic
    9. Reflux
    10. Renal Calculi
      a. Staghorn
      b. Nephrocalcinosis
    11. Renal Failure
      a. Acute
      b. Chronic
  D. Neoplasms
    1. Benign
      a. Renal Cysts
      b. Pseudotumors
    2. Malignant
      a. Hypernephroma
        (Adenocarcinoma,
        Grawitz Tumor)
      b. Nephroblastoma
        (Wilms Tumor)
      c. Bladder Carcinoma

The urinary system is one of four excretory pathways of the body. The other three are the large bowel, the lungs, and the skin. The urinary system consists of two kidneys, two ureters, a urinary bladder, and one urethra. In the male, the urethra is also part of the genital tract.

ANATOMY

The kidneys are bean-shaped organs that lie behind the peritoneum; only the anterior surface is covered with peritoneum. They are not fixed in the abdomen, and they move with respiration.

The kidneys are about 11.25 cm (4.5 inches) in length and can be found around the level of T-12 to L-3. The right kidney is slightly lower than the left one because of inferior displacement by the liver. The inferior vena cava lies medial to the right kidney, and the aorta lies medial to the left kidney.

The renal capsule is the fibrous connective tissue that encloses the kidney. The cortex, or parenchyma, is the pale-colored outer area of the kidney that consists of the columns of Bertin (renal columns) located between the medulla and the columns between the pyramids. The cortex extends from the capsule and the base of the pyramids. The dark-colored inner area of the kidney is called the medulla (Fig. 6–1). It consists of 8 to 12 renal pyramids. These renal pyramids consist of many collecting tubules. Each pyramid is shaped like a triangle with the base towards the cortex. The blunted apex fits into the minor calyx.

The rounded medial ends of each renal pyramid are called the renal papillae. These ends fit into the cup-shaped end of a minor calyx (see Fig. 6–1 inset). Minor calyces are a division of the major calyx. There are as many as 12 minor calyces to one major calyx. One end receives the papilla while the other becomes the major calyx. There are approximately four major calyces per kidney. They are short, fat

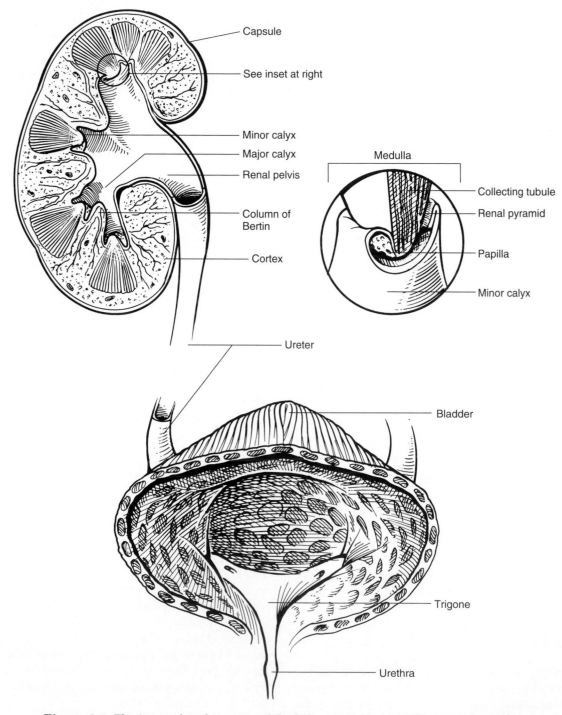

Figure 6–1. The internal architecture of the kidney and bladder. The inset shows the anatomy of the medulla, renal pyramid, and papilla, which drain into the minor calyx.

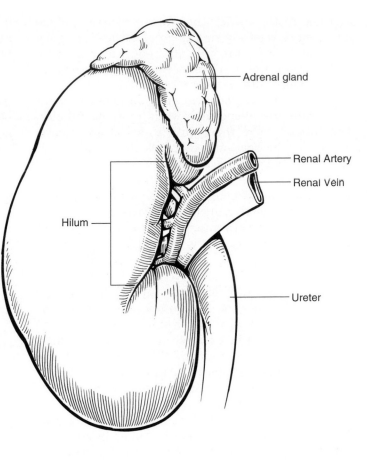

Figure 6–2. The external anatomy of the right kidney. Note that the ureter and renal vessels enter at the hilum. These structures are known as the renal pedicle.

Adrenal gland

Renal Artery

Renal Vein

Hilum

Ureter

tubes that arise from the renal pelvis and are located in the renal sinus.

There is a sac-like collecting portion of the upper expanded end of the ureter known as the renal pelvis. The pelvis is located at the hilum and is found both within and outside the kidney. The point at which the ureter ends and the pelvis begins is called the ureteropelvic junction. Along the medial border of each kidney is a depression called the hilum. The renal artery, vein, nerves, lymphatic vessels, and renal pelvis enter and leave the kidney at the hilum. This group of structures is known as the renal pedicle (Fig. 6–2).

The ureters should number two, one on each side. Anything other than this configuration is an anomaly. Each ureter is a hollow tube that extends from the kidney to the urinary bladder, about 25 to 30 cm (10–12 inches). The ureter has three coats: the outer fibrous layer, the middle visceral muscle, and the lining of epithelium.

The urinary bladder lies posterior to the pubic symphysis and is a sac that is a reservoir for urine. The bladder wall has four coats: the outer mucosal, the submucosal, the muscular, and the inner serosal.

There are three openings into the bladder, one at each ureter and one at the urethra. The triangular area between these three openings is called the trigone. The bladder can hold as much as 500 mL of urine, but 250 mL should be enough to cause distention and discomfort.

The urethra is the single passage to the outside of the body from the bladder. The female urethra is very short, only about 2.5 to 3.8 cm (1–1½ inches) long, while the male urethra extends approximately 20 cm (8 inches) through the prostate gland and penis before reaching the outside. The opening to the outside is called the urinary meatus. What has been presented here is a basic review of anatomy. The radiographer should be familiar with the microscopic anatomy such as the glomerulus and renal tubule makeup. An anatomy and physiology book can provide this information.

PHYSIOLOGY AND FUNCTION

The main function of the kidneys is to excrete urine so that the body maintains its hemostatic state. The functional unit of the kidney is the nephron which contains the Bowman capsule, the glomerulus, and tubules. Over one million nephrons are located in the cortex of each kidney. It is within the glomerulus of the nephrons that the filtration of waste materials from the blood takes place, so they can be excreted in the urine. The waste products include nitrogenous wastes from the breakdown of proteins, toxic substances, mineral salts, and water, both ingested water and that produced during metabolism. In the blood-filtering process, water and solutes from blood in the glomeruli pass through the capillaries and the glomerular walls into the tubules. The tubules have the ability to select substances needed by the body and reabsorb these substances to return them to the blood. If it were not for the reabsorption in the tubules, the body would soon be drained of fluids. Secretion takes place in the distal tubule and collecting ducts. Tubular secretion is the determinate of potassium ion concentration. The speed at which the blood is filtered, reabsorbed and secreted through the kidneys is affected by the blood pressure.

The kidneys also maintain the pH level of the blood so that it does not become too acid or too alkaline. Additionally, they remove excess glucose from the blood to be excreted in the urine. Regulation of the acid-base balance of the body fluids and the maintenance of normal concentrations of electrolytes are functions that are equal in importance to urine production.

When kidney function is damaged, two problems immediately arise. First, there is an excessive accumulation of wastes and poisons in the bloodstream. Second, there is an excessive loss of essential chemicals from the bloodstream. As a result of these abnormalities, the tissues through the body are supplied with blood with an improper chemical balance. If this balance is not quickly restored to normal, the patient will die.

After passing through the tubules, urine enters the collecting ducts of the renal pyramids and then passes through the papillae into the minor and major calyces, the renal pelvis, and finally the ureter, whose only function is to convey urine from the kidney to the bladder. This is accomplished by peristalsis and gravity. The bladder acts as a holding tank for urine until enough has been collected that pressure upon the stretch and tension receptors signal the need to urinate.

In the female, the urethra serves only one function, to convey urine from the bladder to the outside. In the male, it also serves a second function, to convey sperm to the outside.

SPECIAL RADIOGRAPHIC PROCEDURES

Intravenous pyelography (IVP, also known as intravenous ureography) is the most common radiographic procedure for the entire urinary system. This examination is done to determine the presence and location of an obstruction, the cause for abnormal laboratory results, the presence of arterial hypertension, and the location of a mass. For example, if the right kidney is displaced down and laterally, there could be a duodenal, pancreatic, or adrenal mass. In a male patient, a superiorly displaced bladder may indicate a prostate tumor. The contrast agents used, such as Conray or Renografin, are normally excreted and help to determine glomerular filtration. It takes about 15 minutes for an intravenously injected contrast medium to reach its greatest level of concentration in the renal collecting system. Fluid restriction in order to produce some dehydration improves the concentration of the contrast agent. The first portion of the excretory system to be shown by an IVP are the calyces. The postvoid film also gives information, as it shows any reflux of urine from the bladder back into the ureters.

There are some examinations that could be classified as special procedures; however, as they are nothing more than variations of the routine intravenous ureogram, they will only be explained briefly.

Nephrography is a study of the kidneys, with the first radiograph taken immediately after injection to show the blush of the renal cortex. The contrast medium may be introduced via rapid injection into a vein or by infusion.

A bolus **hypertensive intravenous ureogram** provides information regarding kidney function in cases of high blood pressure. In hypertensive patients, there is decreased urinary flow and more concentration of contrast material on the affected side. Rapid injection and films taken at 1 minute intervals for 5 minutes are the usual routine.

Large amounts of contrast medium can be continually dripped into a vein for **drip infusion pyelography.** Such an examination is performed when clarity of the collecting system and ureters is required or when the blood urea nitrogen (BUN) and creatinine levels indicate that the kidneys will not visualize. BUN and blood creatinine determinations can be very useful to the radiologist before an IVP as they indicate not only kidney function but also efficacy of the examination. Together, these laboratory evaluations are sensitive indicators of kidney function. BUN assay measures the nitrogen portion of urea in the blood. It is used as a gross index of glomerular filtration in the production and excretion of urea. A BUN level of 25 mg per 100 mL of blood is considered too high for a routine IVP to adequately show the functioning aspects of the kidneys. Creatinine is the byproduct of muscle metabolism. It is another nitrogenous waste that is also filtered out of the blood and excreted by the kidneys.

Normal creatinine levels are 0.6 to 1.2 mg per 100 mL of blood.

Cystography is the radiographic examination of the bladder to determine cystoureteral reflux caused by an incompetent ureteral valve (Fig. 6–3). This procedure is performed by inserting a catheter into the bladder and filling it slowly with contrast medium. As the bladder fills, the increased pressure on the valves keeps them closed, not allowing any reflux to occur. Valves that are incompetent because of infection can not stop leakage into the ureters. **Voiding cystography** can be performed after films of the bladder have been taken by having the patient void while on the table and taking films during the voiding process. This will visualize the urethra (Fig. 6–4).

A **bead-chain urethrogram** is a type of voiding cystogram that is used to detect abnormalities responsible for stress incontinence in women. A flexible bead chain is inserted into the bladder and the end is taped to the thigh. The length of the ureter is marked on the chain and contrast material is then introduced via a catheter. Once the catheter is removed, the patient is ready for radiographs. The films are taken in the upright anteroposterior and lateral positions while the patient relaxes and again while the patient performs a Valsalva maneuver. The lateral radiographs determine the angle the urethra makes with the posterior part of the bladder.

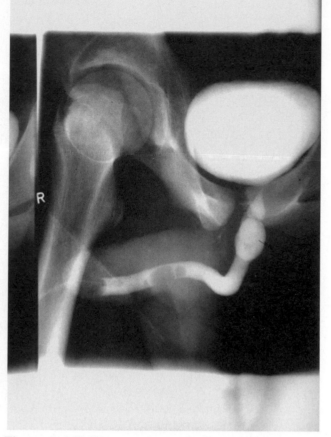

Figure 6–4. Voiding cystogram showing a partial tear of the urethra of a 15-year-old boy.

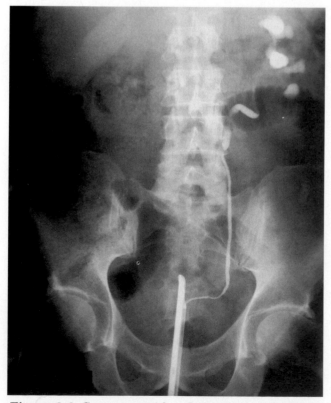

Figure 6–3. Cystogram with reflux into the left kidney.

Retrograde urethrography is performed on men to study the full length of the urethra. This procedure is performed by injecting contrast material into the urethra by a syringe. It does not allow the study of the bladder as a voiding cystogram does.

Retrograde pyelography is performed in the surgery suite after the patient has been sedated. The patient lies on a cystoscopic table in a modified lithotomy position so that the ureterocystoscope can be inserted into the ureter with the tip placed as near the renal pelvis as possible. Contrast medium is injected into the renal pelvis and films are taken (Fig. 6–5).

An examination that can study renal emptying after nephrostomy is called **percutaneous antegrade pyelography (PAP)**. This is performed by direct puncture of the renal pelvis through the posterior lateral aspect. Using ultrasonography or fluoroscopy or both, a needle or a catheter is placed into the renal pelvis and contrast material is instilled. **Percutaneous nephrostomy (PCN)** is a special procedure performed to relieve an obstruction in the collecting system. Following a percutane-

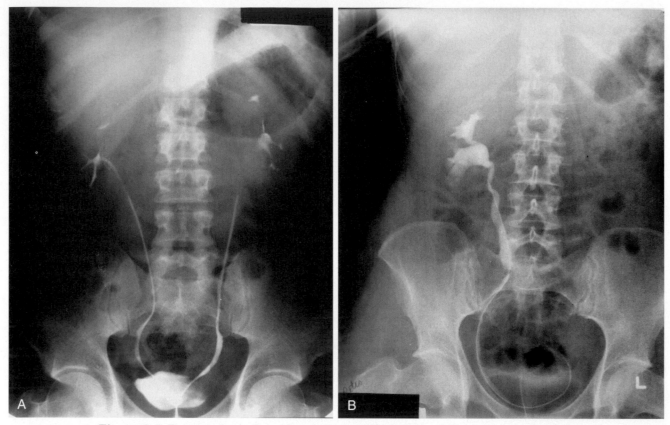

Figure 6–5. Retrograde pyelography. *A,* Essentially negative bilateral study. *B,* Right kidney showing hydronephrosis.

ous antegrade pyelogram, a catheter may be left in place to provide drainage of an obstructed kidney or to allow retrieval of a stone.

Renal angiography is performed to determine vascularity of lesions (Fig. 6–6) or to see lacerations, thrombi, or fractures of the renal parenchyma. Assessment of renal artery stenosis is also accomplished by this procedure which includes placing a catheter into the femoral artery and injecting contrast material into the renal arteries.

Computed tomography and ultrasonography are excellent modalities that are readily utilized to see the anatomy of the kidneys, as well as pathologic conditions. Computed tomography is useful in staging renal and bladder neoplasms or evaluating constricting ureteral lesions. Computed tomography is more useful than ultrasonography in obese patients since fat attenuates sound transmission but enhances the boundaries of the kidney under examination by computed tomography. There are limitations as well. Differentiation between benign cysts, necrotic tumors, and abscesses can be difficult.

Ultrasonography becomes the method of choice for evaluating patients who are allergic to contrast media, have renal failure, have an elevated BUN level, or who are pregnant (during which time radi-

ation should be avoided). Sonography plays a secondary role in the assessment of renal infection, abscess localization, evaluation of a flank mass in children, and distinguishing cystic from solid components in renal masses.

Radionuclide evaluation of the urinary system includes the imaging of structural abnormalities as well as making estimates regarding renal perfusion and function. With the widespread use of ultrasonography and computed tomography, the evaluation of renal anatomy by **nuclear medicine** is diminishing and the role of nuclear imaging is becoming more confined to analysis of function.

Two types of nuclear medicine studies are done for the renal area. An **architectural renal scan** uses a nuclide that localizes in the tubular cells. This is done to differentiate renal masses from pseudotumors. A **dynamic renogram** shows perfusion as well as excretion. It is performed most often to see if a transplanted kidney is functioning poorly because of rejection or tubular necrosis. The renogram can also evaluate renovascular hypertension.

Extracorporeal shock wave lithotripsy (**ESWL**) is a relatively new method used to attack renal calculi. The process uses focused shock waves to disintegrate renal stones while the patient is

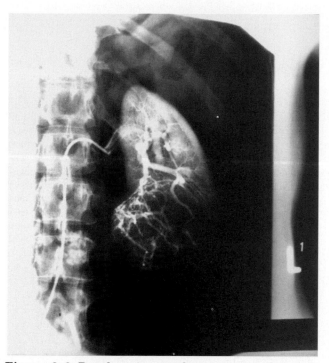

Figure 6–6. Renal angiogram demonstrating the vascularity to the left kidney. There is a mass in the lower pole, which is a Grawitz tumor.

suspended in a special chair within a large water bath. An electrode is located below the patient, and when the electrode is fired, the water surrounding it is vaporized, which creates a shock wave.

Treatment of stones with ESWL requires a close working relationship between the urologist and the radiography department. IVPs and supine abdominal radiographs are done both before and after treatment to assess stone size, configuration, location, and density. An IVP determines whether any obstruction is present distal to the stone that would impede the fragments' passage.

Biplane fluoroscopy is used to position the stone with the focal point of the shock wave. After each 100 shocks, the patient's position is rechecked. The treatment continues until the stone is broken into fragments no larger than 2 to 3 mm. When radiolucent stones are encountered, the use of a contrast agent helps to locate the stone for placement. A maximum of 2400 shock waves are administered per treatment so the potential for renal damage is decreased.

About 10 percent of stones treated by ESWL require a radiologic interventional procedure, chiefly PCN. Stone fragments are irrigated through the PCN tract. This flushes and removes the fragments.

PATHOLOGY

Before various pathologic conditions are discussed, a quick review of definitions should be included.

When a patient experiences a decrease in the amount of urine that is being passed, that patient is said to have **oliguria.** Conversely, too much urine being excreted is termed **polyuria.** If the kidneys fail to function and produce no urine, the patient will experience **anuria,** which is total suppression of urine formation and secretion. Anuria should not be confused with **retention,** which occurs when the bladder does not release urine into the urethra. Material in the urine can be suspicious for disease processes and must be evaluated. Blood in the urine, termed **hematuria,** should be of concern to both the patient and physician. When a blood test reveals toxic wastes in the blood, known as **uremia,** it indicates the kidneys' failure to filter these wastes and secrete them.

Common inflammation problems include inflammation of the bladder, called **cystitis,** and inflammation of the renal pelvis, called **pyelitis** (Fig. 6–7). Both of these conditions are more common in women and are caused by bacteria.

Congenital Anomalies

A **double system (bifid)** can be in the form of a double renal pelvis or ureter or both (Fig. 6–8). The upper ureter is usually the ectopic ureter. It may insert below the trigone in the bladder, outside the bladder in the urethra, or, in the male, into the seminal vesicles. Occasionally, a complete double kidney will appear on one side. Duplication of any part of the urinary system, except the bladder, is the most common congenital anomaly. Usually the condition presents no symptoms and is found only when another condition is being investigated. When anomalies do cause problems, they result in obstruction to the upper pole collecting system or reflux.

Horseshoe kidney is a condition in which both kidneys are joined at their lower poles across the midline of the body (Fig. 6–9A). This causes rotation of the renal pelvis so that they face more forward. The lower calyces will have a medial rotation. Stones are more common in horseshoe kidneys because the horizontal angle of the ureter attachment allows urine to sit for longer periods (see Fig. 6–9B).

Crossed ectopy exists when one kidney (usually the lower one), lies either partially or completely across the midline and is fused with the other kidney at the lower pole (Fig. 6–10), as in a horseshoe kidney. Both kidneys demonstrate various anomalies of position, shape, fusion, and rotation with this condition. Stone formation and reflux are more likely than with normal kidneys.

A floating kidney is termed **nephroptosis.** When a person stands up, the kidney falls down into the

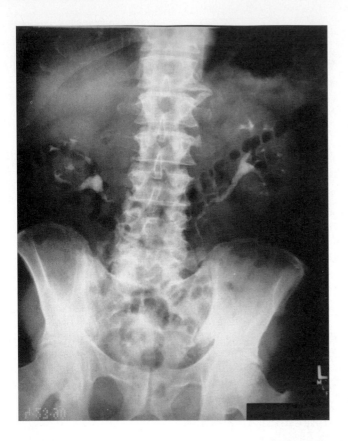

Figure 6–7. Pyelitis. Note the distorted collecting system and the uneven, tortuous ureters.

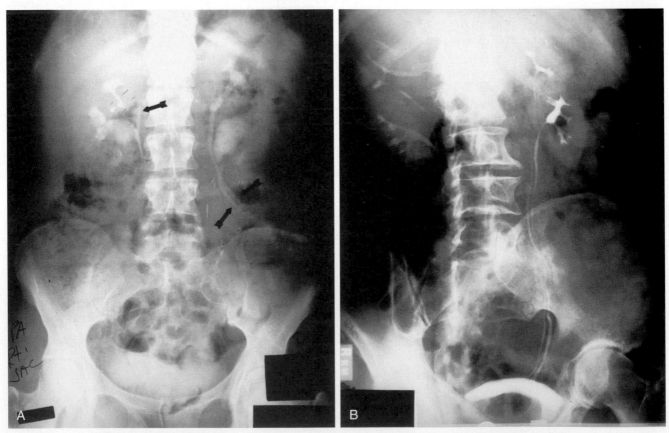

Figure 6–8. Bifid collecting systems. *A,* Posteroanterior view, showing stones on the right side *(single arrow)* and a double renal pelvis and ureter on the left *(two arrows).* *B,* Left posterior oblique view clearly shows the double ureter on the left, coursing down to the bladder. The right side was also duplicated. Note the mass impinging on the bladder.

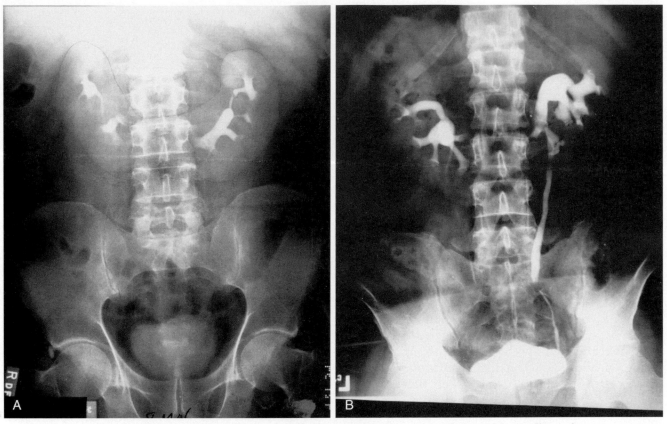

Figure 6–9. Horseshoe kidney. *A,* The lower poles are connected across the midline of the body. *B,* View of the abdomen with the patient in prone position, demonstrating a horseshoe-shaped kidney with radiolucent stones on the right kidney.

Figure 6–10. Crossed fused ectopy. The left kidney is rotated and fused with the lower, medial aspect of the right kidney.

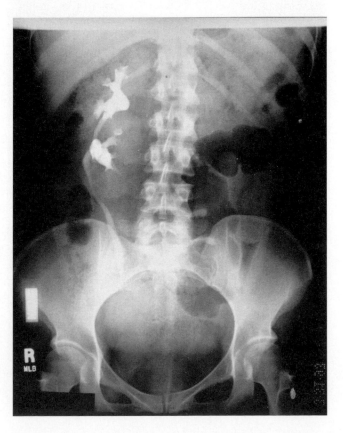

pelvis because of the pull of gravity. Nephroptosis is considered to be a variation of normal anatomy without significance. Descent of several centimeters may normally occur when an individual inspires deeply. As much as 5 centimeters can be expected when the patient assumes the upright position. However, when the kidney is not fixed to the peritoneum, nephroptosis will occur and the kidney will fall quite a distance. This should not be confused with ectopia, wherein a kidney is located below its normal level (Fig. 6–11).

Polycystic renal disease is an inherited renal cystic condition and is the most common cause of enlarged kidneys. This disease affects both kidneys and can be classified into two types. **Infantile polycystic disease** is characterized by dilated collecting tubules bilaterally and smooth renal borders. It can be further delineated into newborn and childhood types of polycystic disease.

The **newborn** type develops in utero and results in oligohydramnios and nephromegaly. Unfortunately, most infants with this disease are stillborn or die within days of birth. **Childhood infantile polycystic disease** occurs between the ages of 3 and 5 years. As in newborn types, the disease is

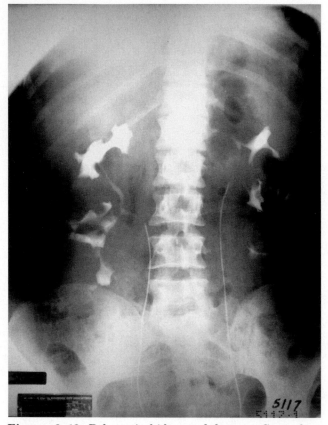

Figure 6–12. Polycystic kidney, adult type. Cysts form the outer margins of the kidney, making the renal outline difficult to see; however, the enlarged size of both kidneys is demonstrated by the placement of the collecting system.

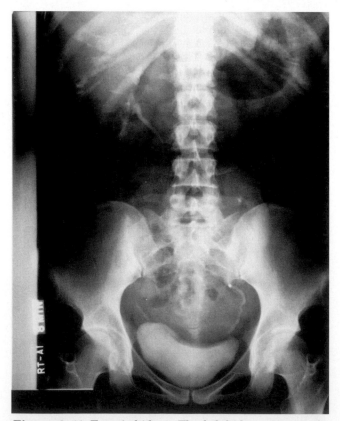

Figure 6–11. Ectopic kidney. The left kidney may not be visible immediately; however, the left ureter can be seen. If the ureter is followed up, the left kidney can be seen overlying the pelvis.

fatal if it is bilateral. If it is unilateral, hepatosplenomegaly, portal hypertension, and esophageal varices are also associated with it.

The second type of polycystic disease is **adult polycystic disease.** In this type, the normal kidney tissue is replaced by many small cysts until hardly any normal tissue is left. These cysts compress the nephrons, causing renal obstruction (Fig. 6–12).

The formation of the cysts begins early in life but progresses so slowly that manifestations do not present until the age of approximately 30 years. An increase in the size of the kidney, hypertension, renal insufficiency, and uremia are manifestations of adult polycystic disease. Often patients with this disease have cysts in the liver caused by bile duct hyperplasia. The pancreas and, less often, the spleen are also involved. Approximately one half of the patients die within 10 years of the onset of symptoms of kidney failure.

The IVP radiographs demonstrate somewhat enlarged kidneys with a lumpy, lobulated border (Fig. 6–13), enlongated renal pelvis, and distortion of the

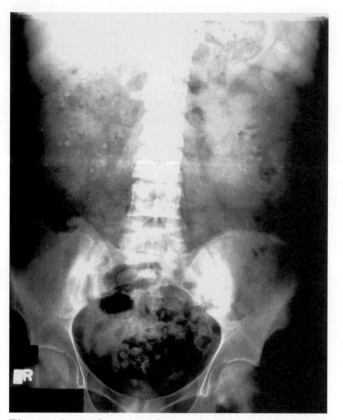

Figure 6–13. Long-standing polycystic renal disease presents with large, lobulated kidney borders. This patient also has nephrocalcinosis.

calyces. Radiolucencies are demonstrated throughout the cortex. Ultrasonography is an excellent method to demonstrate the enlarged, lobulated kidneys filled with cysts. It can also evaluate the liver, pancreas, and spleen for involvement.

Renal agenesis is the total failure of a kidney to develop (Fig. 6–14). This is an uncommon condition that usually occurs unilaterally. **Hypoplasia** describes a kidney that is less developed than normal. Both of these conditions are usually associated with hyperplasia of the opposite kidney. Renal arteriography is used to differentiate hypoplasia from atrophy of the kidney that is the result of disease. **Hyperplasia** is an overdeveloped kidney (Fig. 6–15). Again, this condition is usually associated with renal agenesis or hypoplasia of the other kidney.

Renal ectopia is the condition of a misplaced kidney. Usually, these kidneys are found in the pelvis and are associated with a congenitally short ureter. The short ureter is the determining factor to rule out nephroptosis (Fig. 6–16).

Inflammatory Processes

Bright disease is also called **glomerulonephritis** and is an inflammatory disease of the capillary loops of the renal glomeruli. It may develop after an acute streptococcal infection as a result of antigen-antibody complex being deposited in the glomerulus. It is the most common cause of underdeveloped kidneys in young adults. It is characterized by hypertension caused by the stimulation of the juxtaglomerular apparatus and edema of the face and ankles because of a loss of protein. The patient complains of nausea, malaise, and arthralgia. The urine shows an increase in albumin, BUN and creatinine levels. Pulmonary infiltrates may be present. The majority of patients recover spontaneously, but a small number of patients develop progressive renal failure, and death may be caused by uremia. In other cases, patients experience chronic inflammation. This leads to the fibrosis that results in the shrinkage of the kidney. Along with this, there is loss of renal function with accompanying uremia. The kidneys initially appear larger, especially during the nephrographic phase of the IVP, because of the inflammation. Ultrasonography is usually the diagnostic modality of choice and demonstrates the small kidney size that results from damage to the cortex.

Diverticula of the bladder or ureters or both are abnormal pouches of variable size extending through a defect in the wall. Because urine is apt to lie stagnant in such abnormal areas, stones and infections can develop. The appearance of diverticula of the urinary system is the same as that seen in the gastrointestinal system. These diverticula are best seen on a retrograde ureogram (Fig. 6–17).

Ureteroceles are cyst-like dilatations of a ureter near its opening into the bladder. It is the dilation of the submucosal ureteric segment. Rarely, this dilated portion may evert into the ureter, causing obstruction and simulating diverticula. This configuration has a characteristic appearance on the radiograph, which gives it its nickname of "cobrahead" (Fig. 6–18). As the bladder fills, the ureterocele is progressively diminished in size by the increasing pressure from the urine, making a ureterocele hard to diagnose when the bladder is extremely full. Figure 6–19 shows the different appearances of a ureterocele.

Prostatic hypertrophy describes prostate gland enlargement and subsequent obstruction of urinary output. Almost all men over 50 years of age experience some enlargement of the prostate gland. The early symptoms include reduced urine output but the feeling of a full bladder. The urethra passes through the prostate gland. As the gland enlarges it closes the lumen of the urethra, thus causing diminished urine output. The residual urine retained in the bladder tends to undergo decomposition and becomes infected. Cystitis is a common com-

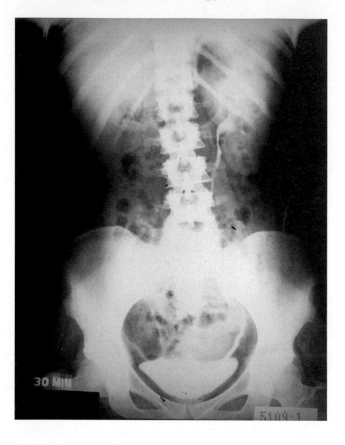

Figure 6–14. Renal agenesis. No ureter can be seen on the patient's right. The left kidney is hyperplastic to compensate for the absence of the right kidney.

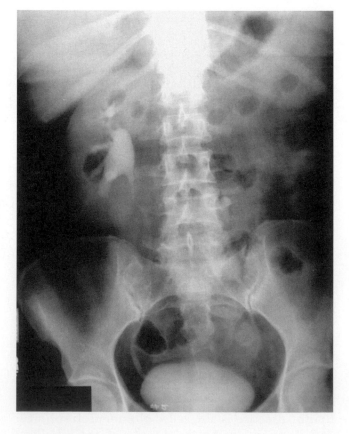

Figure 6–15. Hypoplasia and hyperplasia. This patient has a very small left kidney. The right kidney is hyperplastic because of a compensating workload.

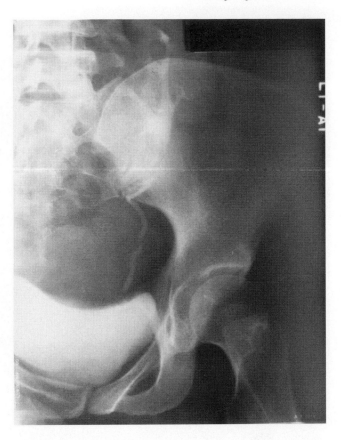

Figure 6–16. Ectopic kidney. The ureter is very short. The left kidney is over the pelvis.

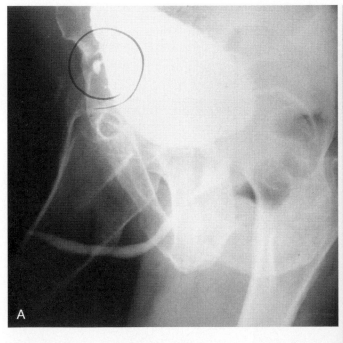

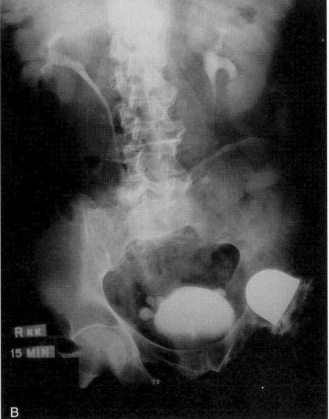

Figure 6–17. *A,* One diverticulum of the bladder is seen on this oblique, voiding cystogram. *B,* Four large ticks are seen on this 15-minute intravenous pyelogram.

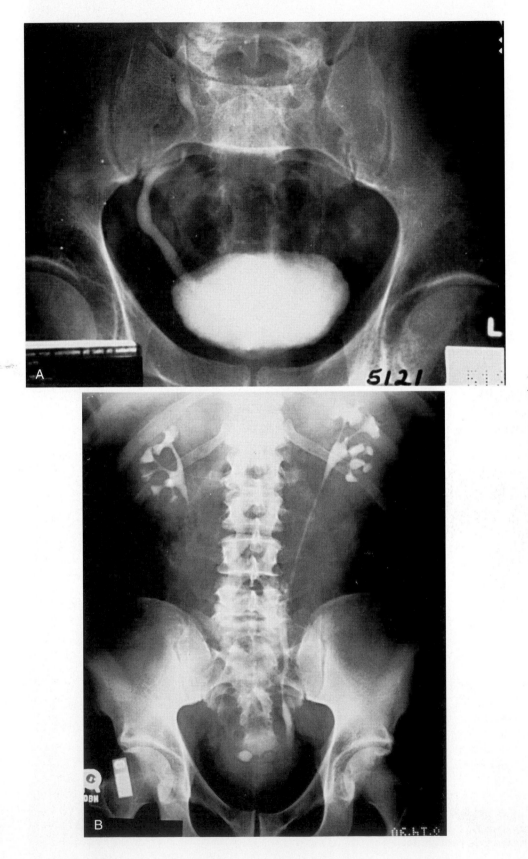

Figure 6–18. Ureteroceles. *A,* This bladder shot shows the "cobrahead" appearance of the dilated right ureter as it enters the bladder. *B,* The bladder is not yet full of contrast medium, thus providing an excellent view of the dilated distal end of the right ureter.

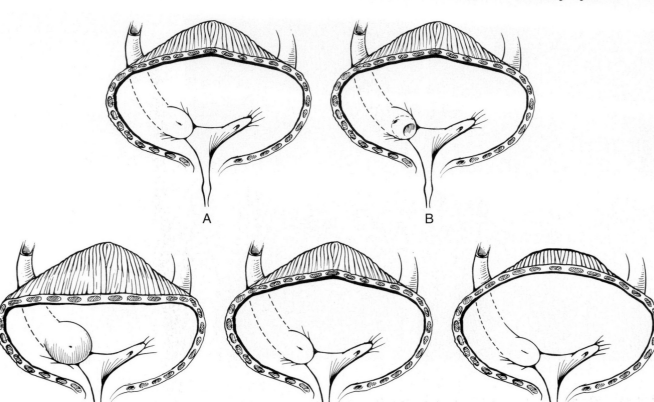

Figure 6–19. A ureterocele is a dilation of the submucosal ureteric segment. Rarely, the dilated portion may slide up into the ureter, causing obstruction *(A)* and simulating a diverticulum *(B)*. *C,* A ureterocele in an empty bladder. As the bladder fills, the ureterocele becomes smaller *(D)* until it is difficult to identify *(E)*.

plaint associated with hypertrophy of the prostate gland. As a result of increased pressure, the trabecular cords on the inner surface of the bladder pull on the wall. This causes the bladder to assume a lumpy, irregular border appearance on the radiograph (Fig. 6–20). Additionally, the base of the bladder has a notched appearance as a result of the enlarged prostate pushing up into the bladder.

Hydronephrosis is a result of some obstruction in the renal pelvis or ureter. It is characterized by dilation of the renal pelvis, calyces and ureter from back pressure of urine that can not flow past the obstruction. The patient experiences hematuria, pyuria, and fever. The radiographs show enlargement above the obstruction with no anatomy demonstrated below the obstruction. The calyces remain sharp, although enlarged (Fig. 6–21). It is possible for hydronephrosis to be present in both kidneys, particularly when the ureters are compressed by a fetus (Fig. 6–22). In this case, the condition of hydronephrosis disappears when the baby is delivered.

Hypertension is the result of a narrowing of one or more renal arteries. In the presence of renal artery stenosis, the kidney releases renin, an enzyme that causes vasoconstriction. Because of the vasoconstriction, the left ventricle of the heart has increased workload. This in turn leads to elevated blood pressure. This is known as primary (essential) hypertension.

Elevated blood pressure may also be the result of glomerulonephritis or pyelonephritis. This form is called secondary hypertension. The hypertensive kidney is so similar in appearance to the kidney in the end stage of glomerulonephritis that it may be impossible to distinguish between the two radiographically. Other names for hypertensive kidneys are arteriolosclerotic kidney (because of the change in the blood vessels) and nephrosclerotic kidney (because the kidney becomes scarred). The kidney that is the source of hypertension is usually smaller, shows delayed excretion, and over-concentrates the contrast agent.

Nephrosis is the tubular degeneration of the

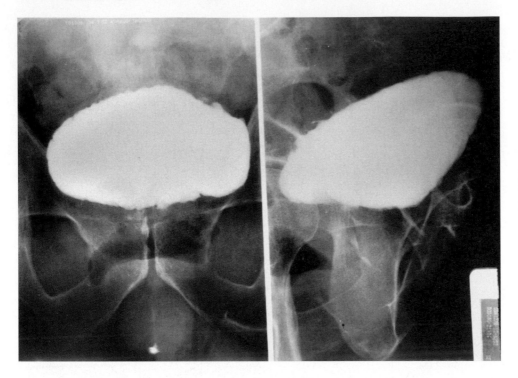

Figure 6–20. Hypertrophic trabeculation caused by hypertrophy of the prostate.

nephron of the kidney. The patient exhibits massive edema and either oliguria or anuria. This condition is more fully explained under the section on acute renal failure.

Pyelonephritis means inflammation of the kidney and renal pelvis. It is the most common single type of renal disease. Acute pyelonephritis is caused by a pyogenic bacteria, most commonly *Escherichia coli,* which invades the renal tissue (Fig. 6–23A). These organisms may enter the kidney through the blood. Other gram-negative bacteria can enter the kidney in a retrograde fashion through the bladder. Pyelonephritis is more common in women than in men because of the higher incidence of urinary tract infections among women. Patients characteristically experience flank pain, bacteriuria, pyuria, dys-

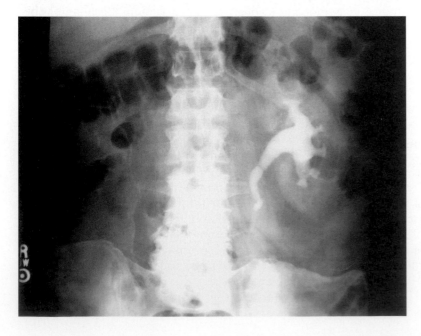

Figure 6–21. Hydronephrosis of the left kidney.

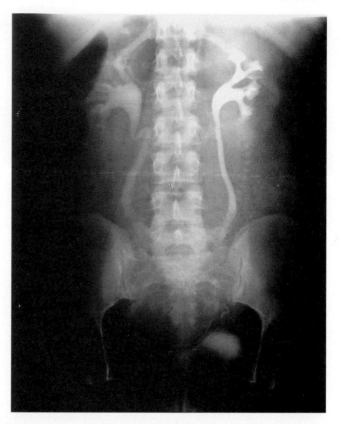

Figure 6–22. Hydronephrosis of both kidneys caused by a fetus obstructing the flow from the ureters.

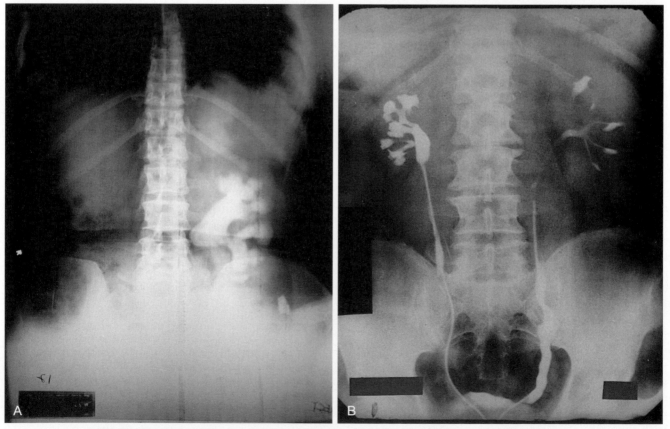

Figure 6–23. *A,* Acute pyelonephritis. Note the blunted calyces. *B,* Chronic pyelonephritis. The right kidney shows conical appearance of calyces with marked narrowing of the neck and infundibuli. The left kidney shows many small cysts.

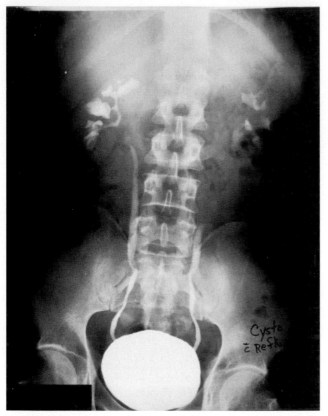

Figure 6–24. Reflux into both kidneys during cystography.

uria, nocturia, and frequent urination. The IVP shows blunted calyces. Chronic pyelonephritis is caused by chronic reflux of infected urine from the bladder into the renal pelvis. The eventual outcome of chronic pyelonephritis is decreased kidney size with destruction and scarring of the renal tissue (see Fig. 6–23B).

Reflux is caused by an incompetent ureteral valve that allows urine to flow back into the ureters and kidneys from the bladder. This condition is best evaluated by a cystogram (Fig. 6–24). Contrast material is introduced into the bladder via a catheter. If the contrast material is seen in the ureter after filling, it is more significant than if reflux occurs during voiding. Voiding and postvoid films are also taken to demonstrate reflux upon straining.

Renal calculi are stones that form in the urinary tract, usually in the renal pelvis (Fig. 6–25), but also sometimes in the bladder. These stones form from urine that contains crystalline materials such as calcium, calcium salts, and oxalates. Under most normal conditions, the minerals can form minute crystals that are passed out of the body along with the urine flow. Sometimes, however, the minerals clump together and cling to the tissue lining the inside of the kidney. There they continue to grow as

new crystals are added. As time passes, they harden. The urine shows elevated crystalline salts, pus, and blood. Calculi are usually asymptomatic until they begin to descend through the ureters (Fig. 6–26) or until they cause an obstruction. Then hematuria and severe flank pain radiating to the groin or genitals are common manifestations. It is important to identify stones because renal failure can occur from an obstruction of the ureter.

A **staghorn calculus** is a large stone that takes on the shape of the pelvicaliceal junction as it completely fills the renal pelvis (Fig. 6–27). This blocks all flow of urine. **Nephrocalcinosis** describes numerous irregular spots of calcium contained in the renal parenchyma (Fig. 6–28A). There may be only a few scattered areas of calcium or there may be numerous densities throughout both kidneys (see Fig. 6–28B). Abdominal radiographs taken prior to injection of the contrast medium are an important part of an IVP, as contrast material may hide some of the smaller calculi.

Although not as commonly as renal calculi, stones do form in the bladder. These stones are either single (Fig. 6–29) or multiple and vary in size (Fig. 6–30). Bladder stones have a tendency to form from stagnant urine that is unable to be passed because of some urethral outlet obstruction.

Acute renal failure is the rapid severe deterioration in kidney function caused by acute degeneration and necrosis of the renal tubules. Causes of acute necrosis include ischemia or toxic injury, especially by alcohol. Necrosis of the renal tubules (nephrosis) rapidly leads to oliguria or anuria. Water and potassium retention results in a life-threatening situation. Other causes of decreased renal function include problems such as obstruction of both renal arteries or of the bladder neck, glomerulonephritis, pyelonephritis, and severe hypertension. The patient exhibits massive edema and uremia. In acute renal failure, the patient undergoes dialysis if there is hope that the kidney function will return to a near normal state.

Chronic renal failure is the slow, insidious, and irreversible progressive loss of renal function. Because of the kidney's role in maintaining water balance and regulating acid-base balance and electrolyte levels, chronic renal failure causes major changes to be noted in all body systems. Hypertension, ventricular tachycardia, congestive heart failure, anemia, generalized edema, nephrocalcinosis, and clotting disorders are some of the manifestations of renal failure. The patient experiences oliguria or anuria and exhibits signs of fluid overload. There is usually extensive scarring and fibrosis of the renal parenchyma resulting in decreased kidney size. With chronic renal failure, the patient under-

Text continued on page 154

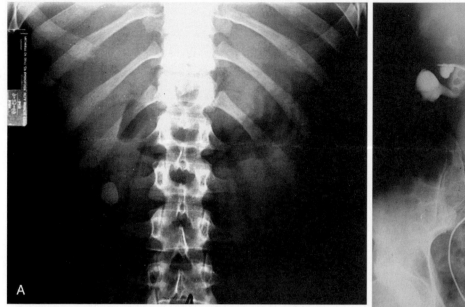

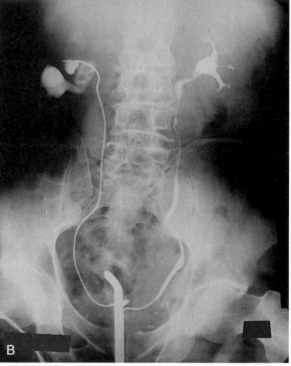

Figure 6–25. Calculi. *A*, Single radiopaque stone in the right kidney. *B*, Retrograde pyelogram reveals radiolucent calculi causing filling defects in the right renal pelvis.

Figure 6–26. Ureteral calculus.

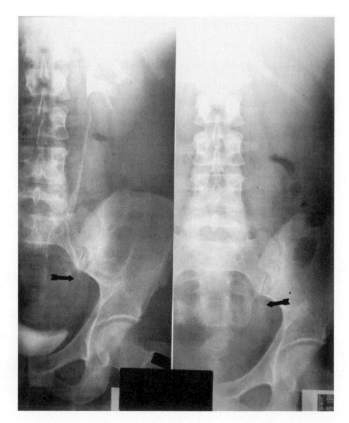

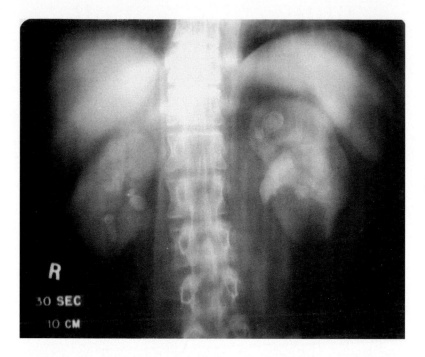

Figure 6–27. Staghorn calculus completely fills the left renal pelvis.

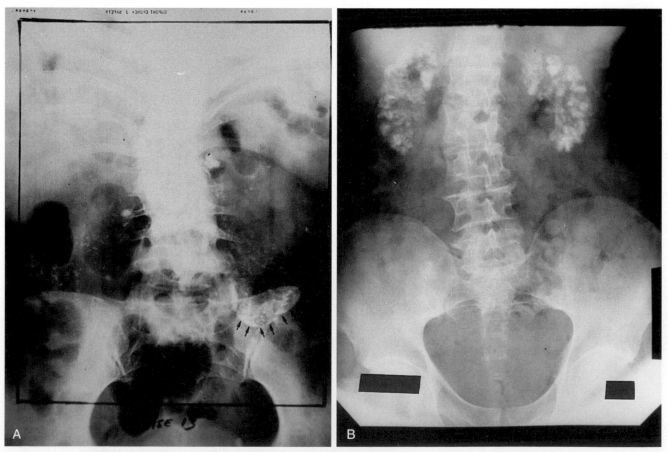

Figure 6–28. Nephrocalcinosis. *A,* A few scattered calcium deposits within the renal parenchyma. *B,* Numerous calcium deposits bilaterally.

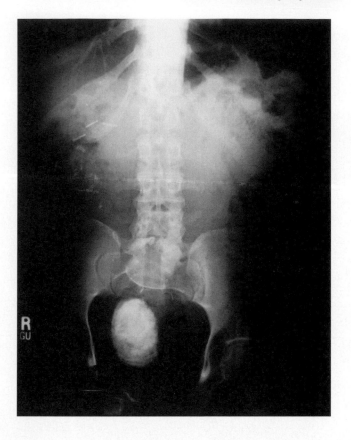

Figure 6–29. Single large bladder stone.

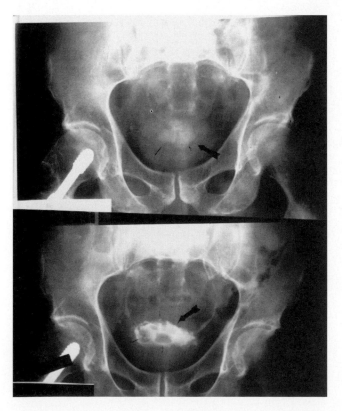

Figure 6–30. *Top,* Multiple calcifications are seen prior to the bladder filling with contrast medium. *Bottom,* The bladder stones create a filling defect within the bladder.

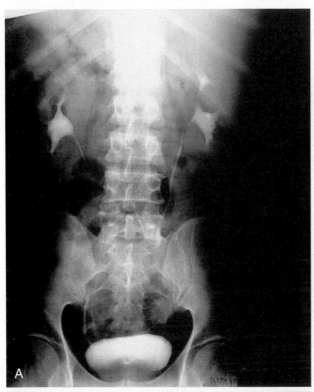

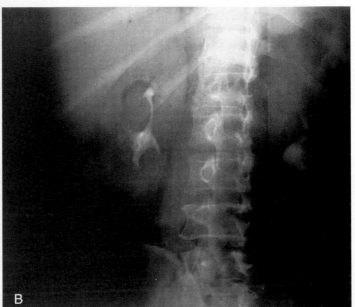

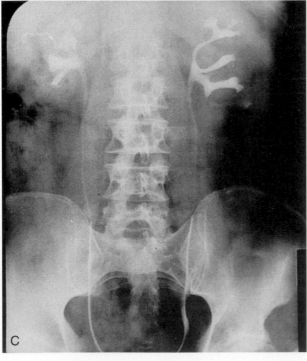

Figure 6–31. Renal cyst. *A,* Left calyces are splayed because of a large cyst. *B,* Oblique view better demonstrates the smooth borders and splayed architecture of the collecting system. *C,* Multiple cysts. This retrograde view shows numerous smooth filling defects causing elongation and distortion of the calyces and infundibuli of the left kidney.

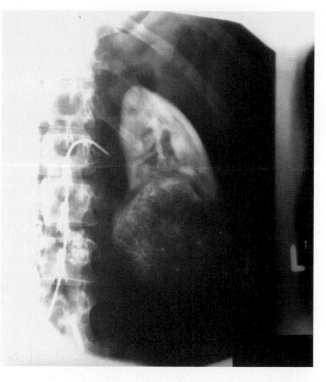

Figure 6–32. Grawitz tumor: large mass in the lower pole, which displaced the collecting system. This angiogram shows the abnormal vasculature of the neoplasm.

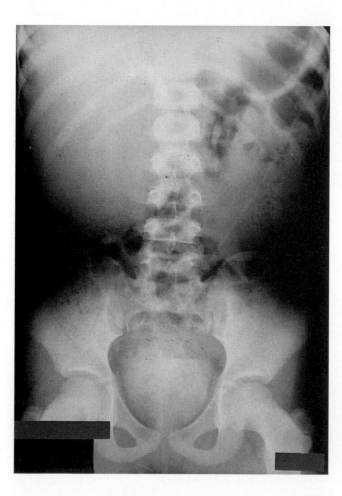

Figure 6–33. Wilms tumor. Retrograde pyelogram showing a large, soft tissue density of the right abdomen, which causes upward and medial displacement of the entire right kidney.

goes regular dialysis on a permanent basis, unless a kidney transplant is undertaken.

In renal failure, the kidneys cannot concentrate well, and large doses of contrast agents are necessary to visualize the parenchyma. IVPs that are performed on patients in acute renal failure demonstrate bilateral renal enlargement and prolonged nephrocortical blush. Tomography is especially helpful in demonstrating the pelvic structures that are poorly visualized. The contrast agent is excreted by the liver when the kidneys fail, and occasionally opacification of the gallbladder is noted.

Because of the large amounts of contrast needed for an IVP, this examination may be deemed detrimental to the patient. Renal failure lengthens the time necessary for excretion of contrast medium or prevents it all together. The longer the contrast medium remains in the body, the more toxic it be-

comes. Ultrasonography is usually the imaging modality of choice, as it does not rely on renal function and can demonstrate the dilation of the system as well as the smooth borders of the kidneys. The size of the kidney can be accurately measured by ultrasonography and is necessary to help determine acute renal failure, which shows enlarged kidneys, from chronic renal failure, with which small kidneys are associated.

Neoplasms

Benign

A **renal cyst** is an acquired condition that usually occurs in the cortex of the lower pole of the kidney. Approximately 50 percent of the population over the age of 50 years have or have had a renal cyst.

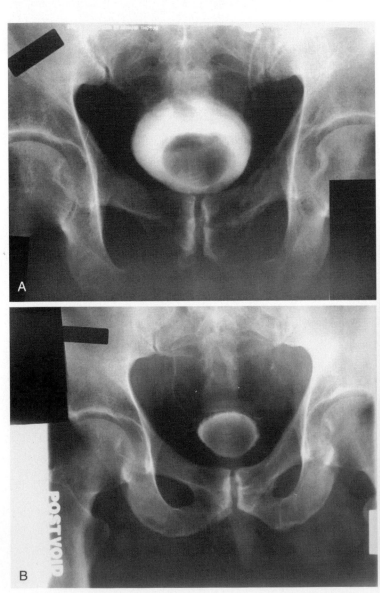

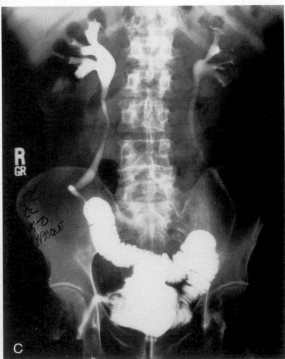

Figure 6–34. Bladder carcinoma. *A,* Large filling defect seen on this intravenous pyelography bladder film. *B,* Film taken after voiding shows the outline of the mass. The ragged edges seen on this film lead to a diagnosis of malignancy. *C,* Following a diagnosis of bladder cancer, the bladder is removed, and the ureters are connected to the small bowel.

Table 6–1.
Clinical and Radiographic Characteristics of Common Pathologies

Pathologic Condition	Causal Factors*	Manifestations	Radiographic Appearance
Horsehoe kidney	Congenital	Stones	Lower poles are fused across the midline
Polycystic kidney	Congenital		
Newborn	Newborn	Oligohydramnios, nephromegaly	Large kidneys
Childhood	3 to 5 years	Hepatosplenomegaly, portal hypertension, esophageal varices	Large lobulated kidneys
Adult	After 30 years	Hypertension, renal insufficiency, uremia	Nephromegaly, elongated renal pelvis, distorted calyces, lobulated borders
Glomerulonephritis	Strep infection, young adults	Hypertension, edema of face and ankles, nausea, arthralgia	Small kidneys
Diverticula	Weak wall of organ	Stones and infections	Outpouchings
Ureteroceles	Weak area of distal ureter allowing dilation		"Cobrahead"
Prostatic hypertrophy	Men over 50 years, enlargement of prostate	Reduced urine output, cystitis	Notched bladder, trabeculation of bladder
Hydronephrosis	Obstruction of renal pelvis or ureter	Hematuria, pyuria, fever	Well-defined calyces that are enlarged, dilation proximal to obstruction
Hypertension	Narrowing of renal arteries	High blood pressure	Small kidney, delayed excretion, hyperconcentration of contrast agent
Pyelonephritis	Pyogenic bacteria	Flank pain, bacteriuria	Blunted calyces, decreased kidney size
Calculi	Clusters of calcium	Hematuria, flank pain	Calcifications, large stone that fills renal pelvis, numerous irregular calcifications in cortex
Staghorn			
Nephrocalcinosis			
Renal failure			
Acute	Ischemia, toxic injury	Massive edema, uremia	Bilateral renal enlargement, prolonged nephrocortical blush
Chronic		Hypertension, ventricular tachycardia, congestive heart failure, anemia	Ultrasonography recommended
Renal cyst	Older than 50 years	Asymptomatic	Calyceal spreading
Hypernephroma	Older than 40 years	Hematuria	Space-occupying lesion
Nephroblastoma	Younger than 5 years	Firm nontender mass	Large abdominal mass, displaces kidney
Bladder carcinoma	Males over 50 years, excessive smoking	Asymptomatic	Filling defect, computed tomography recommended

*Includes age, if relevant.

Renal cysts are generally asymptomatic unless they are quite large, in which case pain or obstruction caused by pressure being excerted from the cyst may be present. The cyst is readily seen on computed tomographic scan and ultrasonogram. Radiographically, the cyst shows calyceal spreading but does not demonstrate the irregular opacification after injection of a contrast agent that a tumor does (Fig. 6–31).

Renal pseudotumors are normal or hypertrophied renal tissues that contain normal vasculature but often produce an intense blush, especially on nephrotomograms. On routine intravenous pyelography, the tissue splays the calyces in the same way a renal cyst does. Ultrasonography can differentiate the pseudotumor from the cyst.

Malignant

Benign tumors of the kidney are rare. The most common renal tumor in patients of any age is the **hypernephroma,** also called **adenocarcinoma,** or **Grawitz tumor.** This malignant tumor is thought to arise from the renal tubule cells. It destroys the kidney and invades the blood vessels, particularly the renal vein and the inferior vena cava, so that secondary tumors are spread to the lungs and bones. The chief symptom is hematuria. This neoplasm has an increased incidence after the age of 40 years and is twice as common in men. The radiograph shows a space-occupying lesion that distorts and displaces the collecting system (Fig. 6–32). The tumor commonly shows an abnormal vasculature as seen on an angiogram. Ultrasonography not only shows the composition of the tumor but also can demonstrate invasion of the renal vessels by the tumor.

Nephroblastoma (Wilms tumor) is the most common malignant neoplasm occurring in children under the age of 5 years. An IVP shows a large abdominal mass that displaces the kidney (Fig. 6–33). It is a firm, nontender mass deep within the flank. When this condition is treated promptly with surgical removal of the kidney, approximately 50 percent of patients survive. However, if this is not diagnosed and treated early, widespread metastasis occurs to the liver, lungs, and brain, and the prognosis is poor.

Bladder carcinoma occurs more often in men over the age of 50. The cause of this type of carcinoma has been related to excessive cigarette smoking, as the carcinogenic metabolites are excreted in the urine. There is also a high incidence of bladder cancer among workers in factories that manufacture aniline dyes. The tumor usually projects into the bladder in a papillary form, causing a filling defect on the ureogram bladder radiograph (Fig. 6–34). However, because most tumors are small and located in the area of the trigone, detection by radiography is not as reliable a method as with computed tomography, which can stage the tumor.

Table 6–1 summarizes the clinical and radiographic characteristics of common pathologies of the urinary system.

Review Questions

1. Draw a coronal section of the interior of a right kidney. Label the capsule, cortex, medulla, pyramids, papillae, minor and major calyces, and the renal pelvis.
2. Describe the blood-filtration process. Where does secretion take place? Why is reabsorption so important?
3. Describe the flow of urine from the tubules to the urethra.
4. List the two variations of an intravenous pyelogram. Indicate what each is done for and how it is performed.
5. What is cystography? Why is it done? How is it performed? What examination can be combined with cystography? What will this demonstrate?
6. Describe each of the following procedures. What will each demonstrate?
   Retrograde urethrography
   Retrograde pyelography
   Percutaneous antegrade pyelography
7. Name two nuclear medicine studies of the kidneys. Why is each of them done?
8. Describe extracorporeal shock wave lithotripsy. Include what it is, where it is done, how it is done, why it is done, and what other examinations are performed in conjunction with it.
9. When is ultrasonography used to image the renal system?
10. Define the following terms:

Anuria	Polyuria
Oliguria	Retention
Hematuria	Uremia
Cystitis	Pyelitis
Nephroptosis	Crossed ectopy
Renal hypoplasia	Renal hyperplasia
Renal agenesis	Renal ectopia

11. Define horseshoe kidney. Describe its radiographic appearance. What condition is common with this condition? Why?
12. Describe polycystic kidney disease. What are the complications of this disease? What do the radiographs demonstrate?
13. Describe glomerulonephritis. What causes it? What may death be caused by? Why is this the

cause of small kidneys? Which procedure is best used to demonstrate this?

14. For each of the following, describe what it is and its radiographic appearance.

Diverticula   Ureteroceles
Prostatic hypertrophy   Hydronephrosis
Pyelonephritis   Reflux
Renal cyst   Hypertension
Hypernephroma   Nephroblastoma

15. Compare and contrast acute and chronic renal failure. (What each is, what they cause, what causes them, what the manifestations are of each). Explain why intravenous pyelography is detrimental to the patient in renal failure. If it is done, how is the contrast material excreted? What other organ can be seen if this occurs? Why? What imaging modality is best suited for a patient in renal failure? What can this procedure demonstrate?

16. List and define the two other names given to the hypertensive kidney.

CHAPTER VII

Reproductive System

Goals

1. To review the basic anatomy and physiology of both the male and the female systems.
2. To become acquainted with the pathophysiology of the reproductive system.
3. To become familiar with the radiographic manifestations of all the common congenital and acquired disorders of both the male and the female reproductive systems.

Objectives

At the completion of the chapter, the radiographer will be able to:

1. Describe the physiology of the male and the female reproductive systems.
2. Identify anatomic structures on diagrams and radiographs of the reproductive system.
3. Define terminology relating to the reproductive system.
4. Describe the various pathologic conditions affecting the female reproductive system and their radiographic manifestations.
5. Describe the various pathologic conditions affecting the male reproductive system and their radiographic manifestations.
6. Describe the special radiographic examinations of the female reproductive system.
7. Explain mammography and its importance in women's health.

I. Anatomy
   A. Female
      1. Uterus
         a. Body (Corpus)
         b. Fundus
         c. Cervix
         d. Layers
            1. Endometrium
            2. Myometrium
            3. Perimetrium
         e. Position
            1. Anteverted
            2. Libo-rotated
            3. Dextro-rotated
      2. Vagina
         a. Fornix
      3. Ovaries
      4. Uterine Tubes (Fallopian Tubes)
         a. Openings
            1. Uterine Ostium
            2. Abdominal Ostium
         b. Isthmus
         c. Infundibulum
         d. Ampulla
      5. Breasts
   B. Male
      1. Scrotum
         a. Testis
         b. Epididymis
         c. Vas Deferens
      2. Ejaculatory Ducts
      3. Seminal Vesicles
      4. Prostate
      5. Cowper Glands
II. Physiology and Function
   A. Female
      1. Ovulation
      2. Menstrual Cycle
         a. Proliferative Phase
         b. Secretory Phase
         c. Menstrual Phase
   B. Male
      1. Spermatogenesis
III. Special Radiographic Procedures
   A. Hysterosalpingography
   B. Mammography
   C. Ultrasonography
   D. Computed Tomography
IV. Pathology
   A. Female
      1. Congenital Anomalies
         a. Position
            1. Retroverted
            2. Retroflexed
            3. Anteflexed
         b. Uterine Aplasia
         c. Shape of Uterus
            1. Unicornuate
            2. Didelphic
            3. Bicornuate Bicollic
            4. Bicornuate
            5. Arcuate
            6. Septate
            7. Subseptate
      2. Inflammatory Processes
         a. Endometriosis
            1. Chocolate Cyst
            2. Adenomyosis
         b. Pelvic Inflammatory Disease
            1. Acute
               a. Pyosalpinx
               b. Tubal Ovarian Abscess
            2. Chronic
      3. Neoplasms
         a. Benign
            1. Fibroids (Leiomyomata, Myomas)
               a. Submucous
               b. Intramural
               c. Subserous (Pedunculated)
            2. Teratoma (Dermoids)
            3. Cystic Ovaries
               a. Single
               b. Multiple
               c. Polycystic
                  1. Stein-Leventhal Syndrome
            4. Fibrocystic Breast Disease
            5. Fibroadenoma (Breast)
         b. Malignant
            1. Endometrial Carcinoma
            2. Cervical Carcinoma
            3. Cystadenocarcinoma
            4. Breast Carcinoma
   B. Male
      1. Congenital Anomalies
         a. Cryptorchidism (Undescended Testes)
            1. Orchiopexy
            2. Orchiectomy
      2. Inflammatory Processes
         a. Prostatic Hyperplasia
         b. Prostatic Calculi
         c. Torsion
         d. Epididymitis
         e. Gynecomastia
      3. Neoplasms
         a. Benign
            1. Hydroceles
            2. Spermatocele
         b. Malignant
            1. Seminomas
            2. Teratomas
            3. Prostate Carcinoma

The reproductive system of the female is studied by radiography more often than is the reproductive system of the male. Subspecialties of radiography such as ultrasonography and nuclear medicine play an important role in demonstrating various pathologic conditions. Many pathologic conditions are quite common and present symptoms that should be familiar to the technologist. The external genitalia of the female are collectively termed the vulva and include the mons pubis, labia major and minor, clitoris, vaginal orifice, and Bartholin glands. The male external genitalia consist of the scrotum and the penis. Although these areas are considered to be a portion of the reproductive system (accessory organs in the male), the external genitalia will not be discussed further.

ANATOMY

Female Reproductive Organs

The female reproductive organs are a uterus, a vagina, a pair of ovaries, and a pair of uterine (fallopian) tubes. The breasts are accessory organs.

The uterus is a thick-walled, hollow, pear-shaped organ that lies in the pelvic cavity between the bladder and the rectum. The upper portion of the uterus, the body, also known as the corpus, has a rounded swelling, just above and between the entry points of the uterine tubes, called the fundus. The lower, narrower portion of the uterus is the cervix. The opening from the cervix of the uterus into the cervical canal is called the internal os, and the opening from the cervical canal into the vagina is called the external os.

The uterine walls are formed of three layers. The internal lining is a specialized epithelial mucous membrane called endometrium. The middle layer, the myometrium, is formed of three layers of smooth muscle, extending diagonally, crosswise, and lengthwise. The external layer is formed of serous membrane, called perimetrium, which covers only a portion of the body of the uterus.

The uterus normally sits in the pelvis at a forward angle, with the fundus of the uterus toward the abdominal wall. There should be an almost 90 degree angle between the vaginal canal and the body of the uterus. This position is known as **anteverted**. Additionally, the uterus can be slightly **anteflexed** and not be considered in a deviated position. When the bladder is filled, the anteflexion becomes less pronounced. Normally, the uterus is located in the midline of the pelvic cavity; however, the uterus may extend to the right or left side of the patient's midline. A uterus that is deviated to the left may be termed **libo-rotated**, while a uterus that is deviated to the right of the patient's midline may be termed **dextro-rotated**.

The vagina is a flattened dilatable canal that enters the cervix at right angles when in a normal position. The vagina forms a cuff around the cervix known as the fornix.

The ovaries lie in the ovarian fossa behind the broad ligament on either side of the uterus. They lie at an angle between the external iliac vein in front and the ureter behind. Each ovary lies beneath the suspended end of a uterine tube but does not come into contact with the tube.

There are two uterine (fallopian) tubes. The proximal ends of the uterine tubes open into the uterus at the isthmus. This opening is known as the uterine ostium. The distal ends, the infundibulum, are funnel-shaped with fringed, finger-like processes called fimbriae. The fimbriated ends are over but not attached to or touching the ovaries. The opening at this end is known as the abdominal ostium. The ampulla is the largest portion immediately adjacent to the infundibulum. Figure 7–1 shows coronal and sagittal sections of the female reproductive organs.

The female breasts are lobulated, glandular structures on the anterior lateral surface of the thorax. The breast is cone-shaped, with the base against the chest wall, and tapers down to the nipple, which is surrounded by a circular pigmented area called the areola. Each breast consists of 15 to 20 lobes that are divided into 20 to 40 lobules, which contain the milk-producing acini cells. These lobules are the basic structural unit of the breast.

Within the lobules are the lactiferous ducts, which unite to drain to the nipple.

The layer of subcutaneous fibrous tissue provides support for the breast. Cooper ligaments extend from the connective tissue layer, through the breast, and attach to the underlying muscle fascia, providing further support for the breast. The muscles forming the floor of the breast are the greater and smaller pectorals, the anterior serratus, the latissimus dorsi, the subscapular, the external oblique, and the straight abdominal muscles.

The glandular and connective tissues are water-dense structures. A young postpubescent person has dense, firm, homogeneous breasts that show little tissue differentiation. During pregnancy and lactation, the breasts become very dense and opaque. After pregnancy, the breasts undergo involution and fatty infiltration. **Involution** is the process of the lobules decreasing in size as well as number. The space left is filled with fat. The tissue regenerates for each pregnancy to a point, but with each succeeding pregnancy, the breast tissue becomes more and more fatty. Menopausal women have almost no density in their breasts because the entire organ is made up of fat.

Male Reproductive Organs

The male reproductive organs are the testes, epididymides, vas deferens, ejaculatory ducts, seminal vesicles, prostate gland, and Cowper glands.

The testes are a pair of egg-shaped glands normally located in a sac-like structure that hangs from the perineal area known as the scrotum. The scrotum, which is divided into two sacs internally, also contains one epididymis and the inferior part of a spermatic cord. Each testicle is enclosed in a fibrous white capsule and is divided into compartments, each of which contains a seminiferous tube that joins into a cluster from which several ducts appear and enter the head of the epididymis. It is in the seminiferous tubules that sperm are formed.

The epididymis is a tightly coiled, tube-like structure about 6 m (20 feet) long. It lies along the posterior border of the testis. The epididymis stores sperm before ejaculation. The vas deferens is a tube that is the continuation of the epididymis. It extends from the epididymis up through the inguinal canal, where it is encased by the spermatic cord, into the abdominal cavity and down the posterior side of the bladder where it connects with the seminal vesicle duct and forms the ejaculatory duct. The ejaculatory ducts pass through the prostate gland and extend to the urethra.

The seminal vesicles are two twisted pouches lying along the bladder's lower posterior surface

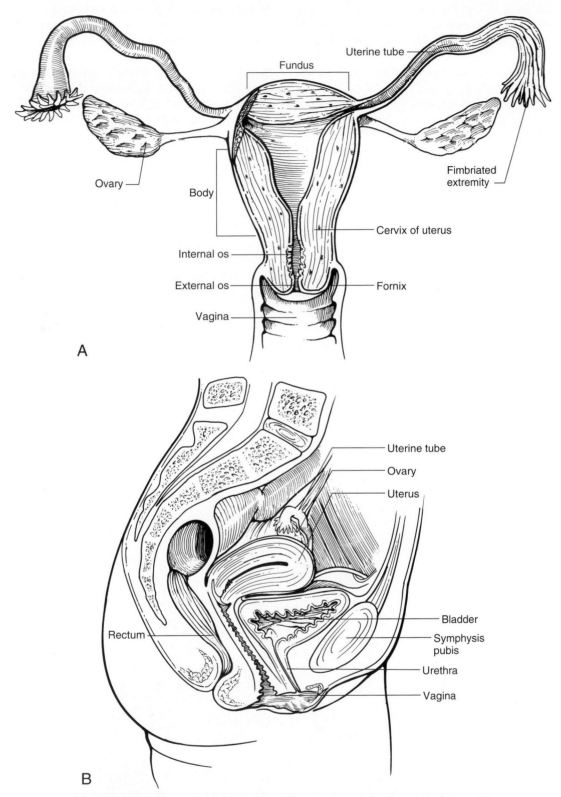

Figure 7–1. Coronal *(A)* and sagittal *(B)* sections of the female pelvic cavity.

and in front of the rectum. They secrete a portion of the liquid part of semen. The prostate gland is composed of smooth muscle and glandular tissue. It surrounds the neck of the bladder and the urethra. The prostate gland secretes a thin, alkaline substance that makes up the majority of the seminal fluid (Fig. 7–2).

Cowper glands (bulbourethral glands) lie on either side of the urethra below the prostate gland. These glands secrete an alkaline fluid similar to that produced by the prostate gland, which protects the sperm from the acid present in the vagina.

PHYSIOLOGY AND FUNCTION

Female

The ovaries are responsible for the production of ova and the secretion of the female hormones estrogen and progesterone. Estrogen is responsible for growth and maintenance of the reproductive organs and secondary sex characteristics. Progesterone and estrogen prepare the endometrium for pregnancy and the breasts for milk production.

Females are born with approximately 200,000 potential ova-containing follicles in each ovary. Menarche usually begins between the ages of 11 and 15. Once each month, around the first day of menstruation, the follicular cells start to secrete estrogen. In most cycles, only one follicle matures and migrates to the surface of the ovary, where it ruptures and expels the mature ovum into the pelvic cavity. The expulsion of the mature follicle is known as ovulation.

The remaining cells of the ruptured follicle enlarge. With the deposit of lutein, the follicle becomes known as the corpus luteum and continues to grow for 7 to 8 days. The corpus luteum secretes progesterone in increasing amounts. If fertilization of the ovum has not occurred, the size and secretions of the corpus luteum gradually diminish until the nonfunctional structure is reduced and eventually disappears. If fertilization does occur, the corpus luteum remains intact throughout the pregnancy.

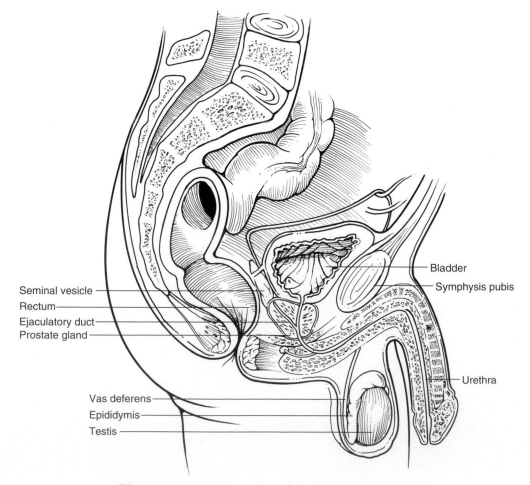

Figure 7–2. Sagittal section of the male pelvic cavity.

The cyclic changes in the ovaries are controlled by a variety of substances secreted by the anterior pituitary gland. Growth of the primitive graafian follicles and ova and the secretion of estrogen are controlled by the follicle-stimulating hormone, whereas follicular rupture, expulsion of its ripe ovum, and the secretion of progesterone are under the control of the luteinizing hormone.

The menstrual cycle refers to the changes in the endometrium of the uterus that occur in women throughout the childbearing years. Each cycle lasts about 28 days and is divided into three phases: proliferative, secretory, and menstrual.

The proliferative phase occurs between the end of the menses and ovulation. The secretory phase occurs between ovulation and the onset of menses. The length of this phase is fairly constant and usually lasts 14 days. The menstrual phase of the cycle is when the actual flow of blood, mucus, and endometrium from the uterus begins and ends. This usually lasts about 4 to 6 days, until the low level of progesterone causes the pituitary gland to again secrete follicle-stimulating hormone and a new menstrual cycle begins.

The reproductive years of a woman terminate with the cessation of the menstrual cycle. This is known as menopause and usually occurs in the late 40s or early 50s.

Male

The major function of the male reproductive system is the formation of sperm, known as spermatogenesis. In addition to sperm cell production, the testes secrete the male hormone testosterone, which is responsible for adult male sexual behavior. Testosterone also helps regulate metabolism by promoting growth of skeletal muscles and is thus responsible for the greater male muscular development and strength. The final maturation of sperm occurs in the epididymis. The sperm spend from 1 to 3 weeks in the epididymis before they become motile and capable of fertilizing an ovum. From the epididymis, sperm are conveyed into the vas deferens where they may remain up to 1 month without loss of fertility. An alkaline fluid is secreted by the vas deferens to maintain viability of the sperm.

Male fertility is related not only to the number of sperm ejaculated but also to their size, shape, and motility. It is hypothesized that sterility results when the sperm count falls below about 50 million sperm per mL of semen. Unlike those for a woman, the reproductive years for a man never end. He is able to fertilize an ovum throughout his life.

SPECIAL RADIOGRAPHIC PROCEDURES

Hysterosalpingography is a procedure that may be diagnostic as well as therapeutic. Diagnostic indications for hysterosalpingography include abnormal bleeding or spotting between menstrual periods, patency of tubes, anomalies, habitual spontaneous abortions, amenorrhea, dysmenorrhea, and a lost intrauterine contraceptive device. Therapeutic indications include restoring patency to the tubes, stretching adhesions, dilatation of the tubes, or straightening of the tubes. Contraindications of hysterosalpingography include pregnancy, pelvic inflammatory disease, vaginal or cervical infection, or menses.

Two types of contrast media are used for hysterosalpingograms. Water-soluble and oily contrast agents each have their advantages and disadvantages. A water-soluble agent may either be in the form of Salpix or Sinografin. This contrast medium is absorbed quickly and leaves no residue. The disadvantage to water-soluble agents is the great deal of pain they produce. Ethiodol is an oily contrast agent that is very opaque and causes little or no pain. Unfortunately, the oil persists in the body.

Besides considering the above advantages and disadvantages when choosing a contrast agent, the radiographer should also keep in mind the time it takes the body to rid itself of the contrast material. It should be either excreted or absorbed rapidly. The contrast agent must also be dense and viscous enough to coat the uterus and not be diluted too easily with the uterine fluids. Finally, it should be nonreactive.

Only about 4 mL is required to fill the uterus. Another 4 mL is used to fill the tubes, if no pathology is present. Carbon dioxide may also be used in addition to the positive contrast agent. About 100 mL is necessary and will be absorbed in approximately 25 to 30 minutes.

The patient assumes the lithotomy position and the cervix is exposed with a speculum. A cannula is placed into the cervical os and is held in place by a tenaculum. The speculum is then removed over the cannula. Contrast material is slowly injected under fluoroscopic guidance. A rubber plug is fixed to the cannula and fits tightly against the external os of the cervix to prevent backflow of the contrast material. Overhead radiographs are usually taken in anteroposterior and oblique projections (Fig. 7–3). If an oily contrast medium was used, a 24-hour delayed film can be taken to check the patency of the tubes.

Mammography is the radiologic examination of the breast, either male or female. Mammography

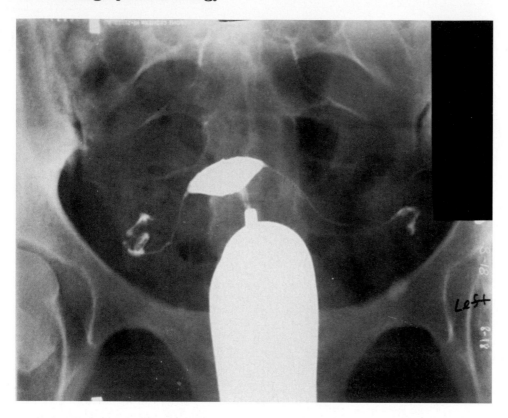

Figure 7–3. Hysterosalpingogram showing normal results.

can show the size of a mass, reveal calcifications, and demonstrate nipple inversion, but the most important function is for early detection and diagnosis of breast cancer. Women have a 90 to 98 percent chance of long-term survival if cancer is detected and treated in its early stages. To ensure early diagnosis, the American Cancer Society advises women to have a baseline mammogram between the ages of 35 and 40. Mammograms are recommended on an every-other-year basis for women 40 to 49 years old and yearly for those over the age of 50. However, decisions for radiographic examinations any sooner than that should be a personal decision between the patient and the physician. All patients with any clinical history such as discharge, nipple retraction, skin thickening, palpable masses, or a family history of breast cancer should undergo mammography.

It has been demonstrated that radiation exposure to the breast can induce breast cancer and that this risk is dose-dependent. Although radiation health professionals consider any radiation dose to be a nonthreshold dose (no safe dose), a maximum of 0.01 Gy (1 rad) has been set as the safe limit of radiation exposure in mammography. The absorption of 0.01 Gy (1 rad) of radiation by the breast raises the chance of cancer from 8 percent to 8.08 percent. In the early 1970s, low-dose film screen systems were introduced so that high-quality mam-

mographic images could be made with low radiation exposures.

In mammography, a single high-resolution intensifying screen and single-emulsion fine-grain film are used. The cassettes achieve almost perfect film-screen contact. Normally, only 0.003 to 0.008 Gy (300–800 mrad) are given at the skin surface, which is well under the 0.01 Gy (1 rad) safety mark. Older nonscreen techniques emitted anywhere from 0.04 to 0.16 Gy (4–16 rad).

Dedicated mammographic units have a molybdenum target to produce low-energy x-ray beams. Filtration is 0.03 mm of additional molybdenum. This is equal to 0.5 mm aluminum. The tube operates only at low kilovoltage. The normal range for mammograms is 25 to 30 kilovolts peak. A small focal spot size, 0.3 to 0.6 mm, is used to improve geometric sharpness, and compression devices help create uniformity of breast tissue as well as improve definition. Cones can be used to prevent scatter and thus fog, to help with compression, and to help to make the position easier to obtain.

Proper classification of breast types and density is essential in choosing the correct factors in mammography. Although breast size may appear similar between patients, the composition and density of the tissue varies. The more fat infiltration the breast has, the easier it is to penetrate the breast radiographically. Young, nulligravida (never been

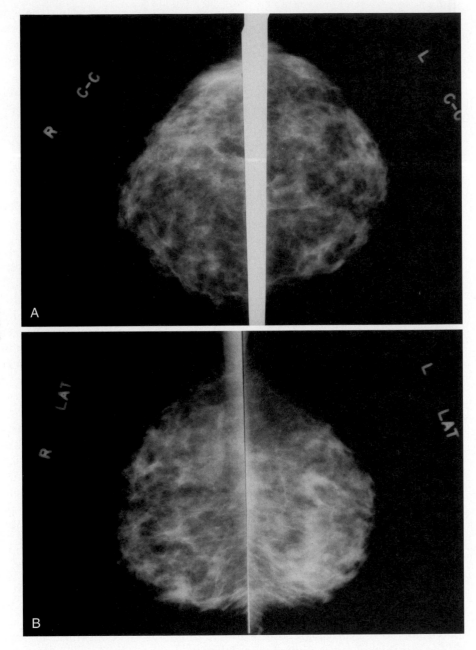

Figure 7–4. Routine mammogram showing normal results. *A,* Right and left craniocaudal view. *B,* Right and left mediolateral view.

pregnant) women have dense, fibrous tissue, making the breast more difficult to penetrate.

For purposes of examination, the breast is divided into five segments: four quadrants and a tail. The greatest amount of glandular tissue lies in the upper outer quadrant. Breast tissue extends from this quadrant into the axilla, forming the tail of Spence. In the axillae, the mammary tissue is in direct contact with the axillary lymph nodes.

Both breasts are examined in the routine positions known as the craniocaudal and mediolateral (oblique) positions (Fig. 7–4). Additional views may be necessary, such as the axillary view to demonstrate the tail of Spence, the axillary tail view (for-

merly called the cleopatra view) to visualize the tail and a portion of the axilla, and the true lateral. In all positions, the breast must be pulled forward to prevent wrinkling of skin. The nipple must be in profile and not folded under. The breast must be free of any clothing and oils. Deodorant and perfume must not be worn during a mammogram as these contain oils and metals, which may simulate a tissue density.

The appearance of a lesion determines its nature. Benign lesions show as a homogeneous, well-described density. Cancer is an area that contains sand-like grains of calcifications (Fig. 7–5).

Ultrasonography can be performed to visualize

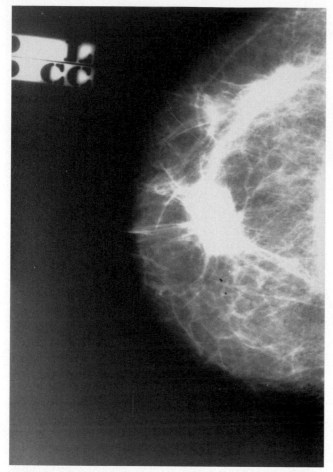

Figure 7–5. Speculated mass lesion, 3.5 cm in diameter, with microcalcifications at the 12 o'clock position. The appearance is consistent with malignancy.

both the female and the male reproductive organs. With the improved resolution of diagnostic ultrasonographic instrumentation, almost all radiographic procedures have been replaced. Ultrasonography is extremely useful in evaluating the female pelvis for both gynecologic and obstetric problems. When combined with clinical and laboratory features, the ultrasonographic findings help to limit the diagnostic possibilities. In obstetrics, ultrasonography is useful in evaluating normal fetal development and positioning and a variety of obstetric complications. Of these applications, those complications arising in the first trimester of pregnancy are by far the most important. No other imaging modality is able to compete with the value of ultrasonography in this respect.

In the male, ultrasonography has been used to evaluate testicular masses and prostatic nodules. Doppler ultrasonography and color flow ultrasonography are excellent means of demonstrating blood flow to the testes.

Computed tomography is very useful in dem-

onstrating the lymph nodes of the pelvis and the invasion of surrounding areas by a tumor. It is particularly advantageous for differentiation of a pathology from bowel. The immediate postoperative patient tolerates examination by computed tomography better than an ultrasonographic examination of the pelvis.

PATHOLOGY

Female

Congenital Anomalies

Congenital anomalies of the female reproductive organs usually are in the form duplications. There are various positions of the uterus that are not considered normal yet are of little consequence.

As was stated earlier, the normal position of the uterus is a slight anteflexion, which means the fundus is anterior to the cervix. It is also anteverted in that the fundus is away from the rectum (see Fig. 7–1B). If the uterine fundus is tipped backward so there no longer exists a 90-degree angle between the vagina, cervix and uterine body, and the fundus is now posterior to the cervix, the condition is known as **retroversion.** If there is backward flexion and the uterine body is now pointing down toward the rectum the uterus is said to be **retroflexed.** Both of these anomalies are quite common and present no significant problems. The fundus of the uterus may also be flexed forward more than it should be. This position is known as **anteflexion.** Figures 7–6 and 7–7 show these abnormal positions of the uterus.

The uterus is made from paired ducts called müllerian ducts that fuse from the lower end up. The lower end fuses to become the uterus and the two top ends of the ducts each become a uterine tube. Congenital anomalies result from varying degrees of failure of fusion of the müllerian ducts (Fig. 7–8). Many of these malformations can be detected by radiographic studies such as hysterosalpingography. If the müllerian ducts do not form in utero, absence of the uterus known as **uterine aplasia** results. If only one duct forms, there can be no fusion. One duct remains as one half of an elongated uterus and only one uterine tube. This is known as a **unicornuate uterus** (Fig. 7–9). A normal vagina is present and successful pregnancy can occur. In most patients, the kidney is missing on the same side as the missing half of the uterus.

A rare condition known as **didelphic uterus** occurs when there is nonfusion of the two müllerian ducts. The result is complete duplication (Fig. 7–10). There are two cervixes and two uterine bodies

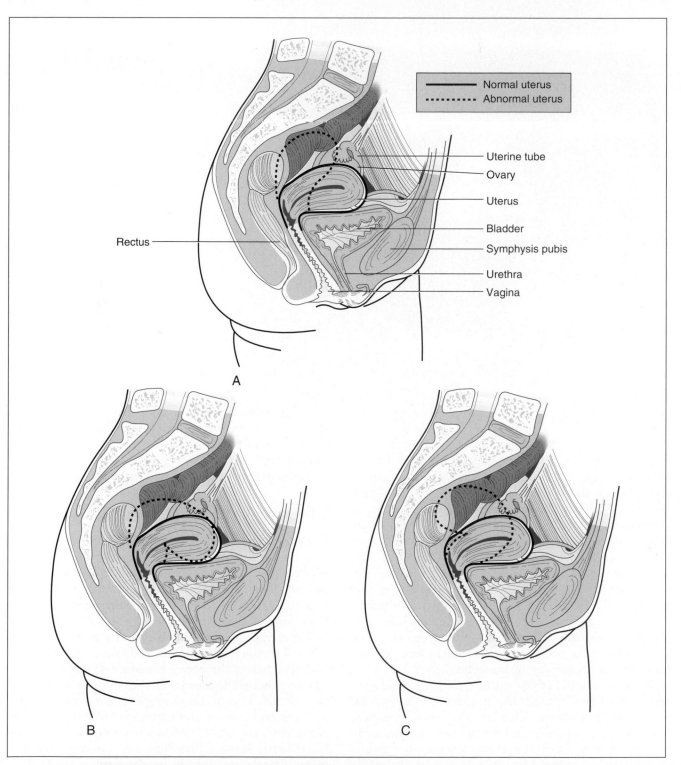

Normal uterus
Abnormal uterus

Uterine tube
Ovary
Uterus
Bladder
Symphysis pubis
Urethra
Vagina

Rectus

A

B

C

Figure 7–6. The dotted lines show the following abnormal positions of the uterus: *A,* retroverted; *B,* severely anteflexed; *C,* retroflexed.

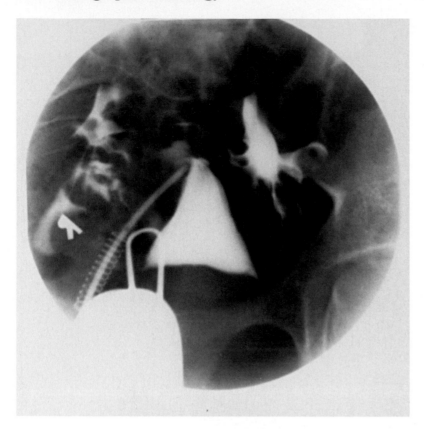

Figure 7-7. Hysterosalpingogram showing a retroverted uterus. Note that the uterus is positioned completely upside down.

but the normal number of uterine tubes. In most patients, the vagina is septate, causing a double vagina. In such cases, the two uterine bodies are often different sizes. A **bicornuate bicollic** uterus (Figs. 7–11 and 7–12) occurs when the ducts fuse to the level of the cervix, creating one vagina, two cervixes, and two uterine bodies. A very common duplication anomaly is called a **bicornuate uterus** (Fig. 7–13), which occurs when the ducts fuse to the level of the body so that there are two fundi. A bicornuate uterus is important in pregnancy in that twin gestational sacs could implant in each horn of the fundus. Twin implantations could also occur wherein one gestational sac is an intrauterine pregnancy and the second one is in one of the horns of the fundus. It is possible for a mass to form in one horn with a pregnancy in the other.

If the nonfusion of the müllerian ducts begins at the level of the fundus, the condition is known as an **arcuate uterus.** This is the most common anomaly and produces only minimal external contour deformity. In the **septate uterus,** a septum extends through the normal uterine body to reach the cervix, dividing the uterus into two complete compartments. A **subseptate uterus** has a partial septum dividing the body only. The septum does not extend to the cervix. For some unexplained reason, twins occur in women with this condition more often (3:1) than women with a normal uterus. Pregnancy

may still occur in many women despite these anomalies. Incidence of complications during pregnancy is considerably increased, however. Complications include abortion, premature delivery, hemorrhages, retained placenta, and breech presentation.

Inflammatory Processes

Endometriosis is defined as the growth of endometrial tissue outside the uterus, usually on the ovary, uterine tube, broad ligament, pouch of Douglas, or retrovaginal septum. This condition is more common in women who have never been pregnant (nulligravida) and are over the age of 30. When the endometrium sloughs off during the monthly cycle, some of the blood and mucus refluxes into the pelvis and attaches to the above mentioned ectopic areas.

Even though the endometrial tissue lies outside the uterus, it still responds to hormonal changes and undergoes a proliferative and secretory phase along with sloughing and subsequent bleeding. Old blood turns brown; therefore, the pockets of endometrial tissue are known as **chocolate cysts.** The blood that escapes each month is brown in color. Sterility may occur if the tubes are badly affected. Symptoms of endometriosis include severe pain with the period (dysmenorrhea) and a dull aching pain the remainder of the month.

Adenomyosis is the ingrowth of endometrium

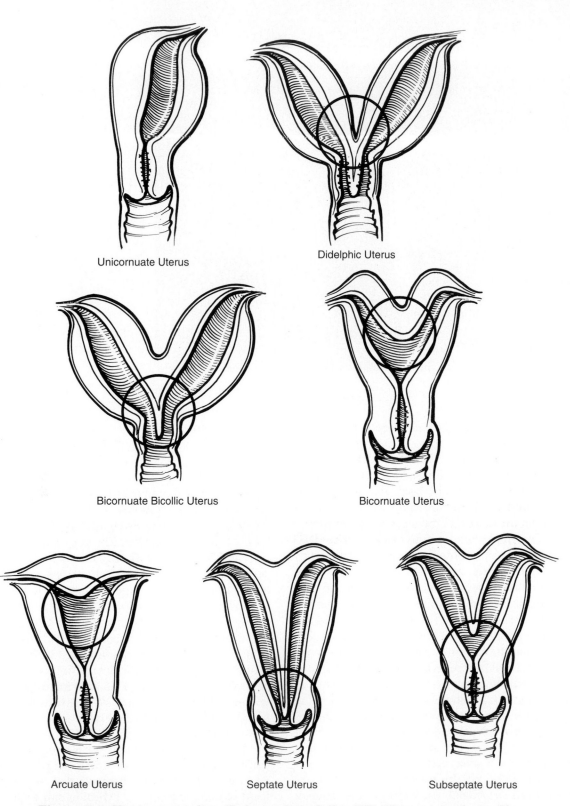

Unicornuate Uterus

Didelphic Uterus

Bicornuate Bicollic Uterus

Bicornuate Uterus

Arcuate Uterus

Septate Uterus

Subseptate Uterus

Figure 7–8. Uterine anomalies. (Redrawn from Callen PW: *Ultrasonography in Obstetrics and Gynecology.* Philadelphia: WB Saunders, 1994; p. 594.)

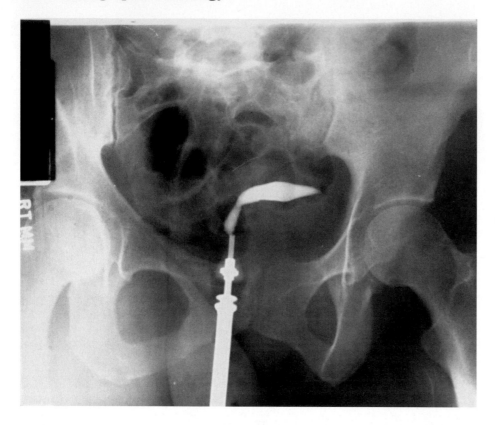

Figure 7–9. Unicornuate uterus.

into the uterine musculature. This condition may coexist with endometriosis.

Pelvic inflammatory disease (PID) is inflammation of the uterine tubes. In 50 to 60 percent of all cases, PID is caused by bacteria that are the result of gonorrhea. Infection may occur by other routes such as an intrauterine contraceptive device and nonsterile abortions or deliveries. **Acute PID** causes slight uterine enlargement. In the early stages, the pelvic sidewall structures can still be identified. Because the uterine tubes open into the pelvic cavity, infection may spread to the ovaries and adjacent structures if the infundibulum is not closed by scar tissue. As the disease progresses, the adnexa become thicker and begins to merge with the sidewall. If left untreated, a **pyosalpinx** (pus in the tube) will develop. This will eventually lead to a **tubal ovarian abscess** (Fig. 7–14). If a tubal ovarian abscess or a pyosalpinx ruptures, peritonitis may ensue, which can be localized in the right upper quadrant under the liver. Free fluid in the cul-de-sac is usually seen with PID.

In **chronic PID,** all the signs of acute PID are gone and the uterus has sharp borders. The adnexa may demonstrate nonspecific thickening because of continued scarring (Fig. 7–15). PID is a common cause of ectopic pregnancy. The fertilized ovum is unable to pass through the scarred, narrow tubes and therefore becomes implanted at this point.

Neoplasms

Benign

Fibroids, also known as leiomyomata or myomata, are composed of connective tissue and muscle fiber. They are the overgrowth of the normal muscular wall of the uterus. They are very common after the age of 35. Fibroids thrive on estrogen; therefore, postmenopausal women do not grow new tumors. If a fibroid exists before menopause, it will atrophy as the estrogen levels drop after menopause.

Fibroids are the most common benign tumor of the uterus. There are three types. The **submucous** type are the least common and grow off the endometrium into the uterine cavity (Fig. 7–16). The most common type is known as **intramural** and grows within the myometrium. The **subserous** type is mostly pedunculated and grows off the perimetrium into the pelvic cavity (Figs. 7–17 and 7–18).

Fibroids can be present with pregnancy and can cause an abortion or an abruptio placentae. They can prevent a normal vaginal delivery if they are located near the cervix. Fibroids can also cause the premature rupture of the membranes.

Teratomas, also known as **dermoids,** are benign "cysts" of the ovary that contain skin, hair, teeth, and fatty elements that derive from ectodermal tissue. About one half contain calcifications,

Text continued on page 177

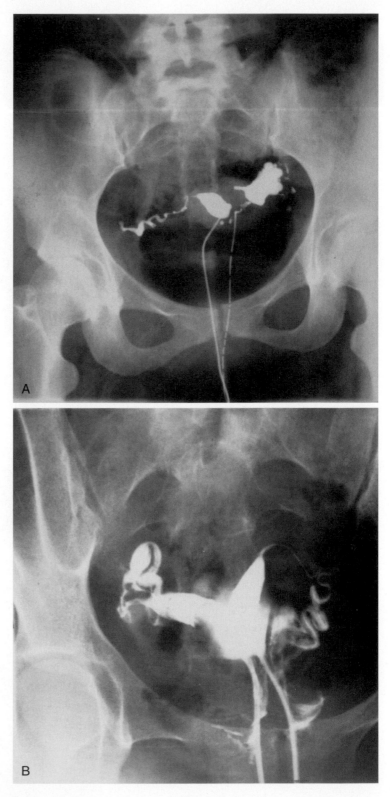

Figure 7–10. Didelphic uterus. *A,* Two complete vaginas, cervices, and uterine bodies. *B,* The complete separation is not seen as clearly, but note the two vaginas.

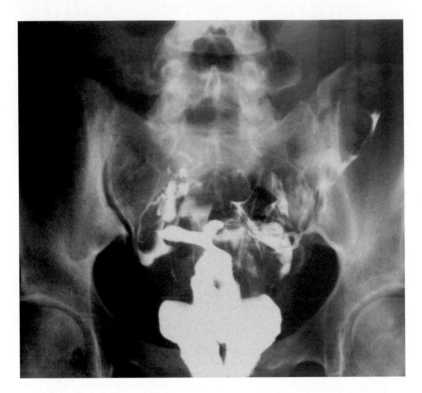

Figure 7–11. Bicornuate bicollic uterus.

Figure 7–12. Retroverted bicornuate bicollic uterus.

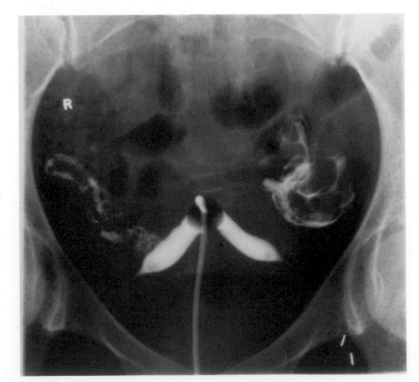

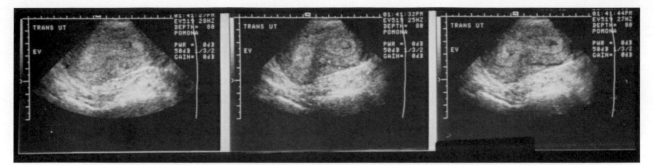

Figure 7–13. Bicornuate uterus. Ultrasonographic transverse view clearly shows the two separate horns of the fundi.

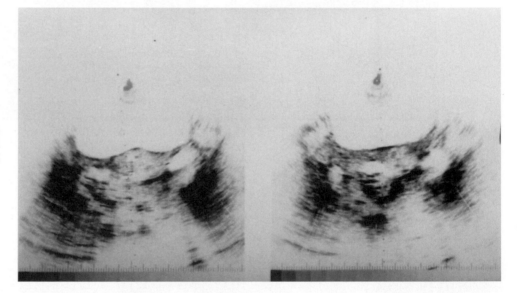

Figure 7–14. Tubal ovarian abscess. Enlarged cystic and solid adnexa are merging with the uterine side wall.

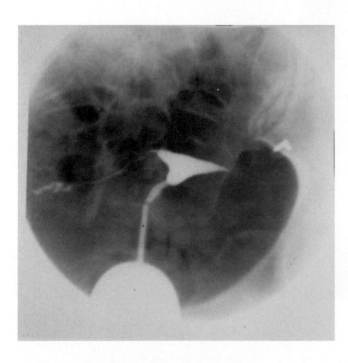

Figure 7–15. Hysterosalpingogram showing complete block of the left uterine tube.

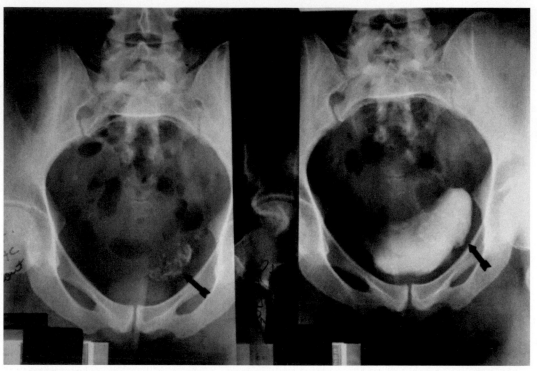

Figure 7–16. Fibroid. *Left,* Before injection, the calcifications are easily seen. *Right,* After injection, the fibroid itself is hidden but a small indentation of the left lateral bladder border can be seen.

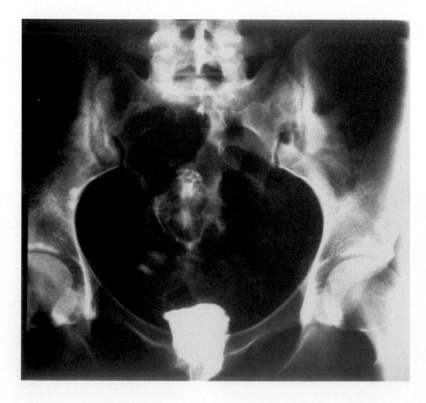

Figure 7–17. The calcified fibroid can be seen as the contrast agent drains after hysterosalpingography has been performed.

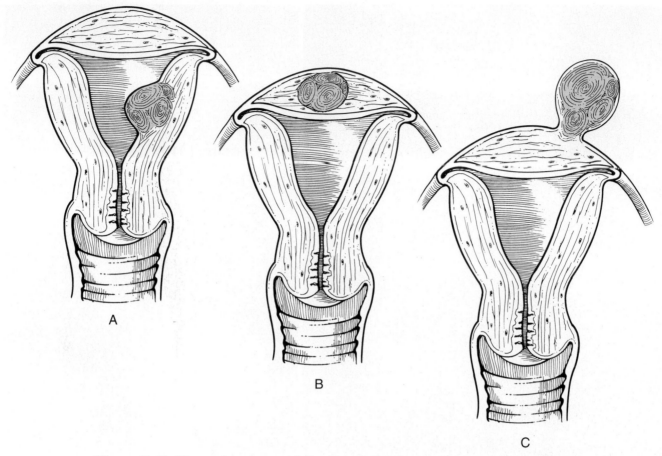

Figure 7–18. The various types of fibroids. *A,* Submucous; *B,* intramural; and *C,* subserous.

usually in the form of teeth, but may include the wall of the cyst (Fig. 7–19). These are of no clinical significance unless they grow so large that they compress adjacent structures. Teratomas account for about 15 percent of all benign ovarian masses.

Single cystic lesions of the ovaries are rarely significant and are usually a follicular cyst or a corpus luteum cyst (Fig. 7–20). Multiple cystic areas may be an indication of endometriosis. **Polycystic ovaries** are enlarged ovaries consisting of many small cysts. This manifestation may be associated with **Stein-Leventhal** syndrome, which is characterized by facial hair, excess weight, amenorrhea, and infertility.

Fibrocystic disease of the breast is a common benign condition occurring in about 20 percent of women who are premenopausal. Fibrocystic disease is a general term that encompasses a variety of changes that occur. The most obvious changes are fibrosis and cystic dilation of the ducts. It is usually bilateral, with cysts of various sizes distributed throughout the breasts, which also contain an increased amount of fibrous tissue (Fig. 7–21). A more important change is hyperplasia of the ducts. This change is thought to be a precursor to cancer. If hyperplasia is present with fibrosis and cystic dilation, the term proliferative fibrocystic disease is used.

A **fibroadenoma** is the most common benign breast tumor (Fig. 7–22). It generally appears as a smooth, well-circumscribed mass with no invasion of surrounding tissue. The masses may be moved around within the breast as they have no attachments to the overlying skin or underlying tissue. Ultrasonography permits differentiation of a solid fibroadenoma from a fluid-filled cyst. Mammography may demonstrate these masses. Fibroadenomas are easily removed and carry no threat of developing into cancer.

Malignant

Adenocarcinoma of the **endometrium** accounts for 90 percent of all uterine malignant neoplasms. It is the most common invasive gynecologic malignancy (excluding breast cancer). It is usually seen

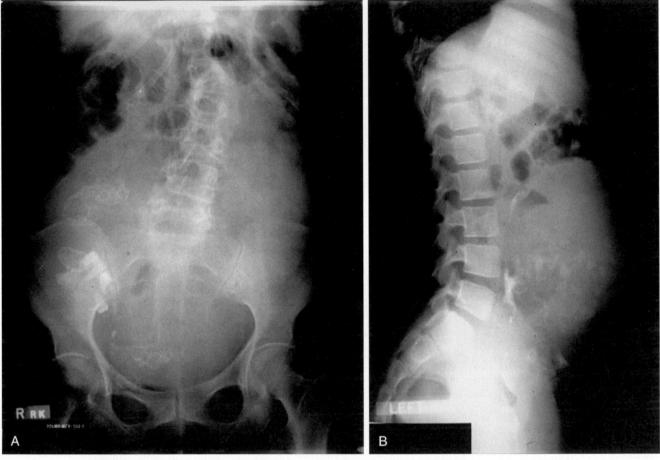

Figure 7–19. Dermoid. *A*, Anteroposterior view shows calcification (teeth) along the right side of the pelvis. Other calcifications can be seen in the pelvis and abdomen. *B*, Lateral view. This dermoid was quite large, giving the patient the outward appearance of advanced pregnancy.

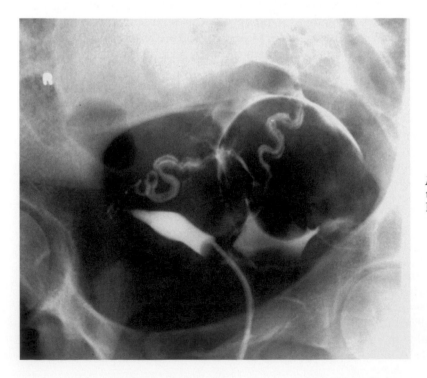

Figure 7–20. Contrast medium from a hysterosalpingogram outlines a huge cyst off the left ovary.

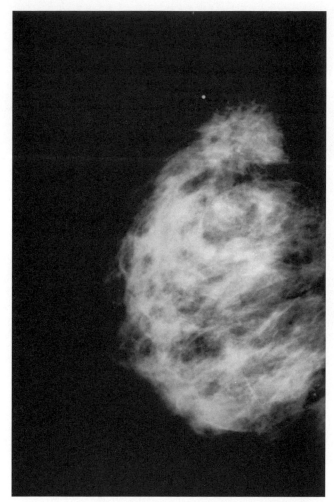

Figure 7–21. Fibrocystic disease. Dense breasts have multiple fibrous areas. The round radiopaque marker at the top of the breast indicates where the patient felt a mass.

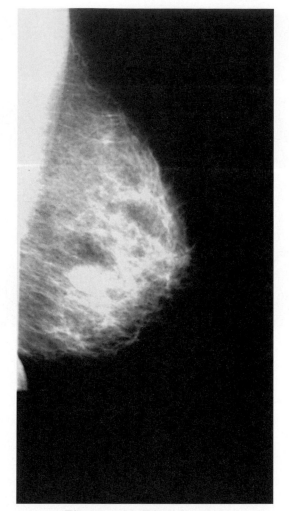

Figure 7–22. Fibroadenoma.

in postmenopausal women who have never borne a viable baby (nullipara). Prolonged estrogen stimulation has been associated with increased frequency of endometrial carcinoma. Clinical symptoms include bleeding, hypermenorrhea, or postmenopausal bleeding. The tumor may project into the uterine cavity (Fig. 7–23) or it may infiltrate the wall of the uterus. An intravenous pyelogram will show the bladder wall depressed by an enlarged uterus. Ultrasonography (Fig. 7–24), computed tomography, and magnetic resonance imaging are all modalities that differentiate endometrium from myometrium, thus accurately locating the tumor. Hysterectomy combined with radiation therapy gives an overall survival rate of approximately 80 percent. This high cure rate is attributed to early detection (bleeding in postmenopausal women is abnormal) and containment of the cancer within the body of the uterus.

Cervical cancer appears to be related to many factors, such as an early onset of sexual activity with multiple partners, multiple pregnancies, chronic irritation, infection, and poor hygiene. A cervical carcinoma arises from epithelial tissue around the neck of the uterus. The intravenous pyelogram demonstrates hydronephrosis in one third of the patients. In fact, the most common cause of death in patients with carcinoma of the cervix is impaired renal function caused by ureteral obstruction. Again, as with endometrial carcinoma, computed tomography, magnetic resonance imaging, and ultrasonography are accurate in the location of tumor cells and any invasion of other organs. With early diagnosis made by regular Papanicolaou smears, this malignancy can be cured with radiation.

Cystadenocarcinoma is ovarian cancer. Although this neoplasm is less common than other malignancies, it is important because it is relatively asymptomatic until the disease has progressed to a stage at which chances for a cure are slim (Figures 7–25 and 7–26).

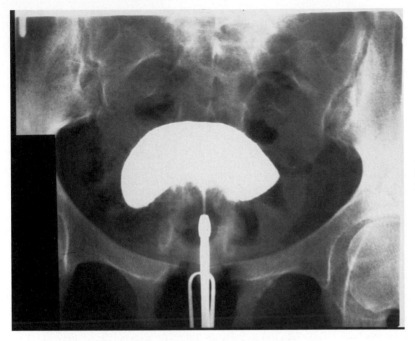

Figure 7–23. Endometrial carcinoma. A tumor in the uterus creates a filling defect during hysterosalpingography.

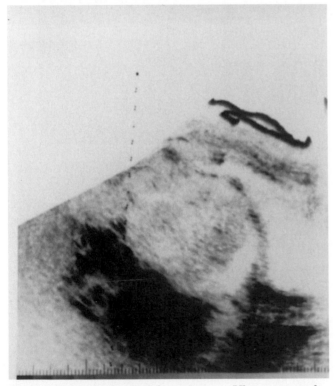

Figure 7–24. Endometrial carcinoma. Ultrasonography demonstrates the large uterine mass.

Breast cancer is the most common malignancy among women. It has the highest mortality rate of any malignant neoplasm in women. If a woman lives to her mid-80s, her overall risk of getting breast cancer is roughly one in eight. Factors that increase the risk of breast cancer include the age at

which a woman has her first full-term pregnancy. Women who delay childbirth tend to have a higher relative risk compared with women who had a first pregnancy at age 17. The relative risk of breast cancer as compared to the age of the first pregnancy is shown in Figure 7–27.

Almost all breast cancers are seen mammographically as a tumor mass (Fig. 7–28), clustered calcifications, or both. Either feature, when clearly demonstrated, is so suspicious of malignancy as to require prompt biopsy, whether the lesion is palpable or not. Secondary changes of breast carcinoma include skin thickening around the areola and nipple retraction.

The typical malignant tumor mass is poorly defined, has irregular margins, and demonstrates numerous fine linear strands or spicules radiating out from the mass. This appearance is characteristic but not diagnostic of malignancy and is in stark contrast to the typical mammographic picture of a benign mass, which has well-defined smooth margins and a round, oval, or gently lobulated contour.

Clustered calcifications in breast cancer are typically numerous, very small, and localized to one segment of the breast. They demonstrate a wide variety of shapes, including fine linear, curvilinear, and branching forms.

Although relatively infrequent, breast cancer also can develop in men. It accounts for only 1 percent of all breast cancers. Male breast cancer is a disease of the elderly and has a somewhat worse prognosis than female breast carcinoma.

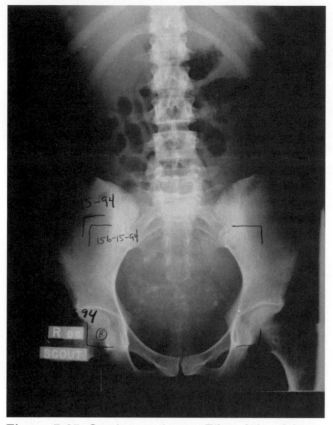

Figure 7-25. Ovarian carcinoma. Film of the abdomen shows multiple calcifications. Patient also has ascites.

Inflammatory Processes

Prostatic hyperplasia is enlargement of the prostate gland (Fig. 7–29). This benign condition is very common in men over the age of 50 and is related to decreased hormone secretions. As the prostate gland enlarges, it pushes on the bladder, which results in an inability to completely empty the bladder. This leads to obstructions, bilateral ureteral dilation, and hydronephrosis. As the urine stagnates in the bladder, urinary tract infections and even pyelonephritis are complications that must be dealt with.

The intravenous pyelogram demonstrates the elevation and smooth impression on the floor of the bladder by the prostate. The elevation of the bladder also causes the elevation of the insertion of the ureters on the trigone. The characteristic J-shape, or "fish hook," appearance of the distal ureters will be demonstrated. A surgical procedure known as transurethral resection of the prostate is performed to relieve the symptoms of obstruction.

Prostatic calculi are small, multiple calcifications found in the prostate gland. Males over the age of 50 are prone to this common condition. The calculi, if dense enough, are visible on plain abdominal radiographs. They are of no clinical significance.

Testicular torsion occurs when the testicle twists over on its pedicle. If this happens, there is

Male

Congenital Anomalies

The testes normally descend from the intra-abdominal area through the inguinal canal into the scrotum near the end of the gestational period. After birth, both testes should be palpable in the scrotum. If one or both are not felt, it must be determined if the testes are absent or ectopic. **Cryptorchidism** is the condition of undescended testes. Ultrasonography is used as a screening mechanism to determine the location of an undescended testicle in the inguinal canal, the pelvis, or the abdomen. If ultrasonography fails to locate the testicle, the patient will be referred for computed tomography or magnetic resonance imaging. Since the rate of malignancy is approximately 40 times higher in males with cryptorchidism, the testicle must be either brought down and surgically fixed in the scrotum by a procedure called **orchiopexy,** or it must be removed **(orchiectomy).** Orchiectomy is performed on those patients who are diagnosed after the onset of puberty.

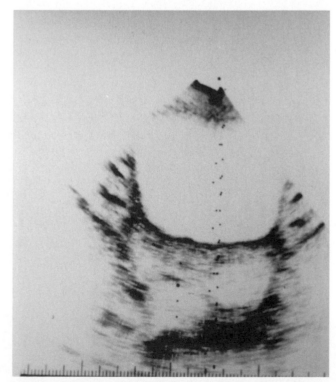

Figure 7-26. Ovarian carcinoma. The ovaries are enlarged. The mass is solid.

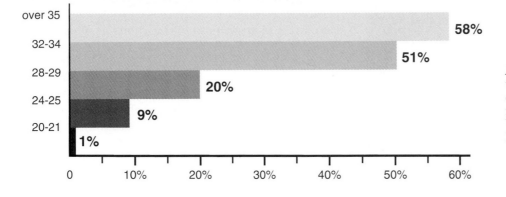

Figure 7–27. Comparison of the relative risk of breast cancer to the age of the first pregnancy. (Data from Brigham and Women's Hospital, Centers for Disease Control.)

a compromise of the vascularity of the testicle. A sudden onset of severe scrotal pain and swelling are the clinical symptoms.

Epididymitis is inflammation of the epididymis and also leads to swelling of the scrotum accompanied by pain and errythemia. Doppler ultrasonography is used to demonstrate the intratesticular arterial blood flow to distinguish between torsion and epididymitis. Arterial perfusion is decreased or absent in testicular torsion, whereas in epididymitis, the blood flow is increased.

Nuclear medicine may also be used to differentiate between the two problems. Similar to ultrasonography, nuclear medicine shows decreased isotope uptake in the affected side in torsion and increased uptake in the testicle involved in epididymitis.

Enlargement of the male breast is known as **gynecomastia.** This proliferation of ducts and connective tissue is the result of estrogen stimulation. A

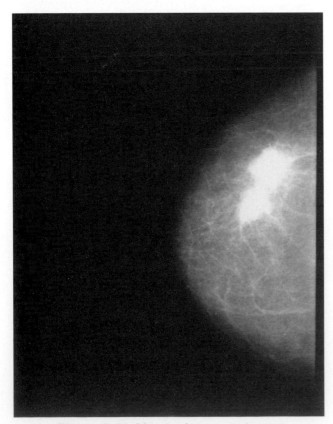

Figure 7–28. Massive breast carcinoma.

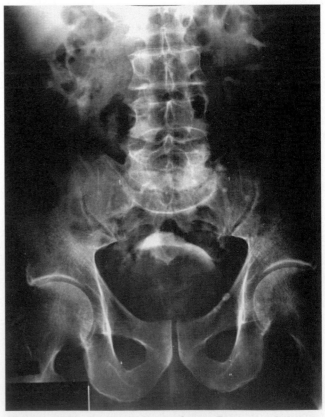

Figure 7–29. Prostatic hyperplasia. Because of the enlarged prostrate gland, the contrast medium does not fill the base of the bladder.

Table 7–1.
Clinical and Radiographic Characteristics of Common Pathologies

Pathologic Condition	Causal Factors*	Manifestations	Radiographic Appearance
Endometriosis	Over 30 and nulligravida	Dysmenorrhea, aching remainder of month	Ultrasonography suggested
Pelvic inflammatory disease	50–60% by gonorrhea	Pelvic pain, foul-smelling discharge	Ultrasonography suggested
Fibroid	Over 30 and nulligravida, estrogen stimulated	Asymptomatic	Ultrasonography suggested
Teratoma	—	Asymptomatic	Calcifications (teeth)
Fibrocystic breasts	Premenopausal	Asymptomatic	Fibrosis bilaterally
Fibroadenoma	—	Asymptomatic, movable mass	Smooth, well circumscribed mass
Endometrial carcinoma	Postmenopausal, nullipara, estrogen stimulation	Bleeding, hypermenorrhea	Depression on bladder wall by uterine mass
Cervical carcinoma	High degree of sexual activity, chronic irritation, infection	Bleeding, pain	Hydronephrosis, ultrasonography or CT suggested
Breast carcinoma	Postmenopausal, delayed childbirth	Nipple retraction, skin thickening, nipple discharge	Tumor mass, clustered calcifications, irregular margins
Prostatic hyperplasia	Males over 50 years, decreased hormones, enlarged prostate	Retention of urine	Hydronephrosis, ureteral dilation, "fish hook" sign
Prostatic calculi	Over 50 years	Asymptomatic	Small multiple calcium deposits near base of bladder
Hydrocele/spermatocele	25–40 years, trauma, inflammation	Swelling of the scrotum	Ultrasonography suggested
Prostate carcinoma	Over 50 years	Retention of urine	Irregular impression on bladder floor

*Includes age, if relevant.
CT, computed tomography.

variety of stimuli can cause males to secrete more estrogen than normal. Cirrhosis, certain neoplasms, marijuana, digitalis, and Klinefelter syndrome are all possible causative agents. Aging, with decreased androgen production, is the usual cause of bilateral gynecomastia.

Neoplasms

Benign

Masses in the testes may be the result of trauma or inflammation, but most commonly are neoplasms. Males between the ages of 25 to 40 are most often afflicted. Benign masses include hydroceles and spermatoceles.

A **hydrocele** is a collection of fluid in the testis or along the spermatic cord. A **spermatocele** is a cystic dilation of the epididymis. Both of these conditions are easily demonstrated by ultrasonography.

Malignant

Malignant tumors of the testes are more common than the benign variety. The two major types are seminomas and teratomas. **Seminomas** arise from the seminiferous tubules. These tumors are extremely radiosensitive and the prognosis is excellent. **Teratomas,** on the other hand, have a poor prognosis. They arise from a primitive germ cell and consist of a variety of structures. Both of these tumors are highly malignant and tend to spread by the lymphatics and the blood to the area of the renal hilum. Testicular tumors are best demonstrated by computed tomography, as this modality will also detect metastasis to the lung, liver, or bone.

Lung cancer is the most common malignancy in men. However, **adenocarcinoma** of the **prostate** gland is a close second. The tumor is rare before the age of 50, but as men age, the risk increases. The intravenous pyelographic examination again demonstrates an elevated bladder. However, unlike hyperplasia of the prostate, which makes a smooth border, carcinoma makes an irregular impression on the bladder floor because of the irregular, lobulated borders of the tumor. It is important to determine carcinoma of the prostate early, as it spreads to the rectum directly. It metastasizes to the bone in 75 percent of all cases.

Ultrasonography, with the use of a transrectal probe, has proved useful in detecting carcinoma of the prostate gland. Magnetic resonance imaging can delineate the prostate and surrounding organs to accurately stage any pelvic neoplasms.

Table 7–1 summarizes the clinical and radiographic characteristics of common pathologies of the reproductive system.

Review Questions

1. List and describe the normal and abnormal positions of the uterus.
2. List the three phases of the menstrual cycle. When do the reproductive years of a female end? What is this stage called?
3. What is the major function of the male reproductive system? Explain the maturation process of the sperm and its life expectancy. What is male fertility related to?
4. List the four reasons a hysterosalpingogram would be done for treatment. What are the seven diagnostic indications for hysterosalpingography? What are the four contraindications?
5. What are the four things to consider when choosing a contrast medium for a hysterosalpingogram?
6. Explain mammography and its importance in women's health.
7. Describe each of the following by stating how it occurs and what it results in.

Uterine aplasia	Unicornuate uterus
Didelphic uterus	Bicornuate bicollic uterus
Bicornuate uterus	Arcuate uterus

8. Define and describe endometriosis. How is adenomyosis related?
9. Describe what happens to the adnexa with acute PID.
10. What are fibroids? Who is more prone to have them? Who is more likely not to have them? Why?
11. What will an intravenous pyelogram show with adenocarcinoma of the endometrium? What will it show on a patient with cervical cancer?
12. Define cryptorchidism. What diagnostic procedure is performed to determine the location of the organs? Why is it important to correct this condition?
13. What two procedures are performed to differentiate between torsion and epididymitis? What will each condition demonstrate on each procedure?
14. What are complications of prostatic hyperplasia? What will the intravenous pyelogram demonstrate with this condition?

CHAPTER VIII

Respiratory System

Goals

1. To review the basic anatomy and physiology of the respiratory system.
2. To become acquainted with the pathophysiology of the respiratory system.
3. To become familiar with the radiographic manifestations of all the common congenital and acquired disorders of the respiratory system.

Objectives

At the completion of the chapter, the radiographer will be able to:

1. Identify anatomic structures on both diagrams and radiographs of the respiratory system.
2. Describe the physiology of the respiratory system.
3. Describe the various pathologic conditions affecting the respiratory system and their radiographic manifestations.
4. Describe the special radiographic examinations of the respiratory system.
5. Define terminology relating to the respiratory system.

I. Anatomy
  A. Nose
  B. Pharynx (Throat)
  C. Larynx (Voice Box)
  D. Trachea (Wind Pipe)
    1. Carina
  E. Bronchi
    1. Lobar Bronchi
    2. Segmental Bronchi
    3. Bronchioles
    4. Alveoli
  F. Lungs
    1. Base
    2. Apex
    3. Lobes
      a. Right
        1. Upper (Superior)
        2. Middle
        3. Lower (Inferior)
      b. Left
        1. Upper (Superior)
          a. Lingula
        2. Lower (Inferior)
    4. Fissures
      a. Right
        1. Horizontal (Minor)
        2. Oblique (Major)
      b. Left
        1. Oblique (Major)
    5. Segments
    6. Pleura
      a. Visceral (Pulmonary)
      b. Parietal
    7. Pleural Cavity
  G. Diaphragm
    1. Costophrenic Angle
       (Sulcus)
      a. Costophrenic Sinus
    2. Cardiophrenic Angle
  H. Mediastinum
    1. Superior
    2. Anterior
    3. Middle
    4. Posterior
II. Physiology and Function
  A. Pharynx
    1. Passage of Air and Food
  B. Larynx
    1. Sound Production
    2. Prevent Solids from
       Entering Trachea
  C. Trachea and Bronchi
    1. Passage of Air to Lungs
  D. Whole System
    1. Take in Oxygen/Rid
       Body of Carbon Dioxide
    2. Ventilation and
       Perfusion
III. Special Radiographic
     Procedures
  A. Chest
    1. Apical Lordotic
    2. Double Exposure
       Inspiration-Expiration
    3. Patient Position
  B. Fluoroscopy
  C. Computed Tomography
  D. Ultrasonography
  E. Bronchography
  F. Laryngography
  G. Tomography
  H. Nuclear Medicine
IV. Pathology
  A. Congenital Diseases
    1. Cystic Fibrosis
    2. Respiratory Distress
       Syndrome (Hyaline
       Membrane Disease)
  B. Inflammatory Processes
    1. Abscess
      a. Embolic
      b. Pneumonic
      c. Inhalation
    2. Adult Respiratory
       Distress Syndrome
    3. Asthma
    4. Atelectasis
    5. Bronchitis
    6. Bronchiectasis
    7. Cor Pulmonale
    8. Croup
    9. Emphysema
      a. Compensating
         (Compensatory)
      b. Centrilobular
         (Chronic Obstructive
         Pulmonary Disease)
    10. Empyema
    11. Hydatid Disease
    12. Pleural Effusion
    13. Pleurisy
    14. Pneumonia
        (Pneumonitis)
      a. Aspiration
      b. Bronchopneumonia
      c. Lobar (Pneumococcal)
      d. Viral (Interstitial)
      e. Pneumocystis Carinii
    15. Pneumoconiosis
      a. Silicosis
      b. Asbestosis
      c. Berylliosis
    16. Pneumothorax
      a. Pseudopneumothorax
      b. Tension
    17. Pulmonary Edema
    18. Pulmonary Emboli
    19. Tuberculosis
      a. Primary (Childhood)
      b. Reactivation
  C. Neoplasms
    1. Benign
      a. Hamartoma
    2. Malignant
      a. Bronchogenic
         Carcinoma
        1. Primary
        2. Metastatic
          a. Nodular
          b. Lymphangitic
          c. Pneumonic
  D. Mediastinal Pathology
    1. Masses
      a. Thymoma
      b. Teratoma
      c. Lymphoma
    2. Pneumomediastinum

The respiratory system consists of the nose, pharynx, larynx, trachea, bronchi, and two lungs. For a detailed anatomic description of the nasal cavity and its related paranasal sinuses, refer to an anatomy and positioning book for radiographers. Anatomy and physiology books give a description of this area, but without the relationship to radiography. The pharynx, larynx, trachea, and bronchi are described in this chapter only briefly. The lungs and mediastinum are more important radiographically and are dealt with in detail.

ANATOMY

The pharynx, also known as the throat, extends from the skull to the esophagus. Both air and food pass through this tube. The larynx, or "voice box," is located between the pharynx and the trachea. The thyroid cartilage makes up a portion of the box-like structure of the larynx, and the epiglottis is the lid to this box.

The trachea, or "wind pipe," is anterior to the esophagus and extends from the larynx to the level of T-5, which corresponds with the level of the sternal angle. The trachea divides here into the right and left main bronchi. The area of bifurcation is known as the carina. Unlike the esophagus, the trachea is not collapsible, because of the rings of cartilage that help to make its walls. The trachea is flattened on its posterior wall, allowing for the expandable esophagus to press into it if need be during swallowing.

The right bronchus is shorter, wider, and more vertical than the left bronchus. Each bronchus enters the lung medially at the hilum. The right hilum should always be lower than the left, as the heart displaces the left hilum upward. The presence of pathology should be considered if this is not the case.

As soon as the main bronchi enter the lungs, they divide into bronchi that go to each lobe of the lung. These lobar bronchi in turn branch into the bronchi that go to each segment of the lobe. The segmental bronchi continue branching until bronchioles (little bronchi) are formed. From these the alveolar sacs (alveoli) are formed, which are the functional units for gas exchange.

The lungs are cone-shaped organs that fill the pleural spaces of the thoracic cavity. Each lung is located in its respective hemithorax. The lungs are separated by the mediastinum. Both lungs should extend from the diaphragm, which is the base of the lung, to just slightly above the clavicle, which is the apex of the lung.

Each lung is divided into lobes by fissures. The right lung has three lobes and two fissures. The right horizontal (minor) fissure separates the upper (superior) lobe from the middle lobe. The right oblique (major) fissure separates the middle lobe from the lower (inferior) lobe. The left oblique (major) fissure divides the upper (superior) lobe and the lower (inferior) lobe. The lower part of the upper lobe of the left lung is called the lingula, and, in some cases, a horizontal fissure can be found between the upper lobe proper and the lingula.

Each lobe of each lung is divided into segments that are the structural units of the lung. The number of segments varies from lobe to lobe. The right lung contains a total of 10 segments, and the left lung contains either eight or nine segments. The number of segments in the lower lobe of the left lung can vary from individual to individual. This accounts for the discrepancy often found between authors as to the total number of segments in the left lung. For radiologic technologists' purposes, segments are not as important as the lobes.

Each lung is encased in a double-walled, serous membrane sac called the pleura. The inner layer is called the visceral, or pulmonary, pleura and actually covers each lung except the hilum. The outer layer is called the parietal pleura and lines the chest cavity. The pleura secretes a thin watery fluid that prevents friction between the visceral and the parietal pleurae. The space between the two pleural walls is the pleural cavity.

The thoracic wall and diaphragm meet at the costophrenic angle, also known as the sulcus. The space this creates is called the costophrenic sinus.

The heart and the diaphragm meet at the cardiophrenic angle. Figure 8–1 demonstrates all the important anatomic aspects of the outward appearance of the thoracic cavity.

Another portion of the thoracic cavity is the mediastinum. It is a compartment separating the two lungs from top to bottom and front to back. Boundaries of the mediastinum are the sternum, thoracic spine, pharynx, and diaphragm.

Four divisions of the mediastinum are used when defining pathology. These are the superior, anterior, middle, and posterior sections. Of these four, only the superior mediastinum is not used in radiography. Located within the mediastinum are the heart and aortic arch, the great blood vessels, the trachea, the esophagus, lymph tissue, the thymus gland, nerves such as the vagus and phrenic nerves, and the main bronchi. Figure 8–2 is a lateral aspect of the chest depicting the four divisions and boundaries of the mediastinum.

PHYSIOLOGY AND FUNCTION

The pharynx, larynx, trachea, and bronchi each have a limited function, but are all indispensable to the main purpose of oxygenating the body. The pharynx acts as a passage for both air and food. Two functions of the larynx are sound production and the prevention of liquids and solids from entering the trachea. The function of both the trachea and the bronchi is to provide a pathway for air to reach the lungs.

The respiratory system as a whole takes oxygen into the body and rids it of carbon dioxide. To carry out the main function of the respiratory system, air must be moved from the atmosphere to the terminal units of the lung, a process called **ventilation,** and gas must pass across tissue from air to blood and blood to air, a process called gas exchange or **perfusion.** The functional units for gas exchange are thin-walled alveoli. Each alveolus is supplied by a terminal pulmonary arteriole, which in turn gives rise to capillaries. Perfusion takes place at this point as each alveolus gives off its oxygen into the blood in the capillary surrounding it. Oxygenated blood can then be sent to various parts of the body to distribute its oxygen.

Since the diaphragm is attached to the thoracic wall, only the dome is able to move. As the dome contracts and pushes down, the abdominal organs are compressed, allowing the lungs to increase in length. At the same time, the ribs are expanded outward, which increases the width of the lung. This change in the shape of the lungs decreases intrapulmonic pressure, causing air to rush into the lungs. At the end of inspiration, the pressure

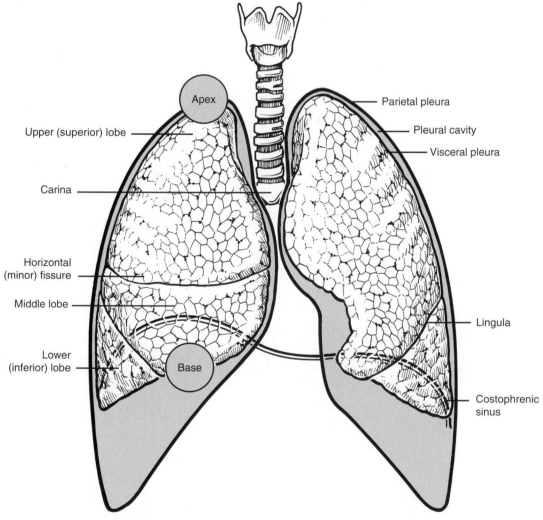

Figure 8–1. Anatomy of the lungs and the pleura.

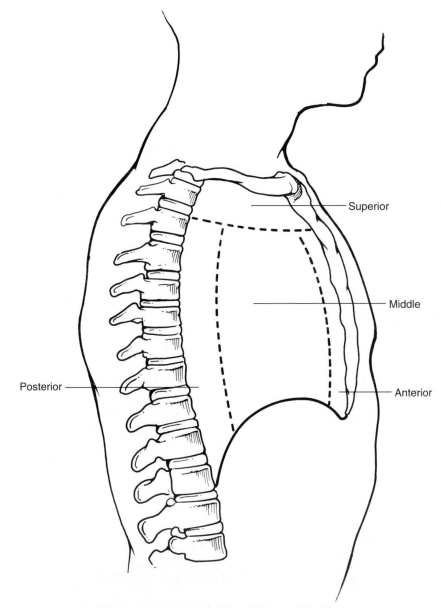

Figure 8–2. Lateral view of the mediastinum.

between the outside atmosphere and the lung is equal.

At expiration, the diaphragm relaxes, and the chest cavity returns to its normal size. Air pressure within the lungs is now greater than outside, so air must be expelled to again equalize the two pressures.

The thorax plays a major role in the function of respiration. It is the changes in size of the thorax that actually bring about inspiration and expiration. The respiratory center in the brain controls the rhythmic movements produced by respiration. The nerves from the brain that pass down the chest wall and diaphragm to control respiration are the vagus nerve, the phrenic nerve, and the thoracic nerves.

SPECIAL RADIOGRAPHIC PROCEDURES

Prior to discussing special procedures that allow the study of the lungs and their bronchi, a short review of the routine chest radiograph will be presented, as the chest is the most complex area examined. Not only are the lungs seen, but so is the lower neck, the soft tissue of the thoracic wall, the mediastinum, the diaphragm, and the upper abdomen. Too much or too little soft tissue could indicate the presence of disease. Bony structures seen include ribs, thoracic spine, lower cervical spine, sternum, clavicles, scapulas, and shoulders.

All these may be present on the film, but if the patient is not positioned properly, good films still will not be obtained. Factors affecting the diaphragm height are rotation of the patient, obesity, scoliosis, loss of lung volume, and abdominal pressure due to a supine position. When the patient is completely upright, the diaphragm moves to a lower position during inspiration. Supine films are unacceptable, as the abdomen contents will raise the level of the diaphragm anywhere from 2 to 4 inches and obscure the lower lung fields. In addition to affecting diaphragm height, rotation will affect the hilar region, magnification of one lung, and heart size. Rotation on a chest x-ray can be demonstrated by asymmetry of the sternoclavicular joint spaces. However, in patients with scoliosis, there are usually unequal distances from the medial ends of the clavicles to the sternum.

Deep inspiration is necessary to evaluate the heart size, as poor inspiration does not allow the heart to assume a more vertical position and chronic heart failure is simulated. On an adult, the eleventh thoracic vertebra should be seen, and on a child, either six anterior ribs or eight posterior ribs should be visualized to verify deep inspiration. Also,

72 inch source image distance is necessary to show true heart size. Other factors that affect cardiac size are posture and blood volume. A chest radiograph taken during the systolic phase causes the heart to appear smaller than it would if the radiograph had been taken during the diastolic phase.

All of these factors show that the "simple" chest radiograph, which is usually the first type students are taught to take, actually has many components that must be remembered in order to make it a good radiograph.

Apical lordotic views of the chest visualize the apices and are performed when a posteroanterior view suggests a possible lesion in that area, but certainty cannot be established because of overlying structures. Two methods of demonstrating the apices are used. The patient can be placed in the anteroposterior position, and the tube can be angled cephalad to project the clavicles superiorly. The other method requires leaning the patient backward against the chest board so that only the scapula touches the board, with the remaining portion of the chest away from it. In this case, the patient has been "angled" so that the clavicles project superiorly; therefore, the tube will remain horizontal and perpendicular to the film.

Double exposure inspiration-expiration films are done for diaphragmatic movement. One film is exposed on full inspiration and then again on full expiration. The kVp factor should be set light enough so as not to "burn out" the diaphragm. However, on the expiration exposure, which should always be done second, the kVp should be increased approximately 8 to 10 kVp (depending on the patient's body habitus) in order to see the diaphragm through the lung fields of the fully inflated lungs. This radiograph should not be viewed for lung radiolucency. It is only to determine the amount of movement that the diaphragm has.

Single exposure inspiration and expiration films may be done sequentially for movement but are less accurate, as the patient may move while the film is being changed or may not breathe as deeply for the second film. Separate single exposure inspiration and then single exposure expiration films are done routinely, however, to rule out a pneumothorax that was not seen on inspiration because of the expansion of the lungs.

Chest fluoroscopy is used to localize a pulmonary lesion, determine the presence or absence of calcium within a pulmonary nodule, evaluate diaphragmatic motion, evaluate a mediastinal mass for expansile pulsation, and evaluate the hila. Since the fluoroscopist controls patient position, definitive information is more often obtained with fluoroscopy than with oblique or lordotic views.

Computed tomography of the chest is most often used in the evaluation of a mass involving the lungs or mediastinum. A central mediastinal mass is often shown better by computed tomography than by plain-film tomography. A computed tomographic examination may alleviate the need for mediastinoscopy in the evaluation of bronchogenic carcinoma. Small subpleural and paramediastinal metastasis can be shown clearly by computed tomography even if the masses are not identifiable on a posteroanterior or lateral chest radiograph or by tomography. Computed tomographic examination following the injection of a radiographic contrast agent helps differentiate an aneurysm from other mediastinal masses. The contrast agent causes a dramatic blush of the aneurysm, which is not found in a mass. Fat has a characteristic appearance on computed tomographic attenuation coefficient. The ability to identify fat has dramatically aided in the evaluation of cardiophrenic angle "masses," which are often accumulations of fat. Diffuse widening of the mediastinum may be caused by the accumulation of fat and fat-containing mediastinal teratomas. These are clearly demonstrated by computed tomography. Both computed tomography and plain-film tomography are useful in evaluating abnormalities of the thoracic cage.

Ultrasonography has limited application in the evaluation of chest disease because of the rapid attenuation of sound by a normal lung. However, the technique is of value in identifying a small pleural effusion and in locating an appropriate site for fluid aspiration.

Bronchography is the radiographic study of the bronchial tree by means of the introduction of a positive contrast medium. It is performed primarily for suspected bronchiectasis, but other indications include obstruction, fistulas, and bronchitis. Contraindications include the presence of a high fever, asthma, severe hypertension, or cardiac problems due to valvular abnormalities. Also, patients who are undergoing therapy treatments to the lung field should not undergo a bronchogram. Bronchial secretions and mucous can cause filling defects during bronchography. To help minimize these secretions, epinephrine or atropine are given to the patient prior to the examination.

Either an iodinated contrast medium or a noniodinated mixture of barium and saline can be used in bronchography. There are two types of iodinated contrast media: aqueous and oily. The advantages of an aqueous contrast medium are the rapid absorption into the blood stream from the bronchi and rapid excretion by the kidneys. However, this is also a disadvantage because filming must be done rapidly and accurately. Another disadvantage is the dilution of contrast material by bronchial secretions, causing decreased tissue contrast. Finally, the aqueous agent is more irritating to the mucosa.

Oily contrast media are more slowly absorbed, which can cause lipoid pneumonia or a granulomatous reaction or both. They are not miscible with secretions, which could give an inaccurate picture of the shape of the bronchi. Small bronchi may be obstructed, which causes a backup of secretions and leads to a fever.

No matter what contrast material is used, the pulmonary function is diminished for a period of time and dyspnea may occur. This requires the use of oxygen. Some reactions to watch for are fever, headache, nausea, vomiting, urticaria, allergic dermatitis, pneumonia, and fatal anaphylaxis. The contrast agent is removed by postural drainage and coughing. These concerns and the rapidly advancing technology in radiography have caused many departments to replace bronchography with computed tomography or magnetic resonance imaging.

Bronchography is usually done on one lung at a time and can be performed on a particular bronchus (selective) or all bronchi (nonselective) (Fig. 8–3). Three procedures are commonly used for introduction of contrast material. A catheter can be inserted either transglotally or through the nose to a position just above the carina. A local anesthetic is given to inhibit the pharyngeal and cough reflexes. Using fluoroscopy as guidance, contrast material is slowly injected and the patient is moved about in order to distribute the material evenly. This procedure allows a "bronchial brush" biopsy to be performed at the same time, if needed. A guide wire with a brush at the end is passed through the catheter into the desired bronchus and a sweep of the tissue is obtained for study. This type of bronchography has been replaced by bronchoscopy performed in the operating room (Fig. 8–4), in which case the physician passes a tube with a scope into the selected bronchus. Fluoroscopic guidance in the operating room is in the form of the C-arm. At this time, tissue samples can be taken for laboratory tests.

A second type of bronchogram requires a percutaneous transtracheal puncture. The patient is sedated before coming to the radiology department, where the neck area is surgically prepped. The circothyroid membrane is pierced by a large (17 g) Teflon needle, which is inserted into the subglottic tracheal space. Selective bronchography can be performed with this method by placing catheters into the desired areas. As with the transglottal type of bronchography, this has been replaced by the more easily performed bronchoscopy in the operating room.

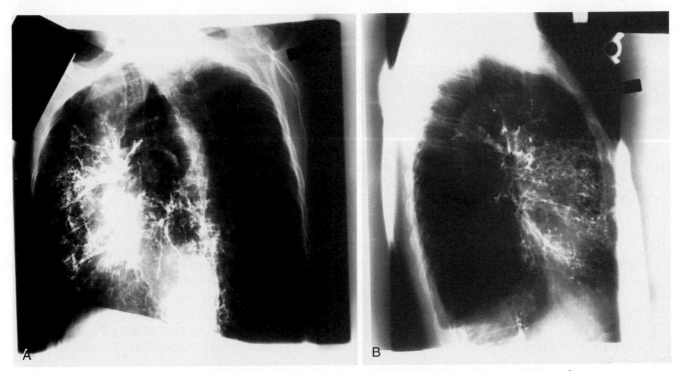

Figure 8–3. Bronchography. Oblique *(A)* and lateral *(B)* views demonstrating the trachea and major bronchi.

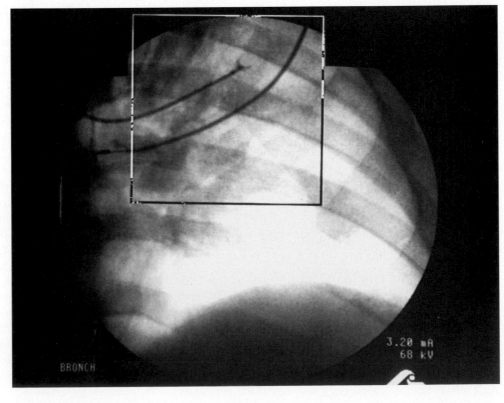

Figure 8–4. Bronchoscopy in the operating room has replaced bronchography in many cases. This image shows the catheter used to obtain a tissue sample.

The easiest method of introduction a contrast agent is aspiration. The patient is seated, the tongue is brought forward, and anesthesia is dropped over the back of the tongue. This causes coughing, which helps to disperse the anesthesia. Contrast material is introduced either in the same manner as the anesthesia, or by a breathing apparatus. The patient is checked under fluoroscopy to see if enough contrast agent has been given before the actual filming is done.

After instillation of the contrast agent by the selected procedure, recumbent anteroposterior and lateral films, as well as an upright posteroanterior chest film are obtained.

Laryngography is the study of the larynx by the injection of a contrast medium through a cannula. Another method of instilling contrast material is to anesthetize the throat and drop an oily medium over the back of the tongue, similar to the method used in bronchography. Fluoroscopy is used, with spot films taken in the anteroposterior and lateral positions.

Plain-film **tomography** is used primarily to evaluate masses involving the lungs, hila, and mediastinum. Localized low-kVp tomography is used to display calcification within a pulmonary nodule if it is not clearly outlined by fluoroscopy. Pulmonary cavities are often better defined by tomography than by plain-film radiography.

Nuclear medicine lung imaging most commonly involves the use of a radionuclide to demonstrate ventilation and pulmonary perfusion. Ventilation scans require the patient to breath in an inert gas, usually xenon. The scan is performed while the patient holds his or her breath. In perfusion scans, a radionuclide material is injected into the venous system. It is carried through the pulmonary circulation around the alveoli where it is picked up by the gamma camera. The information gained from nuclear medicine images helps to differentiate diffuse and regional pulmonary disease. It also forms the basis for a noninvasive diagnostic procedure to diagnose pulmonary emboli.

PATHOLOGY

Congenital Diseases

Cystic fibrosis is an inherited disease of the exocrine glands involving the lungs, pancreas and sweat glands. Heavy secretions of abnormally thick mucus cause progressive clogging of the bronchi and bronchioles, leading to frequent and progressive pulmonary infections. As pulmonary dysfunction progresses, pulmonary hypertension and cor pulmonale often occur. Pulmonary disease with repeated bouts of pneumonia and pancreatic insufficiency are the major clinical manifestations. Recent advances in treatment have extended life expectancy into adulthood. Radiographically, hyperinflation is present, with an interstitial pattern showing thickening around the bronchi and scarring from the pneumonia (Fig. 8–5). The radiograph may also demonstrate atelectasis, bronchiectasis, and consolidation in the middle and upper lungs.

One of the more common indications for doing a chest radiograph on a newborn is **respiratory distress syndrome.** This is also known as **hyaline membrane disease.** A lipoprotein called surfactant coats the alveoli in the lung to reduce surface tension and prevents the collapse of the alveoli. In premature infants there is a deficiency in this surfactant, making inhalation difficult. Chest radiography shows increased density throughout the lung in a granular pattern. Also, there is a well-defined "air bronchogram" sign. An air bronchogram sign is an area of fluid-filled tissue surrounding air in the bronchioles. As the disease progresses, the granular pattern becomes diffuse, presenting a homogeneous opacification of the lungs. Respiratory distress syndrome is the most common cause of death in premature infants.

Inflammatory Processes

Lung abscesses are localized areas of diseased tissue surrounded by debris. **Embolic abscesses** are caused by an infected blood clot being carried to the heart and then, by way of the pulmonary circulation, reaching the lung; a **pneumonic abscess** represents a complication of pneumonia; an **inhalation abscess** is caused by infected material being passed down the trachea into the bronchi. An inhalation abscess is more common in the right lung, which has a more vertical bronchus. Foreign bodies may pass into the lung (especially in children) and cause this type of abscess.

Most lung abscesses are the result of pneumonia or obstruction from foreign bodies breathed into the bronchial tubes. Symptoms of an abscess are like pneumonia; however, the patient's coughed-up sputum is infected. Every time the patient coughs up the sputum (which is the destroyed tissue), a cavity is left. The chest film shows air fluid levels within this cavity with a thick wall surrounding it (Fig. 8–6). In the earlier stages, the radiograph shows a consolidated area of dense pus (Fig. 8–7).

Adult respiratory distress syndrome is sudden respiratory failure because of the inability of the alveolar capillary to exchange air and gases. This occurs in people with healthy lungs and can be caused by acute alveolar injuries such as toxic

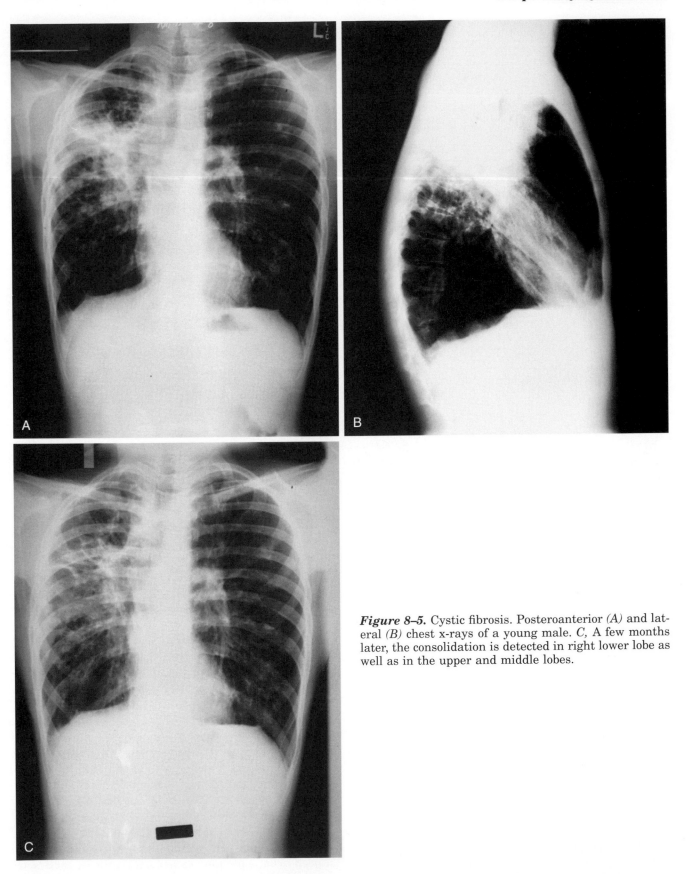

Figure 8–5. Cystic fibrosis. Posteroanterior *(A)* and lateral *(B)* chest x-rays of a young male. *C,* A few months later, the consolidation is detected in right lower lobe as well as in the upper and middle lobes.

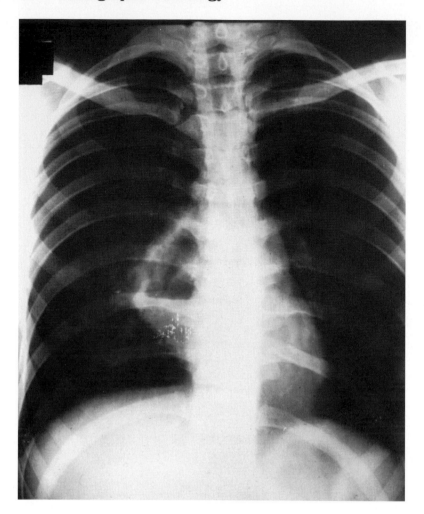

Figure 8–6. Demonstration of air fluid levels found in a lung abscess. The dense areas represent areas of pus.

inhalation, septic shock, and near drowning. The appearance on the radiograph is similar to that of pulmonary edema.

One common reason for obtaining a chest radiograph is a patient history of **asthma.** It is a common disorder that often begins in childhood. Asthma may be caused by a respiratory tract infection, anxiety, exercise, or allergies. As the patient grows older and becomes immune to certain allergies, the asthma attacks may lessen in severity or frequency or both. The episodes are characterized by wheezing, coughing, and a feeling of chest-tightening. There is secretion and edema of the bronchial mucosa and bronchiolar muscle spasm. This narrows the lumen of the bronchi, trapping air in the alveoli and causing labored breathing. When the patient breathes in, the lungs are overdistended because of this trapped air. The diaphragm appears low on the radiograph. The bronchial muscle may become hypertrophied and there is hyperplasia of the mucous glands in the bronchi, which is associated with increased mucous secretions. The overall appearance of the lungs shows as opacity of the lung field because of this increased mucus. In many cases, however, the chest radiograph is normal.

Atelectasis is the collapse of a lung or a portion of it. It is not a disease in itself, but rather a condition caused by another pathology. The lung consists of millions of alveoli, interconnected to each other through small passageways or tubes. When the normal negative pressure within the chest wall is disturbed, either by a puncture wound or through a "blow out" in a weak spot in the lung, a portion of the lung collapses like a deflated balloon. The alveolar walls are opposed to each other and nothing separates them. Since the lung contains less air than normal, it is radiodense (Fig. 8–8). The most common radiographic sign of atelectasis is a local increase in density caused by an airless lung that may vary from thin plate-like streaks to lobar collapse. When only a portion of the lung collapses, the remaining portion expands to fill in the collapsed area. This may cause a shift in the mediastinum. Indirect radiographic signs of atelectasis reflect an attempt by the remaining lung to compensate for the loss of the collapsed portion.

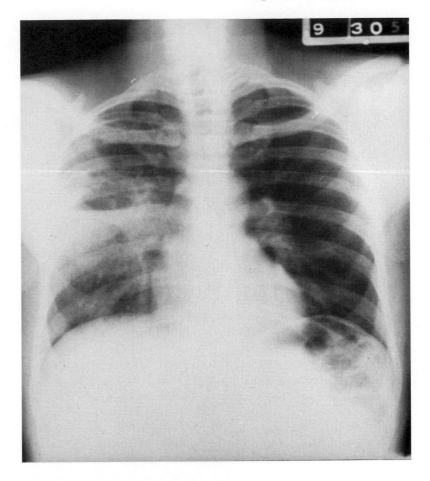

Figure 8–7. Lung abscess. No cavity is seen in the early stages.

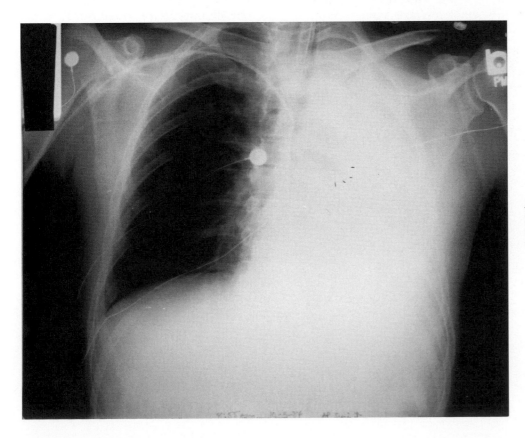

Figure 8–8. Atelectasis. The main bronchus was obstructed, causing the lung to collapse.

These signs include elevation of the hemidiaphragm; displacement of the heart, mediastinum, and hilum toward the atelectatic segment; and compensatory overinflation of the remainder of the lung.

Causes of atelectasis include complete obstruction of a bronchus (Fig. 8–9) or compression of the lung by pleural effusion or pneumothorax. An important iatrogenic cause of atelectasis is the improper placement of an endotracheal tube below the level of the tracheal bifurcation. Lobar atelectasis in the absence of explanations is an important sign of bronchogenic carcinoma.

Bronchitis is a condition in which excessive mucus is secreted in the bronchi. This leads to severe coughing with the production of sputum. Bronchitis may be acute or chronic in form (Fig. 8–10). The acute form usually involves the trachea as well as the larger bronchi. It may be caused by bacteria, dust, or toxic fumes. When the irritant is removed, the inflammation subsides.

To qualify as chronic bronchitis, there must be a cough that produces thick sputum for at least 3 months, and the cough must recur for at least 2 consecutive years. In addition, there may be shortness of breath and wheezing, similar to the breathing problems experienced by people with asthma.

The chief cause of chronic bronchitis is cigarette smoking. Repeated attacks of acute bronchitis may also lead to chronic bronchitis. People who live in smog-plagued areas, especially smokers, are even more susceptible to the disease. Occupational factors, such as exposure to dust or noxious fumes, also increase the risk of chronic bronchitis. The diagnosis is usually a clinical one, but the chest radiograph reveals hyperinflation and increased vascular markings especially in the lower lungs.

Bronchiectasis is the irreversible chronic dilation of smaller bronchi or bronchioles of the lung. The cause of the condition is repeated pulmonary infection and bronchial obstruction. These cause a weakening of the wall of the bronchus, allowing the bronchi to become dilated. Bronchiectasis is also common in lung abscess cases. When the bronchus dilates, it forms an area where pus can collect. This leads to destruction of the bronchial walls. The patient with bronchiectasis typically has a chronic productive cough, often associated with recurrent episodes of acute pneumonia. The cough and expectoration are most often the major clues to bronchiectasis.

Although plain radiographs may suggest bronchiectasis, a bronchogram will accurately diagnose bronchiectasis and show dense pulmonary infiltrate and fibrosis usually occurring in the lower lobes (Fig. 8–11).

Diffuse lung diseases (e.g., emphysema or interstitial fibrosis) may result in an obstruction of pulmonary blood flow and pulmonary arterial hypertension by a combination of two mechanisms: hypoxia with arterial spasm and pathologic obliteration of vascular channel. **Cor pulmonale** is an

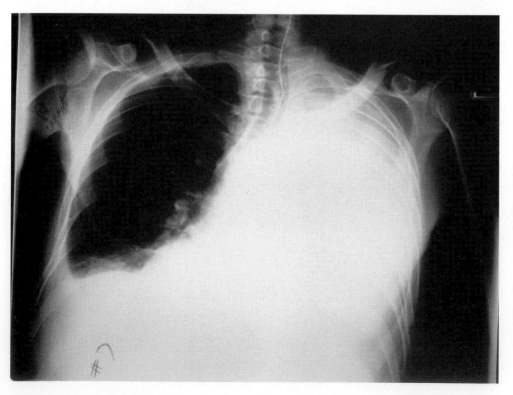

Figure 8–9. Atelectasis. The obstruction in this case was a bronchogenic carcinoma. The collapse has caused a shift of the heart and trachea to the right.

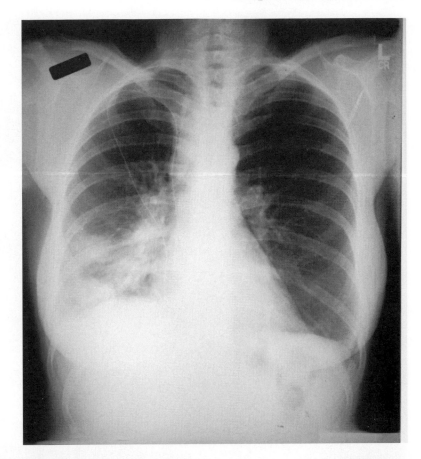

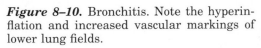

Figure 8–10. Bronchitis. Note the hyperinflation and increased vascular markings of lower lung fields.

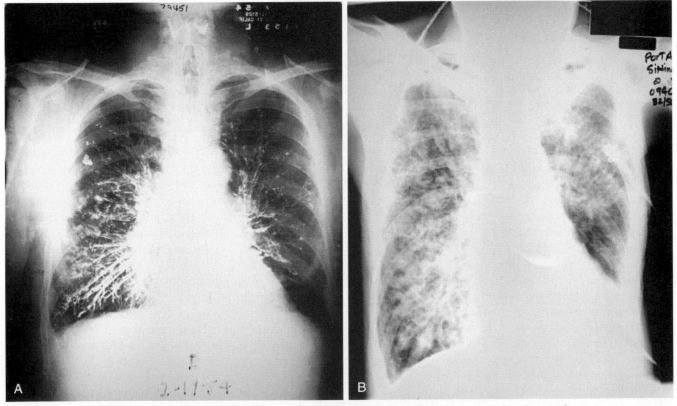

Figure 8–11. Bronchiectasis. *A,* The bronchioles are dilated at the alveoli on the bronchogram. *B,* The large amount of dense pulmonary infiltrates and fibrosis, along with this patient's history, suggested chronic bronchiectasis.

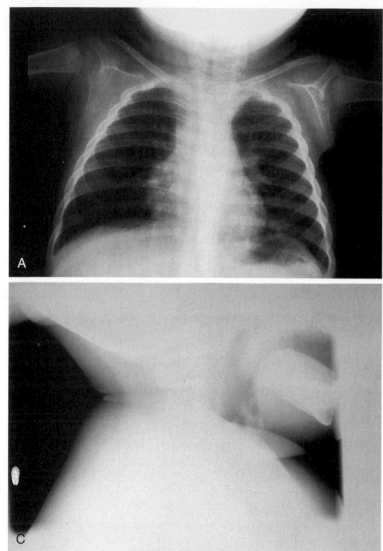

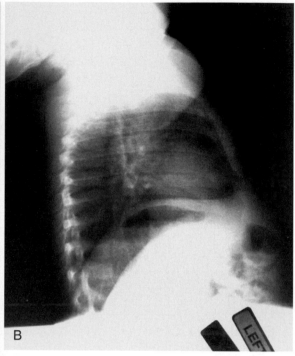

Figure 8–12. Croup. Anteroposterior *(A)* and lateral *(B)* chest radiographs of an infant who presented with a bark-like cough. *C,* A soft tissue neck radiograph was taken to help make the diagnosis of croup.

acute or chronic condition involving right-sided heart failure. In the acute phase, the right side of the heart is dilated and fails, most often as a direct result of pulmonary embolism. In chronic cor pulmonale, a chronic massive disease of the lungs causes gradual obstruction that eventually produces right ventricular hypertrophy, increased stress, and ultimately heart failure. The chest radiograph shows an enlarged right ventricle with widespread pulmonary edema.

Croup is primarily a viral infection, particularly the parainfluenza viruses. It occurs most often in very young children, generally about age 1 to 3 years old. The episode may begin in the evening after the child has gone to sleep. Labored breathing and a harsh, rough cough are characteristic. Fever does not always accompany croup. Soft-tissue anteroposterior and lateral neck radiographs show spasm and constriction of the airway by demonstra-

ting characteristic smooth, tapered narrowing of the subglottic airway (Fig. 8–12).

Chronic obstructive pulmonary disease (**COPD**) is really a process that is characterized by the presence of either **chronic bronchitis** or **emphysema**. These diseases overlap and they share certain causes, therefore, they are under the umbrella of COPD. Emphysema is characterized by increased air spaces and associated tissue destruction leading to hypoxia. The condition causes dyspnea, particularly when the patient is lying down. The patient has a barrel chest and low diaphragm. The radiographer must be careful to include the diaphragm and not to overexpose the lung fields, which can be easily done because of the overdistention of the air spaces with trapped air. Therefore, the technical factors should be decreased when the patient is known to have emphysema.

Emphysema is an irreversible, crippling disease

that is known as "leather lung disease" by pathologists because the lungs become stiff and brittle. The alveoli lose their elasticity and remain filled with air during expiration. This may result in hyperinflation of the lung and reduced expiratory volume, and there is a chance that the alveoli will burst with the pressure of coughing. If a rupture occurs, the alveoli are destroyed, and their numbers are reduced. This will permanently hyperinflate the lung, trapping alveolar gas, essentially in expiration. Gas exchange is seriously compromised. Patients who are receiving oxygen have a very low administration level because their respirations are controlled by the carbon dioxide in their blood.

There are two basic types of emphysema: compensating and centrilobular. In **compensating** (or **compensatory**) emphysema, there is no air trapping. There are no clinical symptoms, and the condition is caused by the removal of one lung, or a portion of it, causing the overinflation of the other lung to compensate for the loss.

Centrilobular emphysema is more common than compensating emphysema and is second only to heart disease as a major cause of death and disability in the United States. This type of emphysema is irreversible and results in airway obstruction and air trapping. It is characterized by an increase in the air spaces of the alveoli with destruction of the alveolar walls. The radiograph

shows a flattened hemidiaphragm, which obscures the costophrenic angle. Also, the heart shadow is elongated because of the diaphragm being pushed down. This causes an appearance of a diminished heart width size. The lung fields are abnormally radiolucent and there is an increase in the retrosternal air space, causing the classic "barrel chest" (Figs. 8–13 and 8–14).

Normally, the pleural cavity is empty. However, when it is filled with pus, it is known as an **empyema.** Fortunately, this is not as common as it once was. Causes of an empyema include a chest wound, streptococcal bronchopneumonia, obstruction of bronchi, and a ruptured abscess of the lung. A chest tube is inserted into the pleural cavity to drain the material away. A chest film shows pleural effusion with air fluid levels (Fig. 8–15).

Hydatid disease may affect the lung as well as the liver. Cysts growing in the lung exert pressure on the bronchus until it finally breaks into the bronchial tree. The cyst can be seen on a radiograph as a rounded opacity.

Fluid in the pleural cavity is known as **pleural effusion.** The term hydrothorax is also used but is an antiquated term. Blood within the pleural cavity is called a hemothorax. The sources of fluid vary; congestive heart failure, infection, neoplasm, and trauma are all possible causes. The most common cause of bilateral or right-sided pleural effusion is

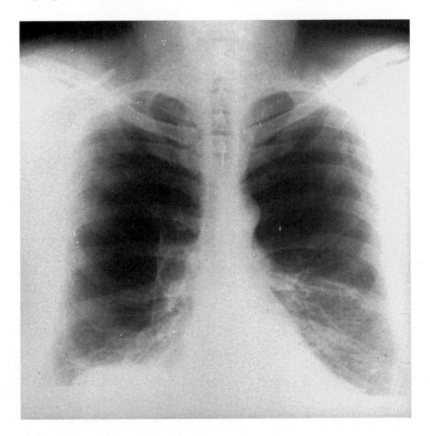

Figure 8–13. Extensive crippling emphysema in a 39-year-old man. Note the elongated heart, radiolucent upper lung fields, and increased markings at the base.

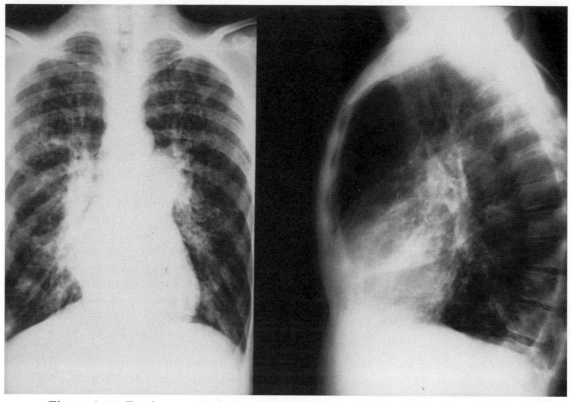

Figure 8–14. Emphysema. *Left,* Posteroanterior view shows marked pulmonary fibrosis and emphysema. *Right,* The lateral view shows marked anterior enlargement of the right ventricle.

congestive heart failure. Isolated left pleural effusion may be caused by a pulmonary infarct, pancreatitis, or a subphrenic abscess.

A large unilateral effusion causes pressure to be exerted on the lung. As pressure builds on the lung, the lung begins pushing on the mediastinum and eventually causes a shift of the heart and mediastinum into the contralateral lung. If enough pressure is applied, the lung opposite the pleural effusion collapses, as it has nowhere to go. All this depends on the amount of fluid that accumulates within the pleural cavity. A large pleural effusion without a mediastinal shift is a significant indicator of malignancy.

Chest radiographs play an important role in the diagnosis of pleural effusion. Pleural fluid first accumulates in the posterior costophrenic angle that is viewed on the erect lateral view of the chest. This is the most dependent portion of the pleural space. On the frontal view, the fluid can be seen on the lateral costophrenic angles. These opacities "blunt" or round off the normally sharp costophrenic angles by displaying an upper concavity known as the "meniscus" sign (Fig. 8–16A). A small amount of effusion is best shown with the patient lying with the affected side down in a lateral decubitus posi-

tion (see Fig. 8–16B). In this manner, the fluid is not superimposed by mediastinal shadows.

Pleurisy is inflammation of the pleura and often accompanies pneumonia and injuries to the chest. The classic symptom of pleurisy is a sharp stabbing pain in the side during respiration. This is caused by the inflammation creating a rough surface on the visceral pleura. When the visceral and parietal pleura come into contact during respiration, the rough surface causes pain. Although this condition can not be radiographically demonstrated, a decubitus chest film can verify pleural effusion, which may be associated with pleurisy.

Pneumonia (pneumonitis) is inflammation of the lungs. The lungs or certain sections of the lung are filled with fluid, causing opacity on the film. In this case, the technologist should slightly increase the technical factors to penetrate the lungs. There are various types of pneumonia, all of which derive their names from the location of the inflammation or its cause.

Aspiration pneumonia results from the aspiration of a foreign object into the lungs, which irritates the bronchi and results in edema. This type of pneumonia occurs in the upper portions of the lower lobes, as this is the most dependent area of the

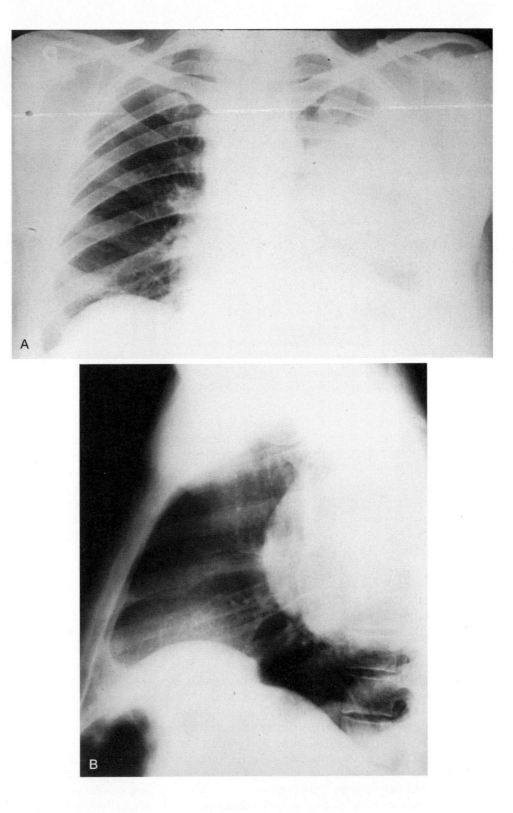

Figure 8–15. A and B, Very large empyema.

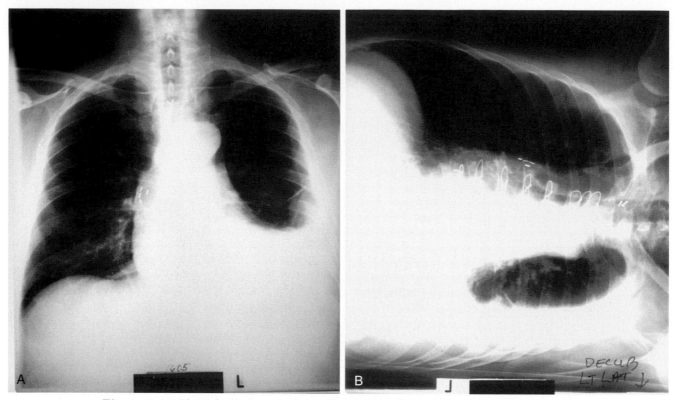

Figure 8–16. Pleural effusion. *A,* Frontal projection showing blunting of the normally sharp costophrenic angles. *B,* In the decubitis view, the fluid goes to the dependent area and is thus not superimposed over other structures.

bronchi in the supine position. Radiographs show multiple areas of opacity in this segment (Fig. 8–17). Small bronchioles containing air may also be visualized as the edema progresses causing the "air bronchogram" sign (Fig. 8–18).

Bronchopneumonia is actually a bronchitis of both lungs, which can be caused by either the streptococcus or the staphylococcus bacteria. The bronchioles fill up with mucus and become infected, which leads to many small abscesses throughout the lungs and is seen as patchy pneumonic infiltrate (Fig. 8–19).

Lobar (pneumococcal) pneumonia involves one or more segments or lobes of a lung and is caused by the bacteria pneumococcus. As in the other pneumonias, the bronchioles fill with fluid. As air in the alveoli becomes replaced by exudate, the affected part of the lung is said to be consolidated. The consolidation is usually confined to one or two lobes; hence the term lobar pneumonia. The patient presents with an upper respiratory infection, cough, chills, and fever. The radiograph shows the affected lobe as a radiopaque area (Fig. 8–20).

Viral pneumonia (also called **interstitial pneumonia**) is inflammation of the alveoli and other supporting structures of the lung. It causes symptoms similar to lobar pneumonia. The patient has a fever and cough and may believe he or she has the flu, hence its nickname of "walking" pneumonia. This virus-induced pneumonia shows infiltrate in the perihilar region.

Pneumocystis carinii occurs in patients with impaired immune systems. Organisms that are normally harmless to the healthy individual cause pneumonia in the patient whose body defense mechanism is unable to fight off the virus. This type of pneumonia is especially dangerous as it is unresponsive to ordinary treatments of antibodies. The pneumonia is widespread and mimics pulmonary edema (Fig. 8–21).

The long-continued irritation of certain dusts encountered in industrial occupations may cause a chronic interstitial pneumonia known as **pneumoconiosis.** The dangerous element in the dust is silica. There are three important types of pneumoconiosis that need to be discussed.

Silicosis is the most widespread and the oldest of all occupational diseases. It is caused by inhalation of crystalline forms of silica and occurs in miners, sandblasters and foundry workers. Very small crystalline particles of silica are carried by phagocytes from the bronchioles into the alveoli. There the dust acts as an irritant, which stimulates the formation of large amounts of connective tissue. At

Text continued on page 209

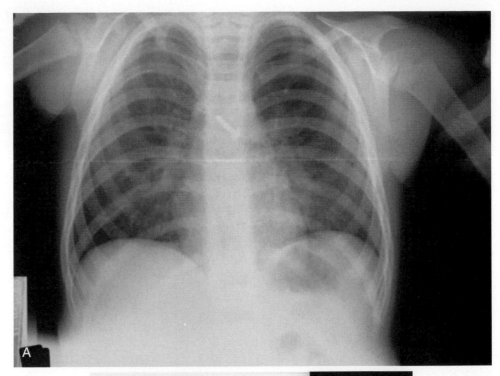

Figure 8–17. Aspiration
pneumonia. Anteroposterior
(A) and lateral *(B)* views of a
21-month-old girl who swallowed then aspirated a
screw. It is blocking the carina, causing both lungs to
become infiltrated.

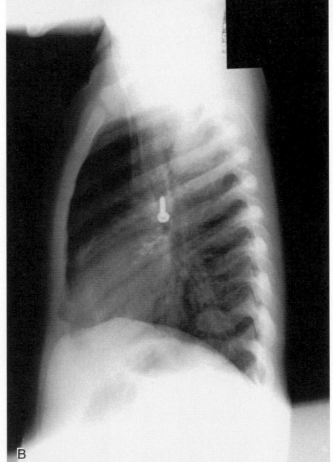

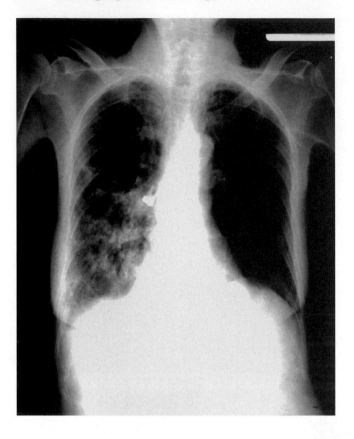

Figure 8–18. This elderly woman aspirated one of her teeth. It is lodged in a major bronchus, causing pneumonia. Note the air bronchogram sign.

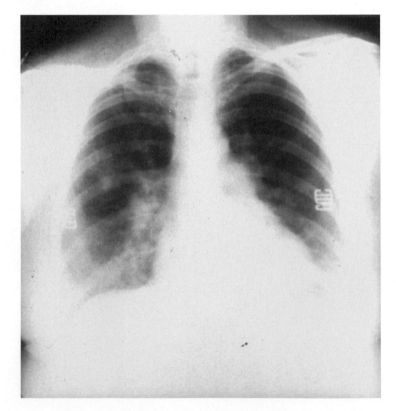

Figure 8–19. Bronchopneumonia involving several lobes on the right in a 57-year-old woman.

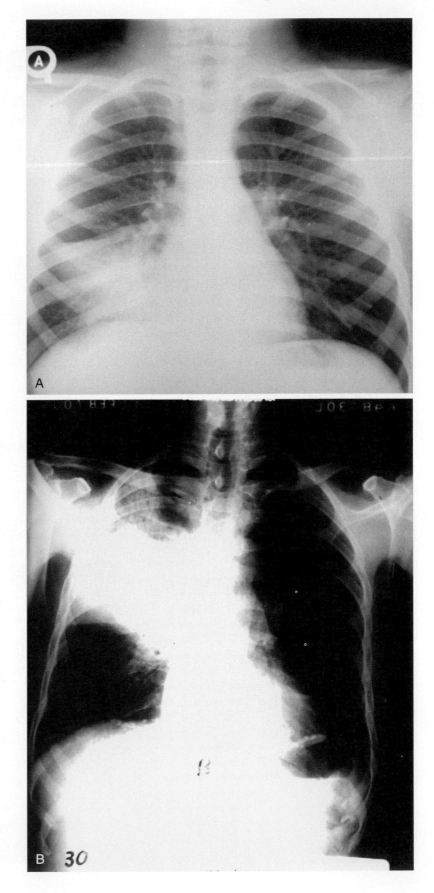

Figure 8–20. Right middle lobar pneumonia in a toddler *(A)* and in an adult *(B)*.

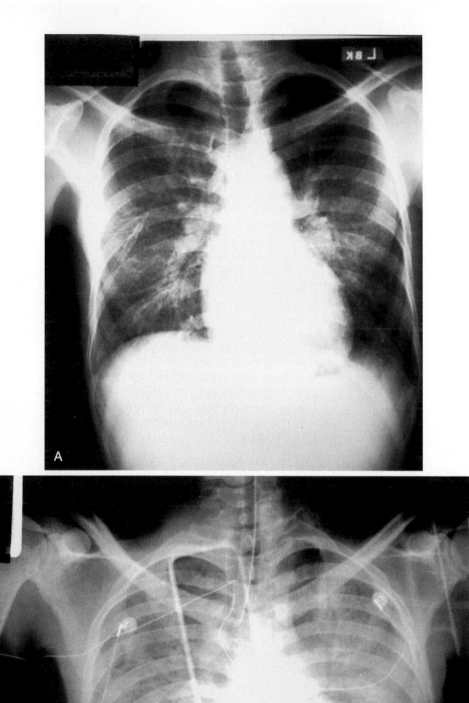

A

B

Figure 8–21. Pneumocystis carinii in a 26-year-old man. *A,* Radiograph taken in the emergency room. *B,* 8 days later in the intensive care unit. Note the compression board for codes under the spine. The patient later died.

first there are discrete nodules of fibrous tissue but, over time, these coalesce to form large fibrous areas. These areas are well circumscribed and of uniform density. The bilateral masses are symmetrical and are almost always found in the upper lung area. Calcium salts are deposited in the periphery of the enlarged lymph nodes. These fibrous areas give rise to the radiographic hallmark sign of "eggshell" which denotes exclusively silicosis.

Asbestosis is an important disease caused by the inhalation of asbestos dust. The disease may be acquired either during the handling and crushing of asbestos rock or in the manufacture and installation of asbestos used in insulation. Asbestosis is associated with pulmonary fibrosis, bronchogenic carcinoma and malignancy of the pleura. The lungs show the same fibrous condition characteristic of silicosis. However, involvement of the pleura differentiates asbestosis from silicosis (Fig. 8–22). The pleura forms thin curved calcifications superior to the diaphragm.

Berylliosis is another form of pneumoconiosis. It is caused chiefly by inhalation of beryllium salt fumes; however, the salt may be absorbed through the skin. Berylliosis may produce acute, diffuse injury or a chronic granulomatous formation reaction.

When free air gets into the pleural space through any route, it is known as a **pneumothorax.** Causes of a pneumothorax include penetrating chest wounds (e.g., stabbing, gunshots, fractured ribs), surgery, and pathologic conditions of the bronchi that cause a spontaneous rupture of an emphysematous bleb. The lung is displaced away from the chest wall.

An upright expiration chest film shows a lung that is not expanded with air, thereby making the pneumothorax more prominent (Fig. 8–23). There are no lung markings seen in the area of the pneumothorax. In the erect position, air rises to the apex; therefore, a small pneumothorax, unless loculated, is first seen at the apex on the upright film with maximum expiration. The boundary of the lung, or "lung edge," should always be identified. On fluoroscopy, the heart seems to "flutter" because of the lack of stabilizing effect from the collapsed lung. The radiographer should take care that excess skin has not folded under on a portable chest radiograph. This produces an artifact known as a **pseudopneumothorax,** as the skin folds mimic a real pneumothorax.

If air enters the pleural cavity during inspiration but does not leave upon expiration, a **tension pneumothorax** exists. The dome of the hemidi-

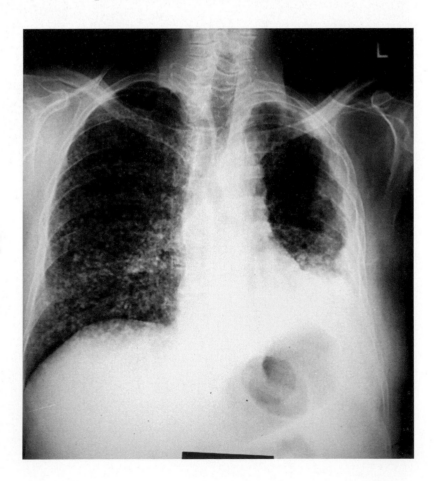

Figure 8–22. Asbestosis. There are dense fibrous areas throughout the pleura of the lungs.

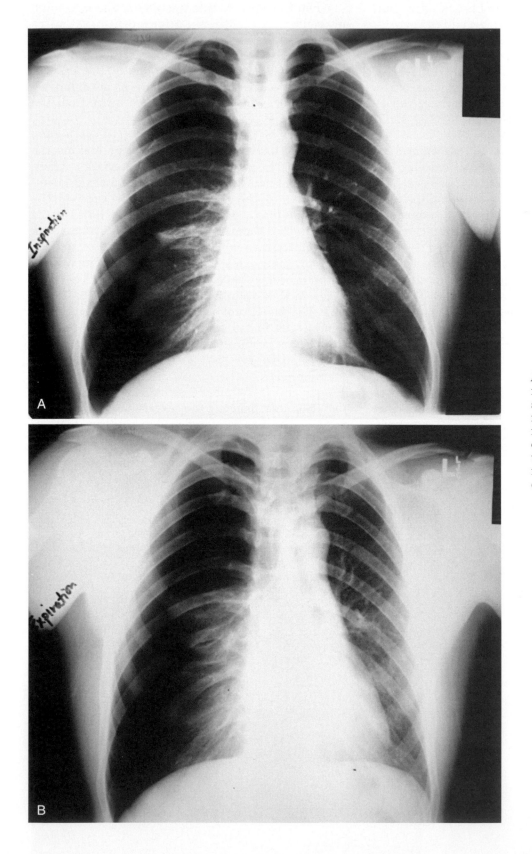

Figure 8–23. Pneumothorax. *A*, Inspiration film shows a large pneumothorax. The lung edge can be identified. *B*, Expiration film of same patient shows the true size of the pneumothorax. The lung edge is now down to the sixth rib.

aphragm becomes depressed or inverted (Fig. 8–24). The resulting mediastinal shift and collapse of the opposite lung because of built-up pressure from air are the same as in pleural effusion.

Chest radiographs for pneumothorax should be taken with the patient in the upright position, as it may be very difficult to identify this condition if the patient is supine. If the patient is unable to be in the erect position, the radiographer should position the patient in a lateral decubitus position with the affected side *up* (not down, as with pleural effusion). In addition to routine full-inspiration films, a posteroanterior radiograph should be obtained with the lungs in full expiration to identify small pneumothoraces. This maneuver causes the lung to decrease in volume and become relatively more dense.

Pulmonary edema means excess fluid within the lung. About threefourths of all cases are caused by pulmonary circulation obstruction. Pulmonary edemas usually occur only when the left ventricle is inadequate to pump blood to the pulmonary vascular system when there is an obstruction beyond the pulmonary capillaries. This causes a backup of blood in the lungs (Fig. 8–25). There is a diffuse increase in density of the hilar regions, which are homogeneous and fade toward the periphery of the lung. A classic radiographic sign is Kerley B lines (see Fig. 9–25A). These are thickened interlobular septa and are shown most clearly laterally above the costophrenic angles. They are fine, perfectly straight lines perpendicular to the chest wall and running 1 to 3 cm from the lung periphery.

Pulmonary emboli are the most common pulmonary complication of hospitalized patients. They are fatal in more than 50 percent of cases. Most pulmonary emboli result in no abnormalities on posteroanterior and lateral chest radiographs. On rare occasions and with a massive pulmonary embolus, a focal hyperlucency may be present in the area supplied by the occluded vessel. The appearance of an infiltrate is usually delayed by 8 to 12 hours after the embolus has occurred. The involvement almost always occurs in the lower lung zones, especially the costophrenic angles. The radiographic appearance of an inverted wedge-shaped area of opacity (Hamptons hump) with the base at the pleural surface and the apex directed toward the hilum is suggestive of pulmonary infarct. The pleural-based nature of the infarct is even more graphically displayed by computed tomography. Nuclear medicine scans will demonstrate which segment of the lung is not receiving blood. This results in a ventilation-perfusion mismatch. Results of the ventilation study are normal, but the perfusion study shows abnormality.

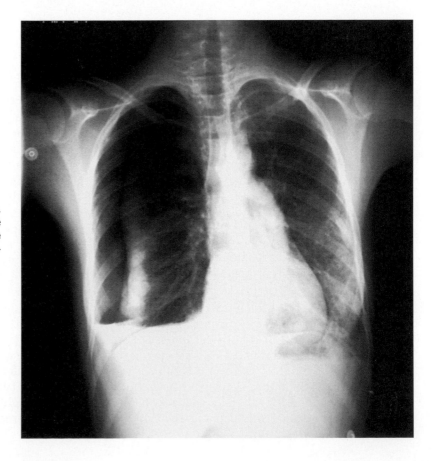

Figure 8–24. Tension hydropneumothorax. The diaphragm has flattened out and the trachea and heart are being shifted to the left, causing pressure of left lower lobe (radiodense).

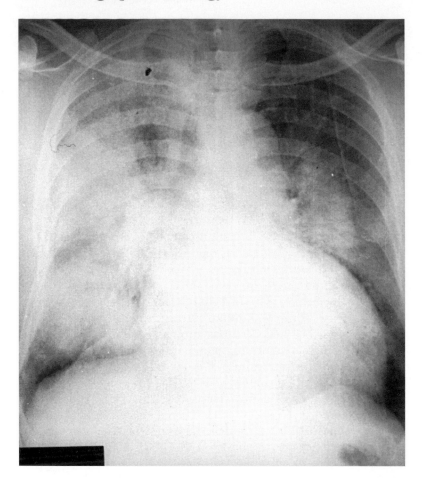

Figure 8–25. Pulmonary edema caused by hypertensive heart disease.

The overall radiographic appearance of a pulmonary infarct may mimic pneumonia. Air bronchograms are often absent in a pulmonary infarct, whereas they are commonly present in pneumonia, which should be a differentiating characteristic.

Tuberculosis is a disease caused by mycobacterium tuberculosis. It is spread through inhalation of infected material from someone who already has tuberculosis. General symptoms include fever, loss of weight, and weakness. Coughing and sputum production depend on the type of tuberculosis the patient has. Until cavities are formed, very little sputum is coughed up. The patient may also experience pain in the side from tuberculous pleurisy.

Although it generally affects the lungs, other areas of the body such as the spine may also be affected. The type of pulmonary tuberculosis determines the site of infection. **Primary tuberculosis,** also known as **childhood tuberculosis,** occurs in someone who has never had the disease before. It used to occur almost exclusively in childhood when tuberculosis was common, hence the second name. The lesions are small focal spots that can be found anywhere in the lung. This contrasts sharply with secondary tuberculosis, which is found in the apices of the lungs. The disease is spread along the lymphatics; therefore, hilar enlargement is an important sign in primary childhood tuberculosis. Again, this contrasts with what is found in secondary infection. Primary infection does not become chronic, nor is there any cavity formation (Fig. 8–26). Recovery is marked by the disappearance of the lesions within the lung and along the lymph nodes, or the conversion of some or all of these lesions into fibrous tissue with calcification.

Reactivation (secondary) tuberculosis usually develops in adults and is almost always found in the upper lobes bilaterally. The right lung is attacked more often than the left. The first radiographic signs of this type of tuberculosis are bilateral infiltrates, which are mottled, and calcifications, which are streaked (Fig. 8–27). As reactivation heals, the hilar region retracts and the lung shrinks in size. Fibrous tissue surrounds and invades the lesion, leaving only a scar with calcification. Cavities commonly develop and are clearly demonstrated on tomography. In either primary tuberculosis or reactivation tuberculosis, tomography or apicolordotic chest views are helpful in demonstrating the cavitation and calcifications.

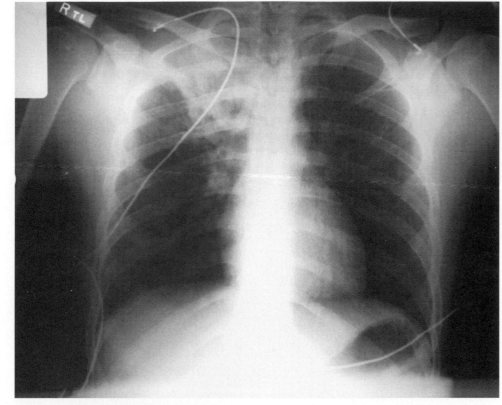

Figure 8–26. Active tuberculosis. No cavity formation has occurred yet in the right apex.

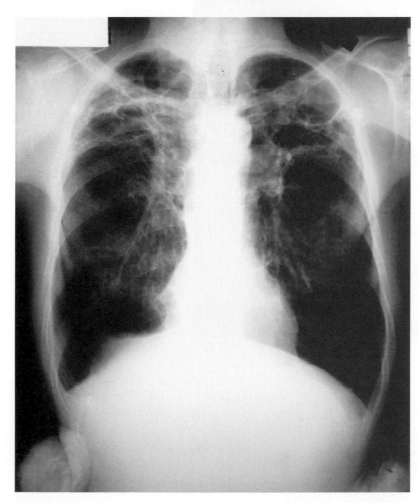

Figure 8–27. Tuberculosis. Scarring and calcification indicate healing.

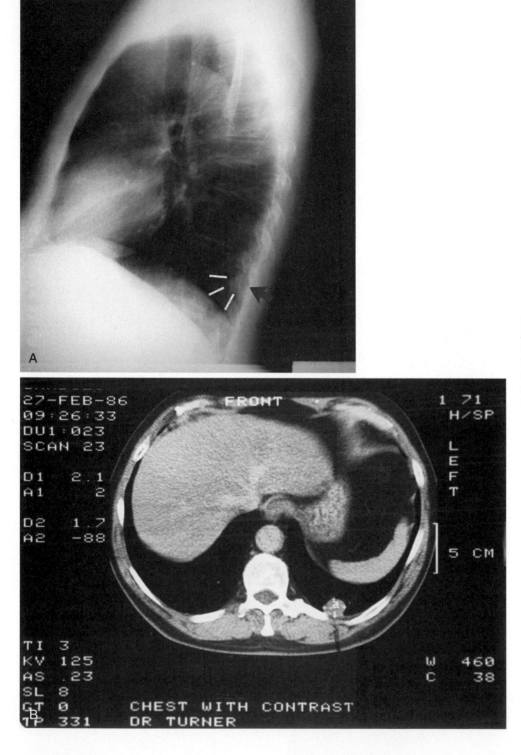

Figure 8–28. Hamartoma. *A,* Lateral chest radiograph shows the single benign neoplasm. *B,* A computed tomographic scan is able to measure the neoplasm's dimensions.

Neoplasms

Benign

A **hamartoma** is the most common solitary pulmonary nodule. It is a mass of tissue without organization usually found in the lung periphery (Fig. 8–28). Most patients with a hamartoma are over 50 years of age. Hamartomas are rarely found in someone under the age of 30. The small mass has a sharp, slightly lobulated outline and does not cavitate. It may calcify and cause a characteristic "popcorn" appearance.

Malignant

Bronchogenic carcinoma does not arise from pulmonary tissue but rather comes from the major bronchus of one or both lungs. It is currently the leading primary malignant tumor in males between the ages of 55 and 60 years. The incidence in women is rising because of the increased number of women who smoke. Smoking is the most important factor in the cause of bronchogenic carcinoma. The tumor grows into and surrounds one of the main bronchi, which results in narrowing and obstruction of the lumen. Obstruction of a bronchus results in atelectasis of the area of the lung that has lost its air supply. A second resulting condition is bronchiectasis and abscess formation. This is caused by secretions in the bronchus that can not escape because of the blockage. The secretions stagnate and undergo putrefaction, causing the walls of the bronchioles to weaken and dilate.

Some of the symptoms include a persistent cough, bloody sputum, dyspnea, and weight loss. The chest film shows a rounded opacity without calcification in the upper lobes of the lung. The opacity represents the radiopaque lung nodule known as a "coin" lesion. Malignant tumors rarely calcify; therefore, calcification in any type of lung tumor usually signifies that the tumor is benign. If the chest shows pleural effusion and adenopathy, the tumor cannot be surgically removed (Fig. 8–29). Left untreated, patients with primary lung cancer survive less than 1 year. A 5-year survival has very low odds even with treatment.

Metastatic carcinomas are more common than primary lung cancer. These are divided into three types. **Nodular metastatic disease** is almost always multiple and appears as round masses of different sizes throughout the lung. These have the characteristic radiographic appearance known as "cotton ball" effect (Fig. 8–30). In women, most often the primary source is uterine cancer.

Lymphangitic is a diffuse form of metastatic cancer that appears as streaks and tiny nodules throughout the lungs. They occur from lymphatic spread from the gastric area. **Pneumonic** processes take on the appearance of localized areas of bronchopneumonia. The alveoli are filled with cancer cells just as they fill with fluid in pneumonia. Breast cancer is commonly the primary source (Fig. 8–31).

Mediastinal Pathology

Mediastinal masses include a variety of benign or malignant tumors. A **thymoma** is usually benign and has a peak incidence in middle life. It is not usually radiographically diagnostic but if it is seen, it should not be mistaken for an enlarged thymus gland. **Teratomas** are also benign masses that occur behind the midsternum in young adults. These contain tissue such as fat, hair, and teeth. **Lymphomas** are related to Hodgkins disease and are located in the middle and anterior mediastinum. The radiographer should look for increased hilar areas.

Air within the mediastinal space (**pneumomediastinum**) may appear spontaneously or as the result of chest trauma, perforation of the esophagus

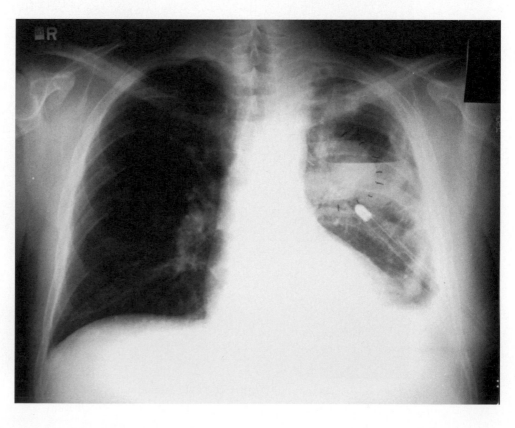

Figure 8–29. Primary carcinoma. Large mass in the left lung and pulmonary edema in the right lung. This tumor is unoperable.

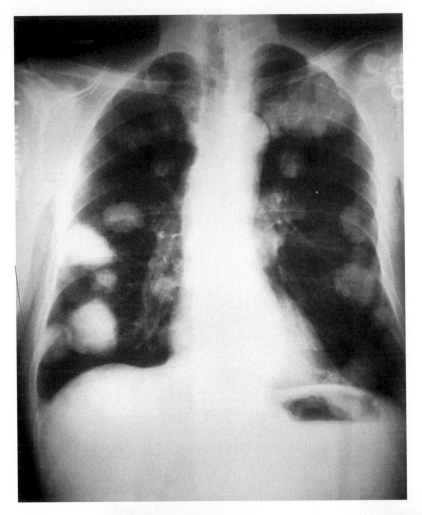

Figure 8–30. Nodular metastasis showing "cotton ball" effect.

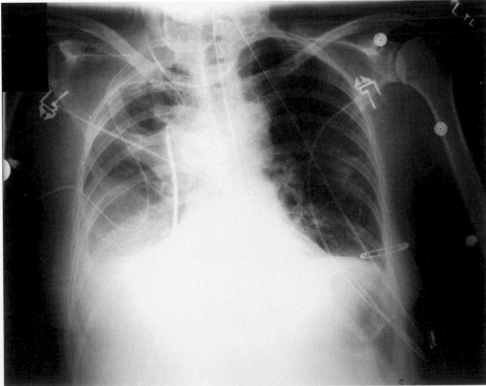

Figure 8–31. Pneumonic metastasis.

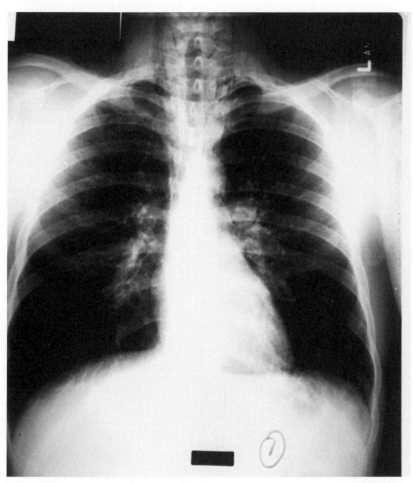

Figure 8–32. Pneumomediastinum. Note the air in the neck.

Table 8–1.
Clinical and Radiographic Characteristics of Common Pathologies

Pathologic Condition	Causal Factors*	Manifestations	Radiographic Appearance
Cystic fibrosis	Newborn, inherited	Repeated bouts of pneumonia, pancreatic insufficiency	Hyperinflation, consolidation in the middle and upper lungs
Respiratory distress syndrome	Newborn, prematurity, lack of surfactant	Difficult breathing	Air bronchogram sign
Abscesses	Embolus, pneumonia, foreign bodies	Coughing, infected sputum	Air fluid levels within a cavity
Asthma	Childhood, allergies, exercise, stress, anxiety	Wheezing, coughing, tight chest	Overall opacity but often normal
Atelectasis	Obstruction of a bronchus, pneumothorax, or pleural effusion	Manifestations due to causative pathology	Local increase in density radiodensity
Bronchitis	Bacteria, dust, cigarette smoking	Cough, shortness of breath, wheezing	Hyperinflation, increased vascular markings
Bronchiectasis	Repeated pulmonary infection and obstruction	Chronic productive cough	Bronchogram to determine dilation
Cor pulmonale	Diffuse lung diseases	Hypoxia	Enlarged right ventricle
Croup	1–3 years, parainfluenza virus	Labored breathing, bark-like cough	Soft tissue-neck view shows spasm and constriction of airway
Emphysema			
Compensating	Older adults, lung removal	Barrel chest, hypoxia, none	Overinflation of remaining lung
Centrilobular (COPD)	Smoking, dust inhalation	Feeling of inability to breathe	Low flat diaphragms, radiolucent lungs
Empyema	Chest wounds, ruptured abscess, obstruction		Pleural effusion, air fluid levels
Pleural effusion	Congestive heart failure, infection, trauma	Mediastinal shift	Atelectasis, blunted costophrenic angles, "meniscus" sign
Pleurisy	Inflammation causes a rough surface of pleura	Sharp, stabbing pain	None
Pneumonia			
Aspiration	Foreign object	Edema	Air bronchogram sign
Bronchopneumonia	Streptococcus or staphylococcus bacteria	Abscesses	Patchy infiltrate
Lobar	Pneumococcus bacteria	Upper respiratory tract infection, chills, fever	Affected lobe is radiopaque
Viral	Virus	Same as lobar	Perihilar infiltrate
Pneumocystis carinii	AIDS	Mimics pulmonary edema	Widespread infiltrate
Pneumoconiosis	Inhalation of dusts		
Silicosis	Inhalation of silica	Fibrous nodules	"Eggshell"
Asbestosis	Inhalation of asbestos	Pulmonary fibrosis	Same as silicosis with involvement of pleura
Berylliosis	Inhalation of beryllium	Granulomatous formation	
Pneumothorax	Penetrating chest wounds	Difficulty breathing, mediastinal shift	No lung markings
Pulmonary edema	Pulmonary circulation obstruction		Kerley B lines
Pulmonary emboli	Inactivity	—	Normal but may show Hampton's hump in pulmonary infarct

Table 8–1.
Clinical and Radiographic Characteristics of Common Pathologies *Continued*

Pathologic Condition	Causal Factors*	Manifestations	Radiographic Appearance
Tuberculosus	Mycobacterium	Fever, weight loss, weakness	
Primary	Childhood		Small focal lesions anywhere in the lungs with hilar enlargement
Reactivation	Adulthood		Bilateral infiltrates in upper lobes; cavities; calcifications
Hamartoma	Over 50 years	Sharply outlined mass	"Popcorn" appearance
Bronchogenic carcinoma	55–60 years, males, smoking	Cough, weight loss, dyspnea	"Coin" lesions
Nodular metastasis	Female reproductive		"Cotton ball" sign
Lymphangitic	Gastric primary		Streaks, tiny nodules
Pneumonic	Breast primary		Same as bronchopneumonia
Pneumomediastinum	Chest trauma	—	Linear opacity parallel to heart border

*Includes age, if relevant.

or tracheobronchial tree, or the spread of air along fascial planes from the neck, peritoneal cavity, or retroperitoneal space. Spontaneous pneumomediastinum usually results from a sudden rise in intra-alveolar pressure that causes alveolar rupture and the dissection of air along blood vessels in the interstitial space to the hilum and mediastinum.

On the posteroanterior chest radiographs, air causes lateral displacement of the mediastinal pleura, which appears as a long linear opacity that is parallel to the heart border but separated from it by the air. On lateral projections, air typically collects behind the sternum, extending in streaks downward and anterior to the heart. Chest radiographs may also demonstrate air outlining the pulmonary arterial trunk and aorta, as well as dissecting into the soft tissues of the neck (Fig. 8–32).

Table 8–1 summarizes the clinical and radiographic characteristics of common pathologies of the respiratory system.

Review Questions

1. Explain the physiology of respiration.
2. List the factors affecting the diaphragm height. On a posteroanterior chest radiograph, patient rotation affects what three things? Why are supine chest films unacceptable? Why is deep inspiration necessary on a chest film? What factors affect cardiac size?
3. Explain two ways to take an apicolordotic view of the chest.
4. Explain the different reasons and procedures for doing single exposure inspiration-expiration

sequential films and double exposure inspiration-expiration chest films.
5. List the two types of contrast media used in bronchography. Explain the advantages and disadvantages of both. How is contrast material removed?
6. List and describe the three most commonly used procedures for introduction of the contrast medium for bronchography.
7. What are three types of lung abscesses? What are these types of abscesses caused by? What happens when the patient coughs up sputum? What will the chest radiograph show?
8. What are the causes of asthma? How does air get trapped in the lung? Describe the radiographic appearance of the lungs and diaphragm.
9. Define and describe atelectasis. What does the radiograph look like? Why? What happens if only a portion of the lung is affected? What are causes of atelectasis?
10. List the three types of metastatic carcinoma of the lung. Describe the appearance of each.
11. Define emphysema. What is usually associated with this disease? What is emphysema characterized by? What manifestations will the patient present with? What must the radiographer be aware of when taking a chest radiograph? Why is this disease known as the "leather lung" disease?
12. List the two types of emphysema. Explain what each is, what the manifestations are, what the cause is, and what the radiographic appearance is. Which is more common?

13. Define pleural effusion. What happens as fluid builds up? Explain how the opposite lung will be affected and why?

14. What does pulmonary edema mean? Explain the classic radiographic sign.

15. List and describe the five types of pneumonia. What is the cause of each, what happens to the bronchi, and what are the radiographic appearances of each?

16. Pulmonary emboli are best demonstrated by what modality? What is the radiographic appearance? What may the overall radiographic appearance of pulmonary emboli mimic? What is the differentiating characteristic? Which pulmonary embolus has this characteristic?

17. Define pneumothorax. Explain how a tension pneumothorax occurs. What does a tension pneumothorax result in? What is a pseudopneumothorax and what causes it? Describe how the chest radiographs should be done to rule out a pneumothorax and explain why.

18. What is the cause and significance of respiratory distress syndrome of the newborn?

19. What causes tuberculosis? How is it spread? Define primary and reactivation tuberculosis.

20. List and describe three types of pneumoconioses.

21. Define each of the following:

Bronchitis	Bronchiectasis
Croup	Cystic fibrosis
Empyema	Hamartoma
Hydatid disease	Thymoma
Teratoma	Pleurisy
Pneumomediastinum	

22. Look at a normal posteroanterior chest radiograph. Identify the following:

apex	trachea
carina	costophrenic angle
diaphragm	cardiophrenic angle
left and right main bronchi	

CHAPTER IX

Circulatory and Lymph Systems

Goals

1. To review the basic anatomy and physiology of the circulatory system and the lymph system.
2. To become acquainted with the pathophysiology of the circulatory system and the lymph system.
3. To become familiar with the radiographic manifestations of all the common congenital and acquired disorders of the circulatory system.
4. To learn the congenital and acquired disorders of the lymph system.

Objectives

At the completion of the chapter, the radiographer will be able to:

1. Describe the internal anatomy of the heart.
2. List the components of the lymph system.
3. Describe the physiology of the circulatory system.
4. Describe the physiology of the lymph system.
5. Describe the various pathologic conditions affecting the circulatory system and their radiographic manifestations.
6. List and define the important pathology of the lymph system.
7. Describe the special radiographic examinations of the circulatory system.
8. Describe the special radiographic examinations of the lymph system.
9. Define terminology relating to the circulatory system.
10. Define terminology relating to the lymph system.

ANATOMY

Circulatory System

The circulatory system is made up of the heart, arteries, arterioles, capillaries, venules, and veins. The heart, a muscular organ, lies in the middle mediastinum with two thirds of it to the left of the midline. It is shaped like a closed fist or inverted cone. The apex of the heart is the rounded tip that is pointed down, to the left, and anteriorly. The base is the large end that points up, to the right, and posteriorly.

The heart has four chambers: the right and left atria found at the base, and the right and left ven-

tricles found near the apex. Each of these chambers is separated by a septum. The interatrial septum is between the two atria, and the interventricular septum is located between the two ventricles.

The heart has 11 openings. Those openings are the right and left atrioventricular opening, the pulmonary opening, the aortic opening, the superior vena cava and inferior vena cava openings, two left and two right pulmonary vein openings, and the coronary sinus opening. Some of the openings have valves within them to prevent retrograde blood flow. There are four that should be known by all radiographers. The left atrioventricular valve, also known as the mitral or bicuspid valve, is located in the opening between the left atrium and ventricle and has two cusps (flaps). The right atrioventricular valve, or tricuspid valve, has three flaps and is found between the right atrium and ventricle. The aortic semilunar valve, located between the left ventricle and the aorta, has three cusps, as does the pulmonary valve, which is found at the pulmonary opening between the right ventricle and the pulmonary trunk.

There are other valves in a few of the remaining openings, but they are not listed here because of their nonfunctional status.

The wall of the heart is made of three separate layers. The endocardium is the lining, the myocardium is the middle muscular layer, and the epicardium is the outer covering. The epicardium is actu-

ally the visceral layer of a membrane known as the pericardium. There is another layer to the pericardium called the parietal layer. This is what makes up the sac in which the heart is located. Figure 9–1 shows the chambers and the valves of the heart. Also seen are the layers of the wall of the heart.

The thick-walled tubes that carry blood away from the heart are the arteries. Arteries are named either for their location or according to direction of blood flow. The major trunk arteries are the aorta, which is to the left of the midline and sends blood to the body tissues, and the pulmonary artery, which arises from the right ventricle of the heart and supplies the lungs with blood. The various ar-

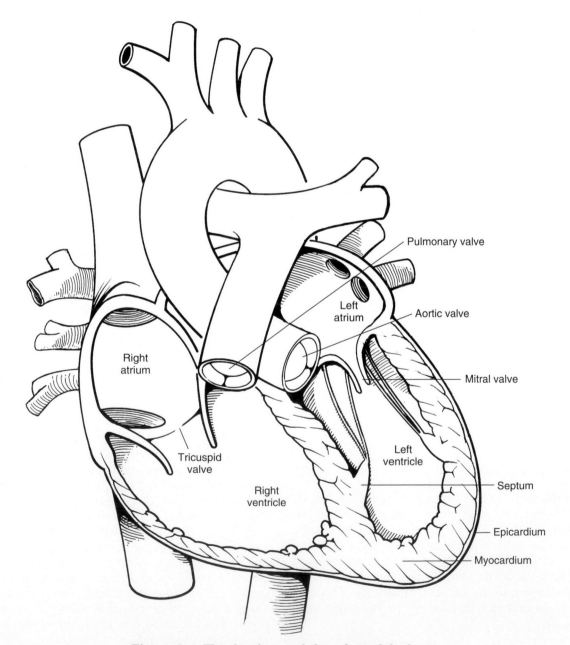

Figure 9–1. The chambers and the valves of the heart.

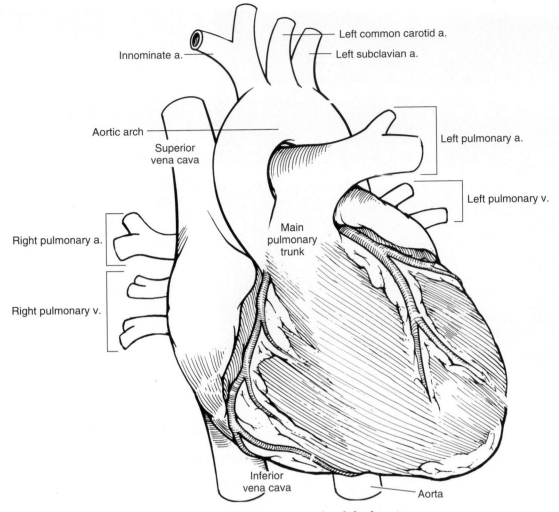

Innominate a.
Left common carotid a.
Left subclavian a.
Aortic arch
Superior vena cava
Left pulmonary a.
Left pulmonary v.
Main pulmonary trunk
Right pulmonary a.
Right pulmonary v.
Inferior vena cava
Aorta

Figure 9–2. The great vessels of the heart.

teries end with short narrow vessels that are found in all tissue supplied by blood. These are called arterioles. From arterioles, the vessels become simple endothelial tubes known as capillaries. These are the minute structures that form the transition from artery to vein. From the capillary system, the vessels again become larger to form the venules, which are the counterpart to the arterioles. Venules converge to form veins, which bring blood back to the heart. The major trunk veins are the superior and inferior venae cavae, which drain the upper and lower body respectively, and the four pulmonary veins, which drain the lungs. Both venae cavae terminate in the right atrium, and all four pulmonary veins empty into the left atrium. Figure 9–2 shows the great vessels of the heart.

Lymph System

The lymph system is considered along with the circulatory system because it comprises lymph and

tissue fluid obtained from blood. The lymph organs consist of the spleen, the thymus, and the tonsils and adenoids. The largest is the spleen, which is located in the left upper quadrant of the abdomen between the stomach and the diaphragm.

The spleen is a highly vascular organ that is composed of splenic pulp encapsulated by connective and muscular tissue. White splenic pulp is made up of lymphatic nodules and diffuse lymphatic tissue that cover the arteries of the spleen. Red splenic pulp is made up of lymphatic tissue that is permeated with sinusoids and flooded with blood.

A blood-forming organ early in life, the spleen is a site for the storage of red corpuscles. It is an important part of the defense system as it has a plethora of blood-filtering macrophages.

The thymus is located in the superior mediastinum, extending upward into the lower portion of the neck, almost to the level of the thyroid. The thymus is relatively large in infants (Fig. 9–3) and

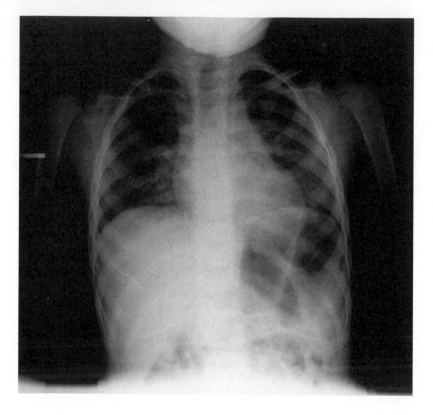

Figure 9–3. Enlarged thymus, which is normal on small children.

continues to grow until puberty. After that, the gland atrophies so that by old age the gland has almost disappeared.

The tonsils and adenoids are small, round masses of lymphoid tissue. They are covered with a mucous membrane. The tonsils are located at the back of the throat (palatine tonsils) and at the base of the tongue (lingula tonsils). The adenoids are actually the pharyngeal tonsils and are located at the back of the roof of the pharynx.

The lymphatic vessels begin as lymphatic capillaries and form a vast network. Every tissue supplied by blood vessels (with the exception of the placenta and brain) has lymphatic vessels. As the capillaries join other lymph vessels, they become progressively larger. These are known as lymphatics. Resembling the venous circulation, the lymphatics are the collecting vessels of the lymph system. They send the lymph fluid through round or oval bodies located in the path of the lymphatics. These bodies are the lymph nodes and are found grouped together by the areas of the body being drained.

As the lymphatics collect lymph from the body, they empty into the right lymphatic duct (which eventually drains into the right subclavian vein) and the thoracic duct. As the major vessel of the lymphatic system, the thoracic duct drains lymph from the rest of the body and empties into the left subclavian vein.

PHYSIOLOGY AND FUNCTION

Circulatory System

The function of the circulatory (cardiovascular) system is to transport blood. To do this, two separate systems are required. The pulmonary system carries blood from the heart to the lungs and back to the heart. The systemic system takes blood from the heart to the body and back to the heart. The trip through the liver to become detoxified is the portal system. The circulation through the heart is the cardiac system. Both the portal and cardiac systems are parts of the systemic circulation.

Pulmonary Circulation

Unoxygenated blood flows through the superior and inferior venae cavae and dumps into the right atrium. By passing through the tricuspid valve, blood flows into the right ventricle. As can be seen in Figures 9–1 and 9–2, the pulmonary trunk originates off the right ventricle and divides into two main branches, the right and left pulmonary arteries. Blood must be pumped through the pulmonary valve into the main pulmonary artery and into the right and left pulmonary arteries. These arteries send blood into the respective lungs, with 60 percent of the blood being sent to the right side and 40 percent of the blood going to the left side. After entering the lungs, the blood receives oxygen in the capillaries that surround the alveoli and returns to the heart through the right and left pulmonary veins. At this point, systemic circulation begins.

Systemic Circulation

The left atrium receives oxygenated blood from the pulmonary veins and sends it through the mitral valve into the left ventricle. The ascending aorta originates off the left ventricle, passes posterior to the main pulmonary vein and anterior to the right pulmonary vein. Superior to this, the aortic arch has three major branches. The brachiocephalic artery is also known as the innominate artery. The left common carotid and the left subclavian artery are the other two branches. The right common carotid artery does not originate off the aortic arch but rather is a branch of the innominate artery.

The left ventricle pumps blood through the aortic valve into the ascending aorta to the arch. At this point, a portion of the blood flows through the three major branches of the arch to supply the upper body with oxygenated blood. The remaining portion of blood flows through the descending aorta to reach the lower body. At about the level of L-4, the abdominal aorta bifurcates into the right and left common iliac arteries. Each common iliac artery descends and divides into the internal and external iliac arteries. Branches from these arteries supply the pelvic organs and muscles. Within the capillaries of each structure of the body, blood releases its vital oxygen and then drains from the body part into either the superior or inferior vena cava. These two veins return venous blood back to the right atrium of the heart, thus completing the systemic circulation.

Portal Circulation

Blood in the vessels of the abdominal digestive organs must go through portal circulation. Blood from veins in the visceral walls and the visceral organs, including the gallbladder, pancreas, spleen, stomach, and intestines, is carried to the liver by the portal vein. Nutrients that are carried to the liver are stored after conversion for later use by body tissues. The hepatic veins carry the blood from the liver to the inferior vena cava, which drains the blood into the right atrium. The blood is now ready for pulmonary circulation.

Lymph System

The lymph system as a whole has a major role in immunity. It moves lymph fluid in a closed circuit with the cardiovascular system. Lymphocytes and antibodies are produced; fat and fat-soluble substances from the intestinal tract are absorbed; phagocytosis is initiated as appropriate; and blood is manufactured when other sources are compromised.

The chief functions of the spleen are the formation of lymphocytes, monocytes, and plasma cells (hematopoiesis); phagocytosis; and the storage of red blood corpuscles. Although the spleen is an extremely useful organ, it can be removed with no detrimental effects.

The lymphatic tissue of the thymus gland helps to produce lymphocytes (T-cells and B-cells), which work to destroy foreign organisms.

The tonsils filter out bacteria and other foreign matter and play a role in the formation of lymphocytes.

The lymph vessels collect protein and water, which are continually filtered out of the blood. Lymph nodes filter out bacteria, particles, or other foreign bodies to remove these from the blood.

SPECIAL RADIOGRAPHIC PROCEDURES

On a normal posteroanterior view of the chest, the right heart border is primarily the right atrium and the lower left heart border is the left ventricle. The right ventricle is seen on the normal lateral view as the anterior portion of the heart shadow. The lateral position shows the left atrium in the posterior, superior area and the left ventricle in the posterior, inferior area. Figure 9–4 demonstrates both a right anterior oblique and a left anterior oblique view. The chambers of the heart have been labeled.

A **cardiac series** is done in conjunction with fluoroscopy and includes four views: a true posteroanterior, a left lateral, a right anterior oblique with a 45-degree obliquity, and a left anterior oblique with the patient in a 60-degree oblique position. The steeper oblique position on the left anterior oblique view allows the visualization of the pulmonary window which is made up of the left bronchus, carina, and the pulmonary great vessels. Usually, barium is used to outline the esophagus to show its reference to the chambers of the heart. However, barium is not used in the left anterior oblique view, as it would obscure the pulmonary window. Through analysis of this series of films, isolated chamber enlargement can usually be identified. Fluoroscopy may be employed to visualize cardiac calcification and chamber motion. Fluoroscopy by itself is of limited value, however, in the diagnosis of heart disease.

Angiography is a general term used to describe

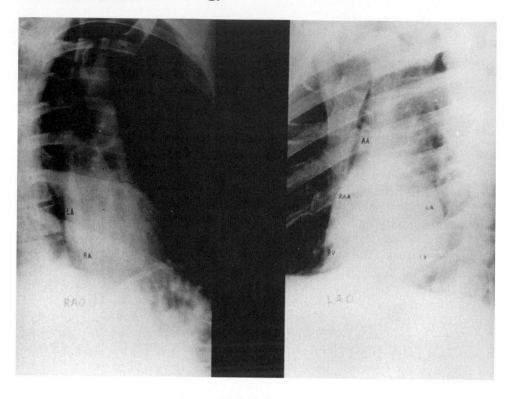

Figure 9–4. Right anterior oblique and left anterior oblique views showing the chambers of the heart.

the radiographic examination of the vessels of the body. Subcategories of angiography include **arteriography** (Fig. 9–5), which is the study of the arterial system of the body, and **venography,** which is the study of venous system. **Aortography** is the study of the thoracic or abdominal aorta (Fig. 9–6), and **angiocardiography,** also called **cardiography,** is the examination of the chambers of the heart. Under sterile technique, a catheter is fed into the femoral or brachial artery of the patient with fluoroscopic guidance. Once the radiologist has been able to place the tip of the catheter into or near the area that is to be studied, a contrast medium is injected under pressure. Radiographs are taken in a timed sequence with a rapid film changer, or more commonly, with cinefluororadiography. This allows the filming of the body part from the moment the contrast material is visualized in the arterial phase through the venous phase and dilution and excretion. The patient is constantly monitored throughout the entire procedure for any abnormal reaction or physiologic changes.

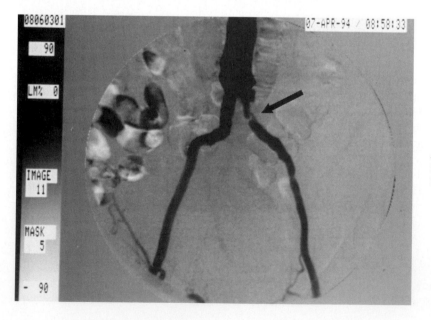

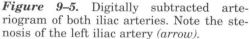

Figure 9–5. Digitally subtracted arteriogram of both iliac arteries. Note the stenosis of the left iliac artery *(arrow).*

It is not the intent of this book to describe in depth the complex procedures of angiography. There are special procedure books that devote entire chapters to that purpose, and the radiographer is encouraged to read up on the subject.

Echocardiography is the use of ultrasonography to visualize the chambers of the heart as well as the contracting and relaxation phases of the heart. Echocardiography is used to study the valves of the heart for motion or prolapse. It is also used to determine any septal defects and to evaluate pericardial effusion and atrial myxoma.

Advances in radionuclide techniques in the form of instrumentation, radiopharmaceuticals and computer applications have revolutionized the noninvasive evaluation of cardiovascular physiology and function. Examinations by **nuclear medicine** now permit the detection and diagnosis of many abnormalities as well as the functional consequences of these diseases.

Nuclear medicine is a complement study that can be in the form of a gated heart scan, which is done to watch motion of the wall of the heart. Incoming information is "gated" into specific intervals from systole to diastole using an echocardiogram. Radionuclide thallium perfusion scanning is the major noninvasive study for assessing regional blood flow to the myocardium. Radionuclide scanning using technetium pyrophosphate or other compounds that are taken up by acutely infarcted myocardium is a noninvasive technique for detecting, localizing, and classifying myocardial necrosis. Other nuclear medicine scans are done to demonstrate myocardial infarction, myocardial ischemia, pericardial effusion, and intracardiac shunts.

Lymphography is a general radiographic examination of the lymph vessels and nodes to assess the extent of lymphoma or to determine the location of obstruction or other impairment of the lymph system (Fig. 9–7). When only the lymph vessels are studied, the term **lymphangiography** is used. This is carried out within an hour of injection of the contrast agent. Delayed radiographs done 24 hours after injection are termed **lymphadenograms** and study the lymph nodes. By this time, all contrast material has left the lymph vessels. This usually occurs within several hours. Nodes, however, can retain contrast material for as long as 1 month. When the nodes are abnormal, the contrast medium can still be visualized for as long as 2 months, thus making further injection unnecessary.

Lymphography is contraindicated in those patients who have advanced stages of pulmonary disease. Because the lungs are already compromised by disease, complications can occur as they receive the overflow of oil from the contrast medium. For similar reasons, patients undergoing radiation therapy should not undergo this study. Prior to the

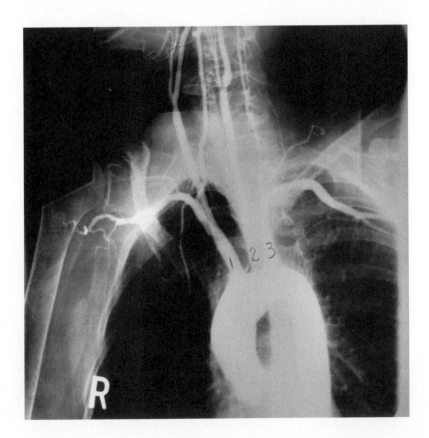

Figure 9–6. Aortography of the aortic arch and its major branches, the innominate *(1)*, left common carotid *(2)*, and left subclavian *(3)* arteries.

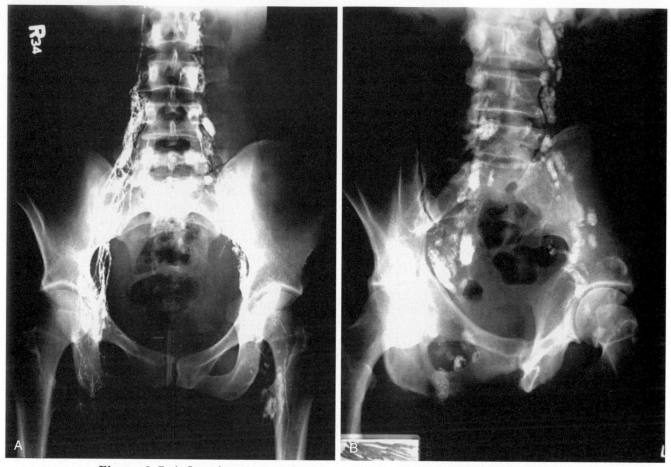

Figure 9–7. *A,* Lymphangiogram demonstrating the lymph vessels and some nodes. *B,* Same patient examined 52 days later. Lymph nodes are clearly seen.

contrast medium's being injected into the lymph vessel, a suitable vessel in the foot must be found. Because these vessels are similar to small veins in appearance, an indicator dye is used to differentiate the two. Chicago Blue 6B, Evans Blue, and Patent Blue AC are several types of indicator dyes available for this purpose. The dye is injected between the first and second toes of the foot about 15 to 20 minutes prior to the examination. This gives the dye time to infuse into the lymphatics.

Once the indicator dye colors the lymphatics, a local anesthetic is injected subcutaneously and a cutdown is made over the top of the foot. A small lymphatic vessel is isolated, dissected away from surrounding tissue, and dilated to make it large enough for cannulation. The contrast medium (Ethiodol or Lipodol) is injected with a special automatic injector that provides low, constant pressure. A total of 6 mL to 8 mL of contrast material is injected over a period of 30 minutes for each lower extremity. After the injection is completed, the needle is removed, and the overlying skin incision is closed with several sutures. The patient is still in the supine position and is now ready for filming.

PATHOLOGY

Circulatory System

Before the various pathologic conditions can be described fully, it is important to review a few terms that will be encountered throughout the study of the circulatory system.

Lipids that are deposited in the arteries cause plaque. The gradual buildup of fatty deposits (mainly cholesterol) on the inner lining of an artery wall is termed **atherosclerosis.** Atherosclerosis progressively narrows the artery, decreasing the blood flow. The process of atherosclerosis begins at an early age. Significant disease may be present in some patients before the age of 20. **Arteriosclerosis** is the hardening of the wall of the arteries, usually due to the plaque formation and calcification (Fig. 9–8). Several other conditions may arise from plaque buildup. The arteries may become narrow. This narrowing is known as **stenosis.** Changes in the wall of blood vessels such as the irregularity caused by arteriosclerosis is the major cause of an intravascular clot known as a **thrombus.**

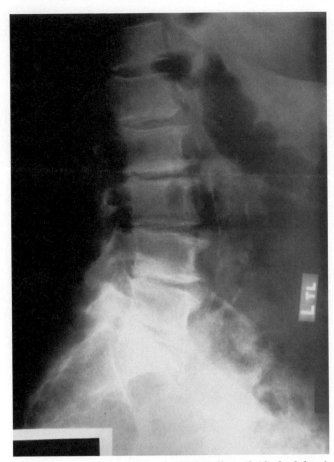

Figure 9–8. Arteriosclerosis. Partially calcified abdominal aorta caused by plaque formation.

A thrombus is a blood clot that has attached itself to the inner wall of an artery or vein. A thrombus may disintegrate spontaneously or it may require medical treatment. Two other factors lead to the development of intravascular thrombosis. Clots tend to form where blood flow is slow. Thrombi especially occur in areas of stasis in patients who are inactive or immobilized, such as after abdominal surgery. If a thrombus remains within the lumen of the vessel, it may occlude the flow of blood, cutting off oxygen that is vital to tissues. Death may result when a thrombus completely occludes a major coronary vessel or a vessel to the brain or lungs.

If one of the coronary arteries becomes completely blocked, that part of the heart muscle will die, resulting in **myocardial infarction.** The major site of involvement is the left ventricle, although some infarcts extend into the right ventricle. Symptoms of myocardial infarctions are variable. Many patients have no symptoms prior to their first myocardial infarction, although a few may experience angina.

Isolated inflammation of the heart wall can occur.

Myocarditis refers to inflammation of the myocardium, and pericarditis is inflammation of the pericardium.

When the muscle fibers stretch, causing the heart to enlarge, the process is known as **cardiac dilation.** When the heart remains enlarged because of a disease process, the term **cardiomegaly** (Fig. 9–9) is used. Shortness of breath, known as **dyspnea,** is often associated with cardiomegaly, as the heart compresses lung tissue.

Various terms are used for malposition of the organs of the body. **Dextrocardia** occurs when only the heart is located on the right side of the body (Fig. 9–10). When all the organs of the body are on the opposite side of normal, the condition is known as **situs inversus** (Fig. 9–11).

When the valves of the heart are affected by some pathologic condition such as thickening or shrinking due to infection, the term **valvular disease** is used. Valvular disease refers to valves that will not operate normally. The valve may be **incompetent,** wherein the valve is normally formed but will not completely close the orifice, which allows retrograde blood flow. A valve that is considered **insufficient** is one that will not operate properly because it is deformed.

Congenital Anomalies

Only the most common congenital defects are described here. Although the radiography student should be familiar with the various conditions that can be seen on a chest radiograph, it is not the intent of this author to cover areas that are rarely seen, or that only a physician can determine.

Coarctation of the aorta is severe narrowing of the aorta (Fig. 9–12) which causes the left ventricle of the heart to suffer an increase in workload in order to push blood through a narrow passageway. The seriousness of the defect depends on the location of the constriction. If the narrowing is severe enough or complete, anastomotic vessels develop in an attempt to compensate for the inadequate blood supply to the lower portion of the body. This results in hypertension in the upper extremities and hypotension in the lower extremities.

There are two varieties of coarctation of the aorta: the adult type and the juvenile type. The most common is the adult type. In an adult, severe hypertension proximal to the coarctation results in dilation of the aortic arch. Rib-notching is an important radiographic sign of coarctation of the aorta (Fig. 9–13). The sign refers to sharply defined bony erosions along the lower margins of the ribs caused by the development of anastomotic vessels that en-

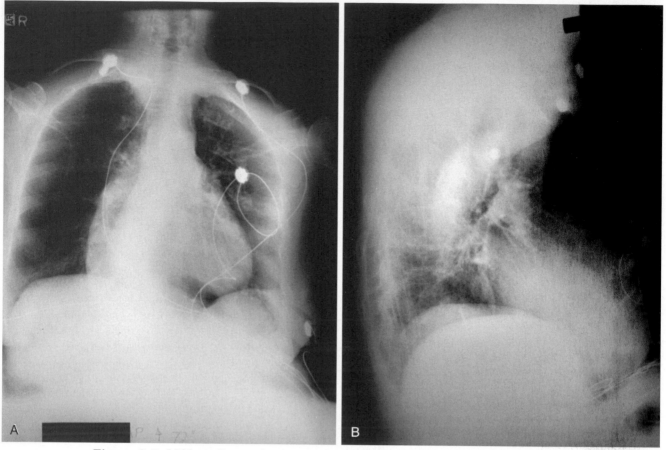

Figure 9–9. Mild cardiomegaly. Anteroposterior *(A)* and lateral *(B)* views, with the patient sitting upright on a gurney.

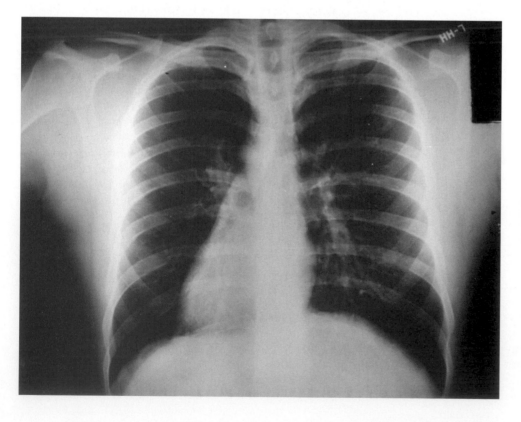

Figure 9–10. Dextrocardia. In this young male patient, only the heart is in reversed position.

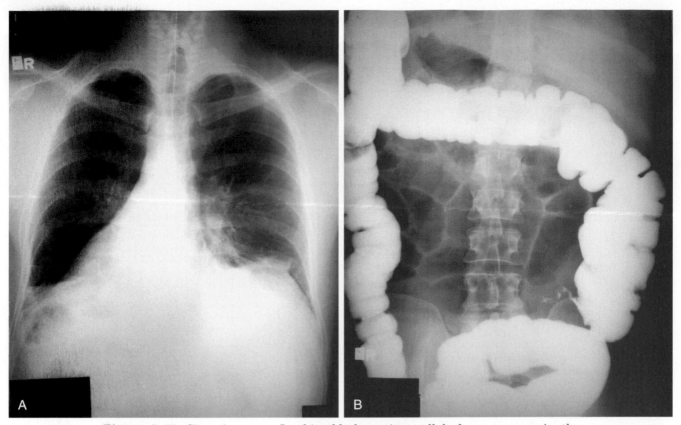

Figure 9–11. Situs inversus. In this elderly patient, all body organs are in the reversed (mirror) position. *(A),* Posteroanterior chest radiograph. *(B),* Anteroposterior barium enema. The splenic flexure on the right and the appendix on the left are positive indicators of situs inversus.

Figure 9–12. Coarctation of the aorta. There is severe narrowing of the aortic arch.

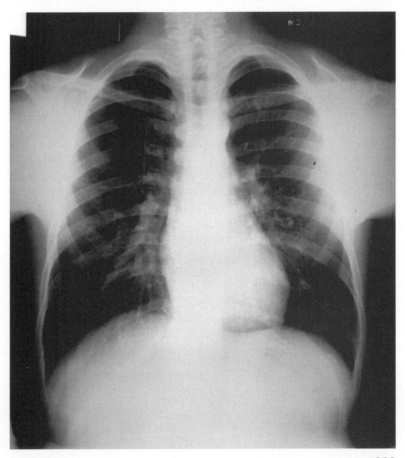

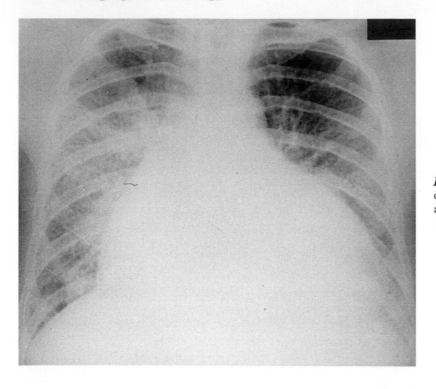

Figure 9–13. Coarctation of the aorta, demonstrating increased size of the left ventricle and rib-notching.

large under their increased volume and cause pressure erosions on the ribs.

Congenital heart abnormalities are the result of inborn defects caused by failure of the heart or major blood vessels near the heart to develop normally during the growth period before birth. The most common type of congenital abnormalities are those in which holes in the heart wall occur. These are known as **shunts** and allow pulmonary and systemic blood to mix. Blood is shunted from the systemic circulation (high pressure) to the pulmonary circulation (low pressure). This causes the lungs to become overloaded with blood. Three major types of shunts are discussed.

Septal defects are small openings in the septum of the heart. Openings in the septum between the two atria are known as **atrial septal defects** and are the most common congenital defect of the heart (Fig. 9–14). Such a defect permits blood flow to mix between the two atria. This is a left-to-right shunt because the pressure is higher in the left atrium than it is in the right atrium. Pulmonary blood flow is increased because of this type of shunt. In addition to overloading the pulmonary bed, the right ventricle experiences an overload. This produces a radiographic appearance of enlargement of the right ventricle and right atrium.

If the defect occurs between the two ventricles, it is known as a **ventricular septal defect.** This defect is more serious than an atrial septal defect because there is a greater pressure difference between the two ventricles than between the two

atria. Some blood flows from the left ventricle to the right ventricle (left-to-right shunt), forcing both ventricles to pump the same blood more than once. The shunting of blood from the left to the right ventricle occurs during systole because of the higher pressure in the ventricle during that phase. The radiograph shows enlargement of the left side of the heart. Usually patients are asymptomatic except for a heart murmur in the first weeks of life. If the septal opening is large, symptoms can be severe. Breathing is rapid; growth is retarded; and the infant has feeding difficulties.

The third major type of left-to-right shunt is **patent arterial duct,** which exists when the arterial duct in a newborn fails to close after birth. The arterial duct is a vessel that extends from the bifurcation of the pulmonary artery to join the aorta just distal to the left subclavian artery. It serves to shunt blood from the pulmonary artery into the systemic circulation during intrauterine life. If it does not close soon after birth, blood will continue to flow through the duct during systole and diastole. Some oxygenated blood is passed back and forth to the lungs instead of going through the aorta to the body. The heart will be overworked in an attempt to balance the supply with the demand for oxygen. Since the heart depends on the lungs for its supply of oxygen, the lungs become overworked in their effort to keep pace with oxygen demands and breathing becomes dyspneic on slight exertion, with resultant fatigue. Chest radiographs demonstrate enlargement of the left atrium and left ventricle

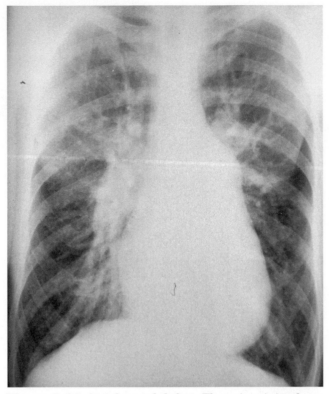

Figure 9–14. Atrial septal defect. There is minimal cardiac enlargement. There is a small aortic knob and large pulmonary arterial vascularity throughout both lungs.

ventricles, arising at a point over the ventricular septal defect. It receives blood from both ventricles, which is a mixture of both oxygenated and unoxygenated blood.

When the right ventricle enlarges, it causes the apex of the heart to become displaced upward and laterally. This is the classic radiographic appearance known as "coeur en sabot." It resembles the curved-toe portion of a wooden shoe (Fig. 9–15). Clinical manifestations include clubbing of fingers and toes, systolic murmurs, and retardation of growth. Corrective surgery is performed after the infant reaches 1 year of age.

Inflammatory and Degenerative Processes

An **aneurysm** is the most common disease, along with atherosclerosis, to affect the adult aorta. An aneurysm is a dilatation of an artery and may be one of three types. A **saccular aneurysm** (Fig. 9–16) is a localized outpouching of one side of the vessel wall, usually located in the cerebral arteries, but it may be in the distal abdominal aorta. A **fusiform** aneurysm is a uniform dilatation of the entire portion of the artery (Fig. 9–17). Such aneurysms are usually found in the distal abdominal

and increased vascular congestion. If the opening does not close within a few weeks of birth, it must be surgically closed.

Tetralogy of Fallot occurs when four conditions exist simultaneously, (*tetra* comes from the Greek word meaning four). There must be pulmonary stenosis, a ventricular septal defect, right ventricle enlargement, and displacement to the right of the aorta or overriding of the aorta above the ventricular septal defect. This combination of defects causes the blood to be unoxygenated, as it does not flow through the pulmonary system. Pulmonary stenosis impedes the outflow of blood from the right ventricle into the pulmonary circulation, causing obstruction of the pulmonary valve. This, in turn, causes an elevation of pressure in the right ventricle and hypertrophy of that chamber as it overworks to pump the blood through the narrow pulmonary valve. Because of the narrowing of the valve, an inadequate amount of blood reaches the lungs to be oxygenated. The ventricular septal defect allows unoxygenated blood in the right ventricle to mix with oxygenated blood in the left ventricle, producing a right-to-left shunt, thus decreasing the amount of oxygen the aorta carries to the body tissues. This gives rise to extreme cyanosis and is the most common cause of "blue baby." The overriding aorta straddles the

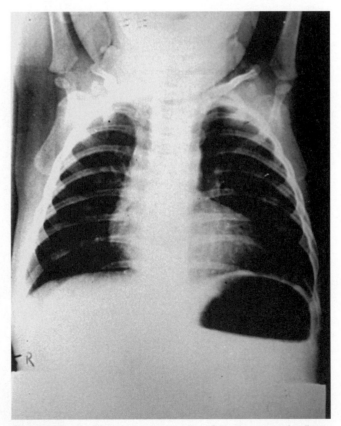

Figure 9–15. Classic appearance of "coeur en sabot" resulting from tetralogy of Fallot.

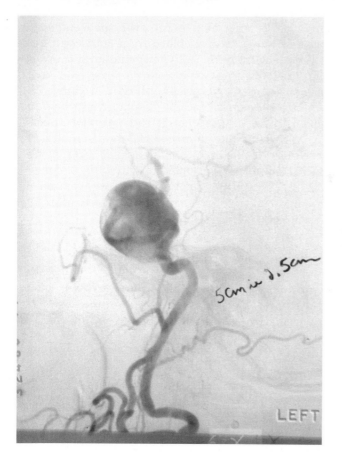

Figure 9–16. Large saccular aneurysm of the common carotid artery.

Figure 9–17. Huge fusiform aneurysm of the lowermost abdominal aorta and left common iliac artery. The abdominal aneurysm measured 16 cm in the craniocaudal dimension and 8.5 cm in the transverse dimension. The iliac aneurysm measured 7 cm in the craniocaudal and 3 cm in the transverse dimensions.

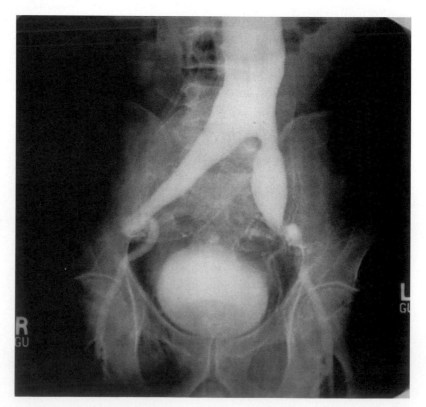

aorta. The third type is known as a **dissecting aneurysm.** This occurs when a hemorrhage occurs between the layers of the wall of the artery. Approximately 75 percent of these aneurysms are found in the arch. Dissecting aneurysms can take on the appearance of a fusiform type as the dissection causes progressive widening of the aortic shadow. The danger of an aneurysm is its tendency to increase in size and to rupture, leading to massive hemorrhage that may be fatal if it involves a critical organ such as the brain. Angiography is the modality of choice to diagnose aneurysms. When a dissecting aneurysm is present, arteriography is used to define the site of extravasation and the extent of the dissection (Fig. 9–18). Ultrasonography is also used, especially if the injection of contrast medium under pressure is determined to be detrimental to the patient. However, if the aneurysm is located within the thoracic cavity, computed tomography may be used if aortography is not indicated.

Atherosclerosis is the major cause of vascular disease. Arteries become narrowed from the plaque buildup. As stated earlier, the plaque can eventually occlude the arteries completely. Plaque formation and stenosis often involve the coronary arteries, causing **arteriosclerotic heart disease** (Figs. 9–19 and 9–20). Arteriosclerotic heart disease is also known as **cardiovascular disease.** It remains the leading cause of death in the United States despite declining mortality rates since the 1960s. In 1992, more than two out of every five deaths were the result of major cardiovascular disease. Coronary artery bypass grafting (CABG) remains among the most frequently performed surgical procedures and will continue to remain so because of hypertension.

Hypertension accelerates the development of atherosclerotic plaques, so it is often found in conjunction with arteriosclerotic heart disease. If enough plaque finally accumulates, the myocardium is damaged. Continual plaque buildup results in a myocardial infarction. Mild cardiomegaly as well as calcification in the coronary arteries can be seen on the radiograph.

Percutaneous transluminal angioplasty with the use of a balloon catheter is now a recognized procedure for the alleviation of symptoms in patients with arteriosclerosis. It is of special value in patients who are extremely ill and in those who would not benefit from arterial surgery.

When the heart cannot supply enough blood at a sufficient rate to meet the metabolic requirements of tissue, **congestive heart failure** results. This can be caused by damage from a heart attack, cardiovascular disease, hypertension, or infection to the heart muscle and damage to the valves. It may affect either the right or left side of the heart. One side of the heart fails while the othe side continues its normal output. When this occurs, there is increased pressure in the pulmonary or systemic veins, or both, resulting in "backing up" of blood. Congestive heart failure is commonly accompanied by pleural effusion. Diffuse cardiomegaly is the classic radiographic sign of congestive heart failure.

Congestive heart failure is divided into left and right heart failure, although both commonly occur together. When there is left heart failure, the left ventricle does not pump a volume of blood equal to that of the venous return in the right ventricle. As fluid builds up, a point is reached at which it has nowhere to go but the alveoli and bronchial tree of the lungs. This produces rales and pulmonary edema. As a result, breathing may become more difficult, and the patient tires easily. Left-sided heart failure is usually caused by hypertension, but can result from coronary heart disease or valvular disease. The radiographs show a congested hilar region of the lungs with increased vascular markings. Left heart failure may lead to right heart failure because increased pressure is transmitted through the pulmonary circulation to the right heart.

Right-sided heart failure causes dilation of the right ventricle and right atrium. The transmission of increased pressure can cause dilation of the superior vena cava, widening of the right superior mediastinum, and edema of the lower extremities. The enlargement of a congested liver may elevate the right hemidiaphragm. Right-sided heart failure can be caused by pulmonary valvular stenosis, emphysema, or pulmonary hypertension resulting from pulmonary emboli. Normally, in a view of the patient in the erect position, the pulmonary vessels in the lower lung zones are larger than those in the apices. With severe pulmonary venous hypertension, there is a redistribution of flow so that vessels in the upper zones are larger than those in the lower lung zones. This change is referred to as "cephalization" of pulmonary blood flow. The chest radiograph of a person with congestive heart failure shows a pulmonary vascular shift, an increase in heart size and, more importantly, "cephalization," which is the hallmark on the radiograph (Fig. 9–21).

The most common cause of congestive heart failure in the older adult is **hypertensive heart disease.** As its name implies, hypertension is a major cause of this disease. High blood pressure over a long period of time causes narrowing of the systemic blood vessels, creating resistance to blood flow. Because of this resistance, the left ventricle must work harder, causing dilation and enlargement of the ventricle. There is often downward displacement of the apex of the heart (Fig. 9–22). Failure of the

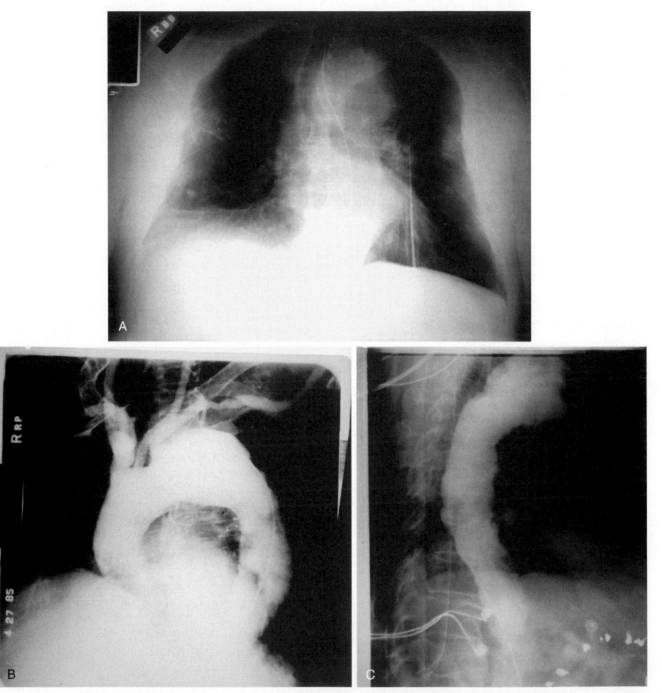

Figure 9–18. Dissecting aneurysm of the aorta. *A,* Chest radiograph shows a large "mass" on left, superior to the heart, that is causing the trachea to become deviated. *B,* Angiogram showing that the "mass" is actually a large dissecting aneurysm of the aortic arch. *C,* Dissecting aneurysm of the thoracic aorta. Note the ragged edges. This is an indication of the hemorrhage between the intima.

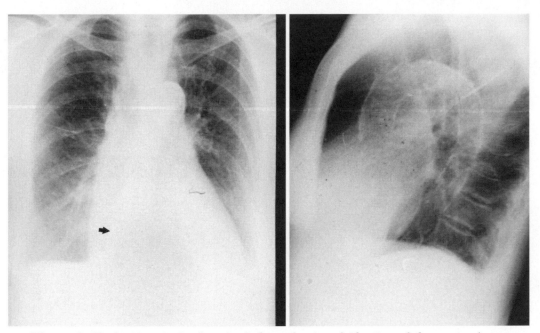

Figure 9–19. Aortic arteriosclerosis. *Left,* moderate calcification of the aorta. Arrow points to the true heart border. *Right,* Lateral view shows marked calcification of the entire aortic arch and thoracic aorta.

Figure 9–20. Arteriosclerotic heart disease with a left ventricular aneurysm.

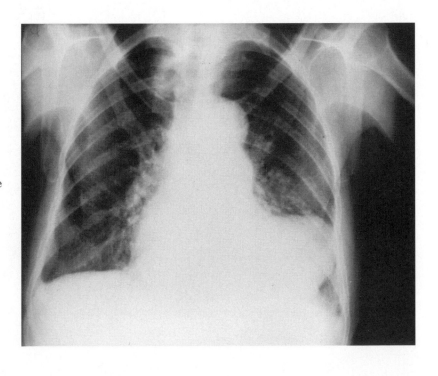

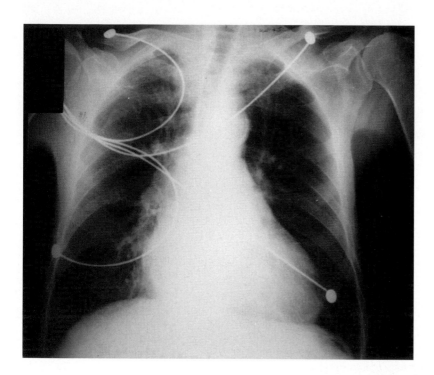

Figure 9–21. Congestive heart failure. Note the cephalization and increased heart size.

Figure 9–22. Hypertensive heart disease. Enlargement of left ventricle by lengthening. The left apex is beneath the diaphragm.

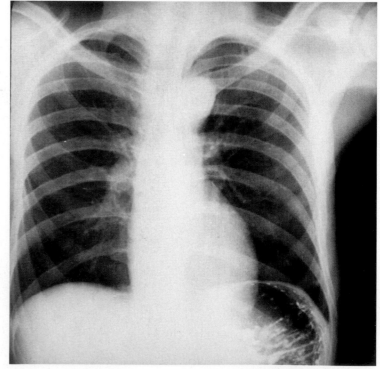

left ventricle leads to increased pulmonary venous pressure and congestive failure. Radiographic signs and symptoms are the same as for congestive heart failure (Fig. 9–23).

Hypertrophy of the separate chambers of the heart may help pinpoint other pathologic processes that are not yet obvious. **Right atrial enlargement** is recognized radiographically by enlargement of the cardiac shadow to the right of the thoracic spine in the frontal view. Malrotation of the patient, scoliosis, or mediastinal shift must be excluded before the appearance can be attributed to right atrial enlargement. Although isolated right atrial enlargement is uncommon, it can be caused by subacute bacterial endocarditis or atrial septal defect.

Right ventricular enlargement is recognized radiographically by encroachment of the cardiac shadow into the retrosternal space on the lateral projection. This is an imprecise indicator, however, owing to the variability of the size of this space. The right ventricle works harder and enlarges in the presence of defects of the pulmonary vascular bed, as with cor pulmonale and pulmonary hypertension. **Cor pulmonale** (see Chapter 8) is the enlargement of the right ventricle secondary to pulmonary malfunction. Usually chronic, but occasionally acute, cor pulmonale results from chronic obstructive pulmonary disease. The alterations in the pulmonary circulation lead to pulmonary arterial hypertension, which imposes a mechanical load on right ventricular emptying. Right ventricular en-

largement is usually associated with right atrial enlargement.

Enlargement of the **left atrium** is seen radiographically as a rounded opacity in the retrocardiac region projecting to the left and right of the spine on the posteroanterior view. The left atrium enlarges in rheumatic heart disease with mitral stenosis or mitral insufficiency.

Finally, **left ventricle enlargement** is demonstrated by the cardiac shadow to the left of the spine, often with a rounded lateral contour projecting below the diaphragm. The left ventricle works harder and longer with each beat when it meets increased resistance to the emptying of blood into the systemic circulation, as occurs with aortic stenosis, volume overload, and systemic hypertension. The ventricle hypertrophies because of the extra exercise, and sometimes it becomes displaced laterally.

Pericardial effusion is fluid in the pericardial sac. Causes of this condition are tuberculosis and viral infection but not myocardial infarction. When there is a rapid increase in heart size seen on the chest films without other signs of heart failure, pericardial effusion should be suspected. An excellent method of demonstrating pericardial effusion is echocardiography. As little as 50 mL of fluid can be detected by this modality, whereas at least 200 mL of fluid must be present before a pericardial effusion can be detected on a radiograph (Fig. 9–24).

The cause of rheumatic fever is unknown, but the attacks are preceded by streptococcal infection.

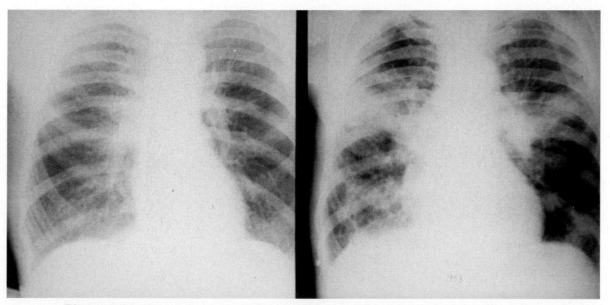

Figure 9–23. Hypertensive heart disease with pulmonary edema. *Left,* No discernible pathology. *Right,* 3 years later, progressive cardiac enlargement is evident. Note the asymmetry of the pulmonary edema.

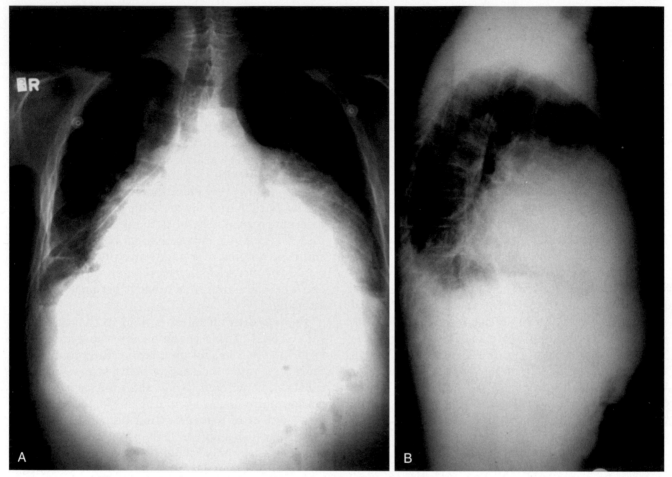

Figure 9–24. Anteroposterior *(A)* and lateral *(B)* views, demonstrating massive heart size caused by pericardial effusion.

Even though the occurrance of rheumatic fever has dropped dramatically because of the antibodies used to fight streptococcal infection, it is still the most common cause of severe valvular dysfunction. The result of one or more episodes of rheumatic fever causes inflammation of the heart valves rather than the myocardium and leads to scarring deformity of the valves known as **rheumatic heart disease** (RHD). Mitral stenosis is the most common heart abnormality of RHD.

At variable times following acute illness, chronic damage to heart valves may become evident. The functional valve damage is produced by stenosis of the valve opening or valvular insufficiency or both. Fibrosis of the mitral valve, the valve most commonly involved, usually leads to left heart failure. The left heart failure results either from backup of blood into the lungs caused by stenosis or from regurgitation of blood back through the insufficient valve. Stenosis and insufficiency of the aortic valve, the other commonly affected valve, cause left ventricular hypertrophy and eventually heart failure (Fig. 9–25).

In addition to heart failure, the valves may be-

come infected, producing infective endocarditis. Calcification of the mitral valve seen on the chest film is one indication of rheumatic heart disease (Fig. 9–26). Kerley B lines are often present (see Fig. 9–25). These lines eventually become permanent.

Subacute bacterial endocarditis (SBE) is caused by organisms living on the heart valves and producing an inflammatory reaction. Bacteria are the most common cause, hence the name bacterial endocarditis. Rheumatic valvulitis is the most common predisposing factor to the development of subacute bacterial endocarditis. Early diagnosis results in treatment that reduces the amount of damage, but the severity of this pathologic process should not be overlooked. The most striking feature of the disease is the formation of large numbers of emboli because of the breaking off of fragments of the vegetations. These travel in the blood stream and stick in various organs where they give rise to some of the characteristic symptoms of the disease.

Lymph System

Because the lymph system has no pumping mechanism of its own, it must depend on the cardiovascu-

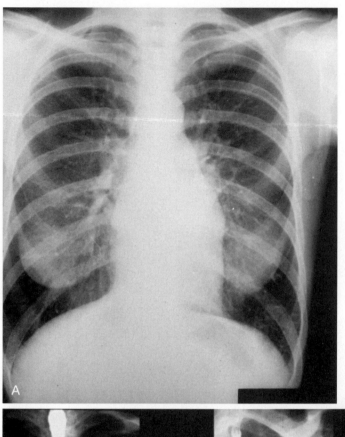

Figure 9–25. Rheumatic heart disease with mitral stenosis. *A,* Bulging of left atrium along left cardiac border. Kerley B lines are evident in the basilar region. *B,* Left, frontal view of a barium swallow. Center, right anterior oblique view visualizes pressure on the esophagus from the enlarged left atrium. Right, left anterior oblique view shows the left atrium appendage projecting behind the esophagus *(arrows).*

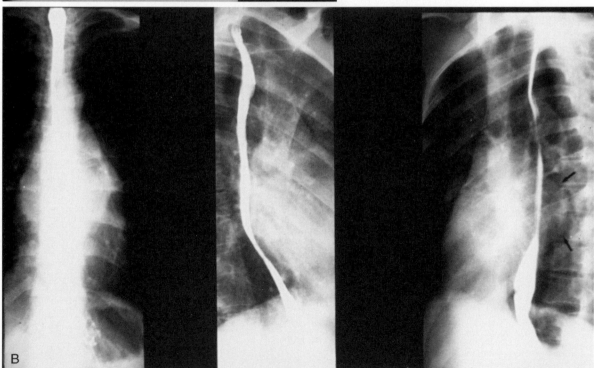

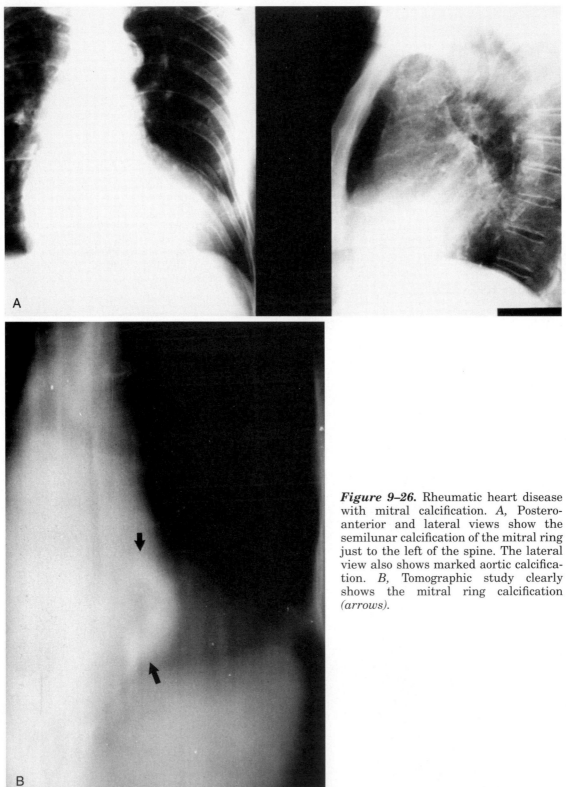

Figure 9–26. Rheumatic heart disease with mitral calcification. *A,* Postero-anterior and lateral views show the semilunar calcification of the mitral ring just to the left of the spine. The lateral view also shows marked aortic calcification. *B,* Tomographic study clearly shows the mitral ring calcification *(arrows).*

lar system for much of its transport. When compared with blood, lymph is sluggish. As lymph fluid volume increases, it flows faster in response to mounting capillary pressure. Any mechanical obstruction will slow or stop the movement of lymph, dilating the system. This is known as **lymphostasis** (Fig. 9–27). If it is obstructed, lymph fluid may diffuse into the vascular system.

Congenital Anomalies

Congenital **lymphedema** is hypoplasia and maldevelopment of the lymph system. It results in swelling and grotesque distortions of the extremities. Obstruction blocks the lymphatic ducts, which causes the edema. The skin does not pit and eventually becomes thickened and tough.

Inflammatory Processes

Acute **lymphangitis** is inflammation of lymphatic channels. It is characterized by pain and possibly fever. **Lymphadenitis** is inflammation of the lymph nodes. This inflammation is usually palpable to gentle touch as swollen lymph nodes.

When the ducts of regional lymph nodes (in particular the axillary and inguinal) have been traumatized, as in surgery, **lymphedema** may occur. As with congenital lymphedema, the overlying skin is thick and feels tough.

Neoplasms

Neoplasms of the lymph system are well-defined and solid. They are divided into Hodgkin and non-Hodgkin **lymphomas** (Fig. 9 28). Hodgkin disease is a lymphosarcoma that occurs in late adolescence and young adulthood. Males are twice as likely to be afflicted as females. There is usually a painless enlargement of the cervical lymph nodes. Occasionally, pressure of the node on other structures produces symptoms.

Splenic abnormalities are rare. When enlargement of the spleen does occur, it is usually the result of some systemic disease process and rarely from any primary splenic pathology. An example is polycystic renal disease, in which **cysts** in the spleen are often found in conjunction with the process. When cysts are found in the liver, there are usually some in the spleen as well (Fig. 9–29).

Table 9–1 summarizes the clinical and radiographic characteristics of common pathologies of the circulatory and lymph systems.

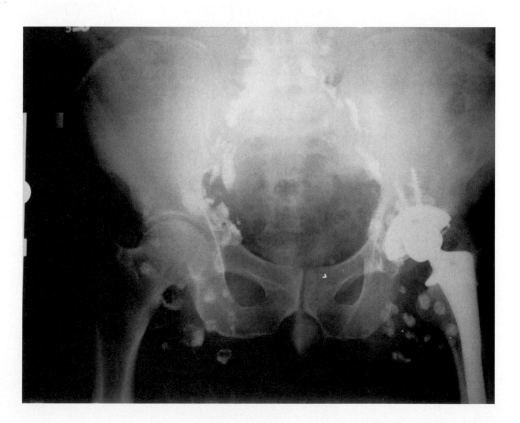

Figure 9–27. Lymphomatosis.

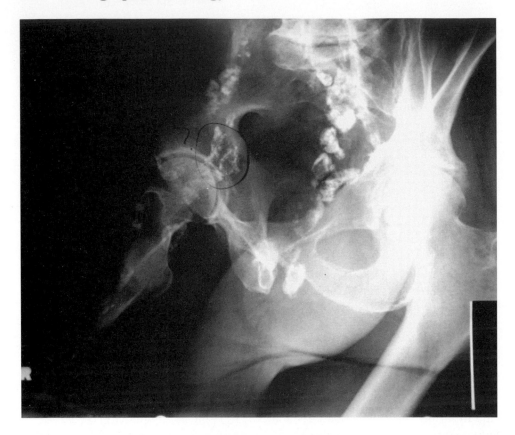

Figure 9–28. Adenoma of lymph node.

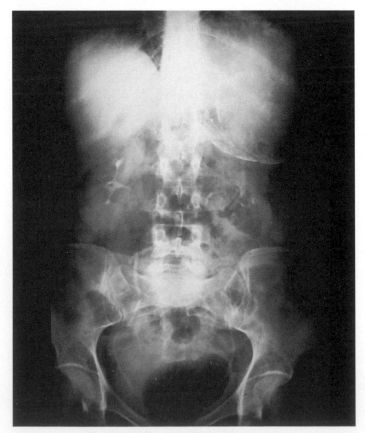

Figure 9–29. Calcified splenic cyst.

Table 9–1.
Clinical and Radiographic Characteristics of Common Pathologies

Pathologic Condition	Causal Factors*	Manifestations	Radiographic Appearance
Atherosclerosis	Early 20s, cholesterol	Narrowing of vessel	—
Arteriosclerosis	Elderly, atherosclerosis	Hardening of wall of vessel	Calcification of vessel
Coarctation of aorta	Narrowing of aorta	Hypertension or hypotension	Rib notching
Atrial septal defect	Congenital	Frequent pulmonary infections	Enlarged right atrium and right ventricle
Ventricular septal defect	Congenital	Heart murmur	Enlarged left heart
Patent arterial duct	Congenital	Asymptomatic	Enlarged left heart
Tetralogy of Fallot	Congenital	Cynosis	Coeur en sabot
Aneurysms Saccular Fusiform Dissecting	Any age, weakened vessel wall	Usually asymptomatic	Localized ballooning Uniform dilation Diffuse enlargement
Arteriosclerotic heart disease	Hypertension	Dyspnea	Calcification, cardiomegaly
Congestive heart failure	Any age (elderly), hypertension	Easy fatigue	Cephalization, cardiomegaly
Pericardial effusion	Any age, tuberculosis, virus	Usually asymptomatic	Rapid increase in heart size
Rheumatic heart disease	Unknown	Endocarditis	Calcified mitral valve, Kerley B lines

*Includes age, if relevant.

Review Questions

1. Name the four chambers of the heart and describe their locations. What is the wall between these chambers called? Name four internal valves of the heart and identify their locations. Name the layers of the heart wall in order from outermost to innermost.
2. Describe blood flow in pulmonary circulation. Describe blood flow in systemic circulation. What are two subgroups of systemic circulation?
3. Describe a cardiac series. What are the four views taken? Explain the obliquity of the patient. What is the pulmonary window? How is it seen? When is barium used and not used in this study? Why? What problem can be identified by this study?

4. Define the following terms:

   Atherosclerosis Arteriosclerosis
   Stenosis Thrombus
   Myocardial Cardiac dilation
   infarction Dyspnea
   Cardiomegaly Situs inversus
   Dextrocardia Myocarditis
   Endocarditis Valvular disease
   Pericarditis Insufficient valve
   Incompetent valve

5. Explain "rib notching." What causes it and when does it occur?
6. What are left-to-right shunts? How do the lungs become overloaded with blood in a shunt? Why is the shunt flow from left to right? Explain fully the three major types of left-to-right

shunts. Be sure to include their names, where they occur, where the blood flows, what the shunt causes, and what the radiographic appearance is.

7. Describe tetralogy of Fallot. What must exist for this condition to occur? What does this combination of defects cause? What type of shunt is produced with this condition? This condition is the most common cause of "blue baby." Why?

8. List and describe the appearance of the three types of aneurysms. What is the danger of an aneurysm?

9. What is congestive heart failure? What causes it? What happens to the heart in left-sided heart failure? What happens to the heart in right-sided heart failure? What is the radiographic appearance of each?

10. What is pericardial effusion? What causes it? When should this condition be suspected? What modality is best suited for pericardial effusion? Why is it the best?

11. How is hypertension related to atherosclerosis?

12. What are the complications of one or more episodes of rheumatic fever?

13. What causes subacute bacterial endocarditis? What is a predisposing factor?

14. Name the major components of the lymph system.

15. What is the function of the lymph system?

16. Define the following:

    Lymphostasis   Lymphangitis
    Lymphadenitis   Lymphedema

17. What is lymphography? How is it performed? What are a lymphangiogram and a lymphadenogram?

CHAPTER X

Nervous System

Goals

1. To review the basic anatomy and physiology of the central nervous system and the peripheral nervous system.
2. Describe the anatomic components of the central nervous system.
3. To review the imaging modalities for the nervous system.
4. To become familiar with the radiographic manifestations of all the common congenital and acquired disorders of the nervous system.

Objectives

At the completion of the chapter, the radiographer will be able to:

1. Describe the physiology of the nervous system.
2. Describe the anatomic components of the central nervous system.
3. Name and describe the imaging modalities for the brain and the spinal canal.
4. Define terminology relating to the skull, brain, and spinal cord.
5. Describe the various pathologic conditions affecting the skull and nervous system and their radiographic manifestations.

I. Anatomy
  A. Central Nervous System
    1. Brain
      a. Forebrain
        1. Cerebrum
        2. Diencephalon
          (Interbrain)
      b. Midbrain
        1. Mesencephalon
      c. Hindbrain
        1. Cerebellum
        2. Pons
        3. Medulla Oblongata
      d. Ventricles
        1. Lateral
        2. Third
        3. Fourth
        4. Foramen of Monro
        5. Aqueduct of Sylvius
        6. Foramen of
          Magendie
    2. Spinal Cord
      a. Meninges
        1. Dura Mater
        2. Arachnoid
        3. Pia Mater
      b. Spaces
  B. Peripheral Nervous System
    1. Cranial Nerves
    2. Spinal Nerves
  C. Autonomic Nervous System
    1. Sympathetic
    2. Parasympathetic
II. Physiology and Function
  A. Central
    1. Cerebrum
      a. Sensation
      b. Thought
      c. Memory
      d. Judgment
      e. Reason
      f. Management of
        Functions under
        Voluntary Control
    2. Midbrain
      a. Correlate Optic and
        Tactile Impulses

      b. Auditory Reflexes
      c. Regulation of Muscle
        Tone, Body Posture,
        Equilibrium
    3. Cerebellum
      a. Integration and
        Correlation of Nerve
        Impulses
    4. Medulla Oblongata
      a. Regulates Heartbeat
      b. Controls Rate of
        Breathing
      c. Regulates Diameter of
        Blood Vessels
III. Special Imaging Procedures
  A. Plain Radiography
  B. Computed Tomography
  C. Magnetic Resonance Imaging
  D. Ultrasonography
  E. Nuclear Medicine
  F. Angiography
  G. Myelography
  H. Discography
IV. Pathology
  A. Congenital Abnormalities
    1. Brain
      a. Anencephaly
      b. Microcephaly
      c. Hydrocephaly
        1. Internal
          (Noncommunicating)
        2. External
          (Communicating)
        3. Compensatory
    2. Spinal Cord
      a. Spina Bifida
        1. Spina Bifida
          Occulta
        2. Meningocele
        3. Myelocele
        4. Myelomeningocele
          a. Arnold-Chiari
            Syndrome
  B. Inflammatory Processes
    1. Abscess
      a. Epidural
      b. Brain

    2. Aneurysm
    3. Cerebrovascular Accident
      (Stroke)
      a. Ischemia
      b. Infarct
    4. Transient Ischemic Attack
    5. Empyema
    6. Encephalitis
    7. Hemorrhage (Hematoma)
      a. Subarachnoid
      b. Intracerebral
        (Intraparenchymal)
    8. Meningitis
      a. Bacterial
      b. Viral
      c. Chemical
    9. Osteomyelitis
  C. Head Injuries
    1. Concussion
    2. Contusion
    3. Fractures
      a. Linear
      b. Comminuted
      c. Depressed
      d. Basilar
    4. Hemorrhage
      a. Epidural (Extradural)
      b. Subdural
  D. Neoplasms
    1. Gliomas
      a. Astrocytoma
      b. Glioblastoma
      c. Medulloblastoma
    2. Meningiomas
    3. Pituitary Adenomas
    4. Craniopharyngiomas
    5. Pineal Tumors
      a. Teratoma
      b. Germinoma
    6. Metastatic Carcinoma
    7. Chordomas
    8. Acoustic Neuromas
  E. Spinal Cord Disease
    1. Meningiomas
    2. Neurofibromas
    3. Slipped Disc

The nervous system can be compared to a telegraph system. The brain acts as the main office and relays messages by way of the spinal cord through nerve fibers of the peripheral nervous system that radiate to every structure in the body. Sensory nerves bring information, or impulses, from the various organ systems, while motor nerves carry impulses from the central coordinating point to the muscles or glands, which need to respond so that the body can adjust for its own safety and welfare.

ANATOMY

The nervous system is divided into central, peripheral, and autonomic systems. The central nervous system includes the brain and the spinal cord; the peripheral nervous system is composed of the cranial and spinal nerves; and the autonomic nervous system comprises the sympathetic and parasympathetic systems. A subsystem of the peripheral nervous system, the autonomic nervous system is often discussed independently, as it controls and harmonizes the work of the vital organs. The nervous tissue is composed of cells and fibers of many types collected together into one central axis and many peripheral strands.

Central Nervous System

The central nervous system comprises the brain and the spinal cord together with the nerve trunks and fibers connected to them. This system is also referred to as the cerebrospinal system. The brain and spinal cord are both protected from injury by the bony components of the skull and the arched vertebrae of the dorsal body cavity.

The brain is the greatly enlarged and modified part of the central nervous system. It accounts for about 98 percent of the entire central nervous system. It contains about 11 billion neurons, which are the cells of the nervous system.

The divisions of the brain are the forebrain, consisting of the cerebrum and diencephalon; the midbrain, or mesencephalon; and the hindbrain, which is composed of the cerebellum, pons, and the medulla oblongata. The term brain stem refers to the midbrain, pons, and medulla.

The cerebrum, sometimes called the forebrain, occupies most of the brain cavity, covering all the other parts. It is divided into two hemispheres called the cerebral hemispheres. The hemispheres are arbitrarily divided into four lobes, each named after the cranial bone to which it is related: frontal, occipital, parietal, and temporal.

The diencephalon is the part of the brain between the midbrain and the cerebrum. It contains the structures called the thalamus and the hypothalamus. The cavity of this part of the brain contains the third ventricle. The midbrain, or mesencephalon, is the upper part of the brain stem, above the pons. It connects the lower brain centers to the higher centers.

The second largest division of the brain is the cerebellum, also known as the little brain. It is situated just above the medulla, which it overhangs, and beneath the rear portion of the cerebrum. The pons lies anterior to the cerebellum and between the midbrain and medulla.

The medulla oblongata is the most posterior part of the brain. It is really an extension of the spinal cord at the point where the central canal of the spinal cord enlarges to form the fourth ventricle. This large cavity secretes some of the cerebrospinal fluid and contains openings (foramina) that connect the cavity with the subarachnoid space with the lateral ventricles in the cerebral hemispheres.

The ventricles of the brain are located within the brain hemispheres and are a series of intercommunicating cavities. They contain cerebrospinal fluid and communicate with the subarachnoid space surrounding the brain and spinal cord and with the central canal of the spinal cord. The ventricular system consists of four cerebral ventricles: two lateral ventricles and two others called the third and the fourth ventricles. The two lateral ventricles are located within the right and left cerebral hemi-

spheres, while the third and fourth are midline structures.

Each lateral ventricle projects an anterior horn into the frontal lobe of the cerebrum, a posterior horn into the occipital lobe and an inferior horn into the temporal lobe. The cerebrospinal fluid is formed in the lateral ventricles, along with the third and fourth ventricles. Each lateral ventricle connects on each side with the third ventricle by a narrow channel known as the interventricular foramina (foramina of Monro).

The third ventricle is a slit-like cavity located in the midline of the skull. It lies just below the level of the bodies of the two lateral ventricles. The cavity of the third ventricle extends downward to where it widens posteriorly and laterally to form the fourth ventricle. The connection between the third and fourth ventricles is known as the aqueduct of Sylvius. The lateral openings from the fourth ventricle into the subarachnoid cistern are known as the foramina of Luschka. The fourth ventricle also connects with the subarachnoid of the cerabellomedullary cistern medially through an opening called the foramen of Magendie. Through these medial and lateral recesses, the fourth ventricle communicates with the subarachnoid spaces of the brain and spinal cord. The relationship of the ventricles to each other and to the foramina can best be understood if first visualized in the lateral aspect, as depicted by Figure 10–1. Figure 10–2 is a superior view of the ventricles and foramina, and Figure 10–3 demonstrates the ventricular system from the front as it lies within the brain tissue. Figure 10–4 is a group of pneumoencephalograms. Although this study is no longer performed, these films demonstrate the actual ventricles within the brain.

The spinal cord, lodged within the vertebral canal, is directly continuous superiorly with the medulla oblongata. It begins at the great foramen and terminates at the junction of the first and second lumbar vertebrae. The end of the spinal canal, called the cauda equina, is located from the second lumbar vertebra to the fifth vertebra.

It is through the spinal cord that the brain maintains intimate association with all the peripheral organs. This is accomplished by the attachment of 31 pairs of spinal nerves along its lateral aspects. This will be discussed further under the section on the peripheral nervous system.

Like the brain, the spinal cord has three coverings known as meninges. They are composed predominantly of white fibrous connective tissue. The dura mater is the outermost layer and is the hardest, toughest, and most fibrous of the three. The middle membrane is called the arachnoid; it is much less dense and is weblike in appearance. The

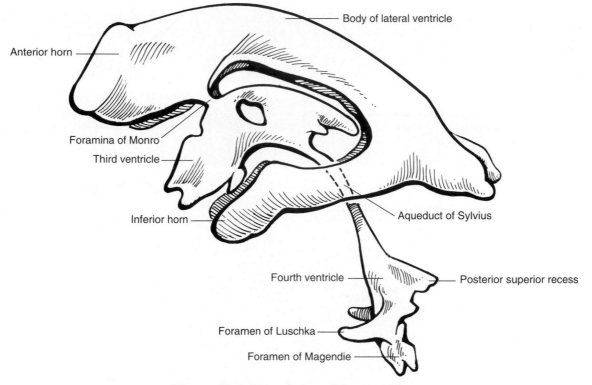

Figure 10–1. Lateral view of the ventricles.

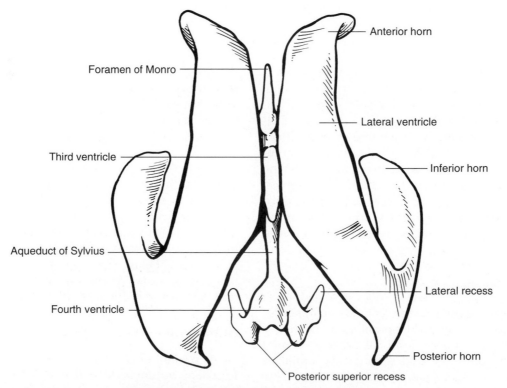

Figure 10–2. Superior view of the ventricles.

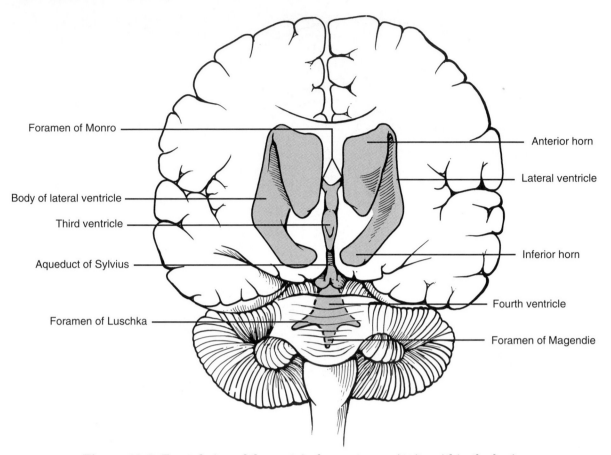

Foramen of Monro

Body of lateral ventricle

Third ventricle

Aqueduct of Sylvius

Foramen of Luschka

Anterior horn

Lateral ventricle

Inferior horn

Fourth ventricle

Foramen of Magendie

Figure 10–3. Frontal view of the ventricular system as it sits within the brain.

pia mater is the thin, compact membrane that is closely adapted to the surface of the central nervous system. The pia mater is very vascular and supplies the blood for the central nervous system. Frequently, the pia mater and arachnoid are considered as one membrane called the pia-arachnoid or leptomeninges. The space between the pia mater and the arachnoid is referred to as the subarachnoid space, and that space between the arachnoid and the dura mater is the subdural cavity. The area between the dura mater and the vertebral canal is the epidural space.

Peripheral Nervous System

The peripheral nervous system is made up of nerves outside of the brain and the spinal cord. There are 31 pairs of spinal nerves and 12 pairs of cranial nerves. Both voluntary and involuntary impulses are conveyed through these nerves.

The 12 pairs of cranial nerves are attached to the brain. Each leaves the skull through a foramen. In general, the cranial nerves are voluntary, except those going to the heart, lungs, salivary glands,

stomach, and eyes. The spinal nerves send involuntary muscle fibers to the smooth muscles of the gastrointestinal tract, genitourinary tract, and the cardiovascular system. The spinal nerves that go to the muscles of the trunk and extremities are voluntary.

The spinal nerves are attached to the spinal cord. After leaving the spinal cord, the nerves are named after their corresponding vertebra. The first eight are cervical; the next 12 are thoracic; and there are five lumbar, five sacral, and one coccygeal. The lower spinal nerves supply the lower extremities and extend below the level of the spinal cord in parallel strands, resembling a horse's tail; therefore, the group of them is called the cauda equina.

Autonomic Nervous System

As its name implies, the autonomic nervous system functions automatically. It is divided into the sympathetic and parasympathetic systems. The sympathetic portion arises from all the thoracic and the first three lumbar segments of the spinal cord. The parasympathetic portion arises from the third, sev-

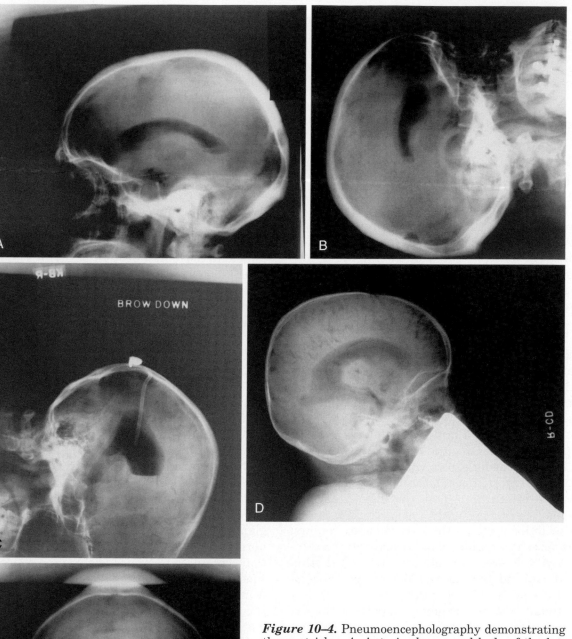

Figure 10–4. Pneumoencepholography demonstrating the ventricles. *A,* Anterior horns and body of the lateral ventricles. The third ventricle is somewhat evident as well. *B,* The anterior horn and a portion of the body of the lateral ventricles. *C,* Clear view of the posterior horn and inferior horns of the lateral ventricles. *D,* Lateral view demonstrating all portions of the lateral ventricles. *E,* Anterior horns and portions of the bodies of both lateral ventricles. The third ventricle is seen in the midline.

enth, ninth, and tenth cranial nerves and from the second, third, and fourth sacral segments of the spinal cord. The parasympathetic system is more advanced structurally and functionally than the sympathetic system.

PHYSIOLOGY AND FUNCTION

The cerebrum's functions are concerned with sensation, thought, memory, judgment, reason, and the initiation or management of the functions that are under voluntary control.

The midbrain contains the optic reflex centers and serves to correlate optic and tactile impulses. Auditory reflexes are located in the midbrain, and it is the center for regulation of muscle tone, body posture, and equilibrium.

The chief function of the cerebellum is to bring balance, harmony, and coordination to the motions of the body initiated by the cerebrum. To carry out its functions, it acts as an organ of integration and correlation of nerve impulses. It has connections with the motor neurons of the brain and spinal cord, and through these connections the muscles receive impulses to react.

The pons serves as a bridge to connect the other three parts of the brain, the cerebellum, the cerebrum, and the medulla oblongata. It is concerned with the control of facial muscles, including the muscles of mastication and the first stages of breathing.

The medulla contains three vital reflex centers: the cardiac center regulates the heartbeat; the medullary rhythmic area controls the rate and rhythm of breathing; and the vasoconstrictor center regulates the diameter of blood vessels.

The spinal cord is extremely important for the maintenance of homeostasis, as it conducts impulses in directions between the brain and the periphery. It also serves to coordinate reflexes.

The function of the autonomic nervous system is to activate the involuntary smooth and cardiac muscles and glands. It also serves the vital systems that function automatically, such as the digestive, circulatory, respiratory, urinary, and endocrine systems.

The two divisions—sympathetic and parasympathetic—oppose each other in function and thus maintain balanced activity in the body. For example, the sympathetic system dilates the pupils, and the parasympathetic system contracts them. The sympathetic system causes the blood vessels of the skin and viscera to contract so that more blood goes to the muscles where it is needed for fight or flight under stress. The parasympathetic system dilates the blood vessels when the need has passed. The sympathetic system causes contractions of the sphincters to prevent the emptying of bowels or bladder; the parasympathetic system relaxes these sphincters so that waste can be removed. Similarly, they regulate the body temperature, salivary digestive secretions, and the endocrine glands.

SPECIAL IMAGING PROCEDURES

A skull radiograph may be requested along with a cervical spine radiograph in trauma cases. It is very important that the radiographer know how to obtain excellent radiographs, even if the patient is unable to move in a desired position. The radiographer must be able to utilize his or her knowledge of the anatomy of the skull combined with tube angulation to obtain radiographs that will demonstrate the anatomy that is critical to determining any underlying pathology. Correct patient position and tube angulation is essential to avoid superimposition of anatomic features. Air-fluid levels must be demonstrated on certain radiographs. If the patient's condition does not warrant an erect film, the radiographer must be prepared to obtain cross-table lateral films with a horizontal beam. Since skull films display the calvarium but not the brain itself, pathologic processes in the brain are made apparent by their effects of the calvarium, by the presence of abnormal calcifications or fat within the brain, or by displacement of the normally calcified pineal gland or choroid plexus. A thorough knowledge of normal anatomy that is visualized in each projection is required in order to determine abnormalities. Blood vessel fissures can often look like a fracture. A calcified pineal gland is normal in 60 percent of the adult population. The sella turcica may be various shapes, but it should be symmetrical.

With **computed tomography** (CT), the brain itself can be imaged. The enhanced contrast resolution of computed tomography allows visualization of fresh blood as an opaque substance. The localization of blood may be within the brain itself, in the subdural space, within the subarachnoid cisterns, or in the epidural space. Computed tomographic scans allow evaluation of the ventricular size or an infarct as well as the presence of blood. Computed tomography of the spine offers a noninvasive technique to evaluate the vertebrae, spinal canal, and paravertebral soft tissues. A herniated disk is often shown clearly, since its density is greater than the normal contents of the spinal canal.

Magnetic resonance imaging (MRI) provides detailed spinal cord anatomy without the use of contrast agents. In addition, it is "blind" to bone, allowing a clear demonstration of various cranial structures. Although computed tomography is excellent for spinal cord defects, magnetic resonance imaging is better for soft tissue. Computed tomography can miss a soft tissue lesion that magnetic resonance imaging will pick up.

Because the skull limits the usefulness of ultrasonography on adults, the procedure is best performed on infants before the fontanelles close. This small "window" allows the soft tissue of the brain to be imaged without the radiation involved with computed tomography. An examination known as echoencephalography is an excellent, noninvasive, diagnostic tool that can be performed on adults as well as children. It is especially valuable in those hospitals that do not have easy access to computed tomography. Its major value is to identify the patient who has a space-occupying intracranial lesion, which may require immediate surgical intervention. It is also a valuable complementary technique to technetium brain scanning and for ruling out tumors as a cause of certain organic brain disorders and psychiatric disturbances. The method is also useful in assessing ventricular size when hydrocephalus is suspected.

Nuclear medicine radionuclide cerebral imaging generally consists of two phases: a dynamic or angiographic study composed of rapid sequence images of the arrival of the nuclide in the cerebral hemispheres; and static images obtained approximately 1 hour after the dynamic study to provide a record of the distribution of the nuclide in the brain. Pathologic processes often affect the blood-brain barrier and result in a focal area of increased radioactivity. Radionuclide studies will indicate an abnormality but will not point to a specific cause.

Angiography can locate and evaluate an aneurysm, an intracranial mass, abnormal cranial vessels, hemorrhages, and malformations. Intravenous digital angiography has been used to evaluate extracranial carotid disease.

The preceding imaging techniques have been touched upon only lightly here, as it takes extra training and skills to perform those diagnostic procedures. Knowledge of the radiographic appearance of the various pathologies comes from the detailed study of those modalities and is beyond the scope of this text. The one remaining special procedure that has not been entirely replaced by computed tomography or magnetic resonance imaging is myelography. This procedure can be performed by "nonspecialized" technologists and is a part of the routine schedule in many hospitals.

Myelography is employed to confirm or exclude the presence of an intraspinal lesion, to determine the location and characteristics of a lesion before operation, and to exclude multiple lesions. This procedure can demonstrate posterior protrusion of herniated intervertebral discs as well as spinal cord tumors. The procedure involves the introduction of a contrast agent into the spinal subarachnoid space, either in the lumbar region (Fig. 10–5) or at the C-1 level of the cervical region. Myelography should be preceded by careful, high-quality plain-film studies, since accurate interpretation of myelograms is often dependent on associating findings with those from conventional radiographs.

Negative contrast studies use air or oxygen. Gas is exchanged for cerebrospinal fluid a few milliliters at a time. A larger amount of gas is injected than fluid removed so that the subarachnoid space is distended. Negative studies are most useful in examinations for intramedullary lesions, atrophy of the spinal cord and for detailed anatomy of the conus medullaris.

In positive contrast studies, a radiopaque agent is instilled, usually after a few milliliters of cerebrospinal fluid have been withdrawn for testing. The contrast agents most widely used today are the aqueous contrast media, which permit relatively low kilovoltage and often provide excellent visualization of nerve roots and axillary sleeves. The contrast agents are directly injected into the subarachnoid space. Indications for a subarachnoid myelogram are encroachment of a disk, a space-occupying lesion, central nervous system degenerative disease, or a suspected spinal cord malformation. There are times when an epidural myelogram is more desirous. Indications for an epidural myelogram include encroachment on the disks or a herniated disk in the lower thoracic or upper lumbar region. Contraindications for either type of myelogram are a known sensitivity to iodine or increased intracranial pressure or both.

The site of the injection may vary. A lumbar puncture is made in the lower lumbar spine to reduce any possibility of cord damage. If the myelogram is mainly concerned with lumbar anatomy, the needle is placed at the L-2/L-3 level. If the cervical or thoracic region is of more concern, the needle puncture is made at the L-3/L-4 or the L-4/L-5 level. If a lumbar puncture is not possible, a cisternal puncture may be made into the cerebellomedullary cistern. This area is continuous with the subarachnoid space of the spinal canal and is located at the base of the cerebellum. When an epidural myelogram is indicated, the puncture site may be in the sacral hiatus. The thoracic region is never utilized as a puncture site in myelography,

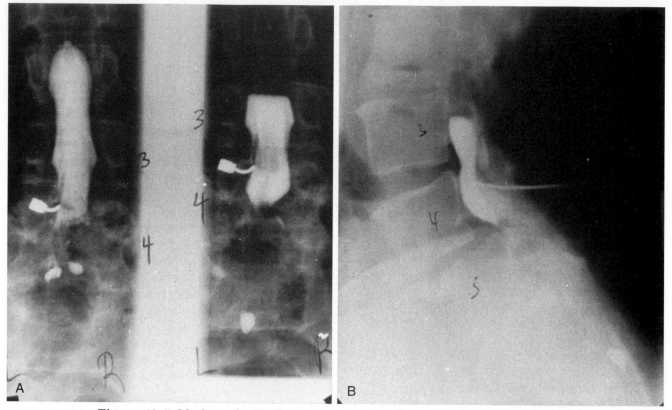

Figure 10–5. Myelography. *A*, Posteroanterior view demonstrating a complete block at the L-4/L-5 interspace. *B*, A lateral view of the same patient reveals a peculiar distortion of contrast at the site of an unusual spondylolisthesis between the fourth and fifth lumbar vertebrae.

as the space is much too narrow for a needle to enter safely.

Cervical myelography is performed at the C-1/C-2 level approximately 4 to 6 mm anterior to the spinolaminar line into the subarachnoid space. A 22 gauge spinal needle is utilized to inject the contrast medium. Cervical puncture may also be used for a thoracic or lumbar myelogram when the lumbar puncture sites are unsuccessful because of stenosis or infection.

A few comparisons between cervical and lumbar punctures bear looking at.

Cervical Puncture	Lumbar Puncture
Evaluates upper blocks	Impeded by blocks
Fewer side effects	2 to 3 times more side effects
Control of contrast material	Little control of the contrast material
Target delivery	Manipulation of patient
Contrast material concentrated	Contrast material diluted by cerebrospinal fluid
Less material needed	More material needed

Anteroposterior and lateral projections are rou-

tine in positive contrast myelography; additional views are selected as needed. Oblique views are of value for lumbar disc herniations, since most occur anterolateral to the nerve roots. An oblique projection also shows an epidural defect to the best advantage. Lateral views with flexion and extension of the cervical spine are important to demonstrate a significant epidural ridge. These maneuvers also aid in distributing the contrast material throughout the cervical subarachnoid space.

Discography best demonstrates the individual intervertebral disc. This procedure involves injecting a contrast medium such as Hypaque meglumine 60%, Renografin 60%, or air into the individual disk. Anterior protrusion or a ruptured nucleus palposis will be clearly seen by this examination. Discography may be performed separately, or it may be combined with myelography (Fig. 10–6). Once the needle has been removed, the patient is adjusted so as to be in the supine position with the legs flexed in the lithotomy position. Frontal projections are taken with a 20-degree cephalic angulation of the central ray. Lastly, the patient is placed in the erect position for flexion and extension weight-bearing lateral projections of the disks.

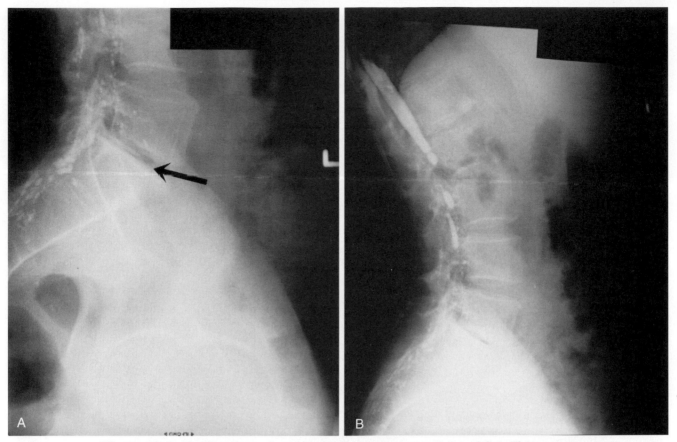

Figure 10–6. Air discogram. *A and B,* Air injected between L-5 and S-1. This patient underwent myelography with iophendylate (Pantopaque) many years prior to the discogram.

PATHOLOGY

Congenital Abnormalities

Developmental abnormalities are more important in the brain than in any other single organ, with the possible exception of the heart. Developmental abnormalities of the central nervous system are usually divided into malformations and destructive brain lesions.

Anencephaly is a severe malformation in which the cranial vault is absent and the cerebral hemispheres are either missing or markedly reduced in size (Fig. 10–7). Almost all infants with anencephaly are stillborn or die soon after birth. There are limited cases of infants surviving until the age of 2 or 3. **Microcephaly** means the infant is born with an exceedingly small head (Fig. 10–8). This occurs when there is failure of the cerebrum to develop properly.

Hydrocephaly literally means water brain, and it may occur congenitally or arise from a variety of causes at any time after birth. In hydrocephalic individuals, the ventricles enlarge as a result of a block in the flow of cerebrospinal fluid at some level.

The most common type of congenital hydrocephalus is stenosis of the aqueduct of Sylvius, which causes enlargement of the lateral and third ventricles with a normal-sized fourth ventricle. If the obstruction occurs at the level of the foramen of Monro, the lateral ventricles enlarge, leaving the third and fourth ventricles at normal size. Enlargement of the entire ventricular system indicates an obstruction at the level of the roof of the fourth ventricle, either the foramen of Magendie or the foramen of Luschka. As the ventricles expand with accumulated cerebrospinal fluid, the head may enlarge enormously, so that normal vaginal delivery of the live infant is impossible (Fig. 10–9). This type of hydrocephalus is known as **internal** (fluid in the ventricles only). This has also been called **noncommunicating hydrocephalus,** as an obstruction in the ventricles does not allow the cerebrospinal fluid to flow through the ventricles into the subarachnoid space and into the spinal canal.

In older children and adults, the cause of hydrocephalus is more often tumors that block the flow of cerebrospinal fluid or meningeal scarring secondary to meningitis or hemorrhage. As the tumors

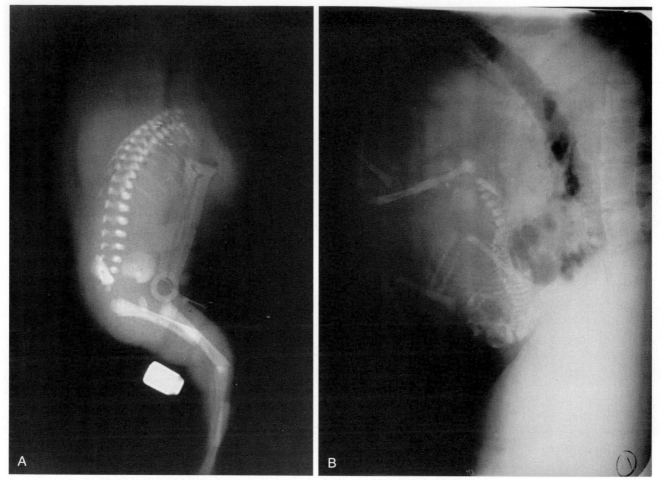

Figure 10–7. Anencephaly. *A,* Radiograph of a stillborn fetus missing the entire cranium. *B,* Radiograph of fetus in utero in normal position. There is only minimal formation of the base of the cranium.

grow, they may press on the aqueduct, force the brain stem against the openings, or interfere with the reabsorption of cerebrospinal fluid by the arachnoid. Usually more than one of these processes is at work. When the blockage is below the ventricular level, so that there is free flow of cerebrospinal fluid between the ventricles and the subarachnoid space, or the cause is faulty reabsorption of the fluid, the hydrocephalus is known as **external, or communicating.** In this case, the head does not usually enlarge because the skull is well formed; rather, the increased pressure from the accumulated fluid in the ventricles causes pressure atrophy of the surrounding white and gray tissue, resulting in mental deterioration. Because the cranium can not get smaller, there is a compensatory increase in fluid within the spinal canal and the spaces that the atrophy of the brain creates. This is referred to as **compensatory hydrocephalus.** If the increased pressure is not relieved, the brain may herniate toward the great foramen. The most effective treatment is a shunt, which is placed either between the

lateral ventricles and the cardiac atrium (ventriculoatrial shunt) or between the lateral ventricles and the peritoneum (ventriculoperitoneal shunt) (Fig. 10–10).

Computed tomography and MRI provide excellent visualization of this disorder and have replaced the use of pneumoencephalography and ventriculography (Fig. 10–11). Ultrasonography may be used to diagnose hydrocephaly in the newborn; however, once the fontanelles close, ultrasonography is of no use in the diagnosis of hydrocephaly.

Approximately 2500 newborns a year in the United States are diagnosed with **spina bifida.** This is one in every 1000 live births. The disorder is characterized by an opening in the spine, the result of a defect in the neural tube in which the posterior arches and spines of some vertebrae fail to close or are absent. The cause is not clear, but it is believed that genetic and environmental factors work together. This defect is often discovered incidentally on x-rays or by ultrasonography of the fetus in utero.

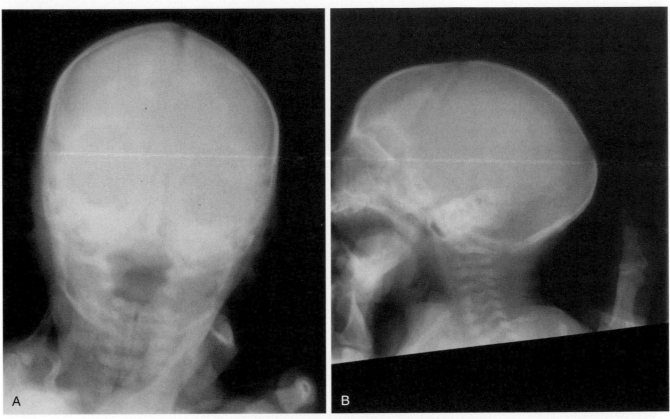

Figure 10–8. Microcephaly. Anteroposterior *(A)* and lateral *(B)* views.

Figure 10–9. A 40-year-old mentally retarded woman who was born with hydrocephalus. Her parents refused treatment for her. Computed tomography showed a 99 percent fluid-filled cranium. Only 1 percent brain tissue remains at the brainstem. Magnification in this radiograph is minimal.

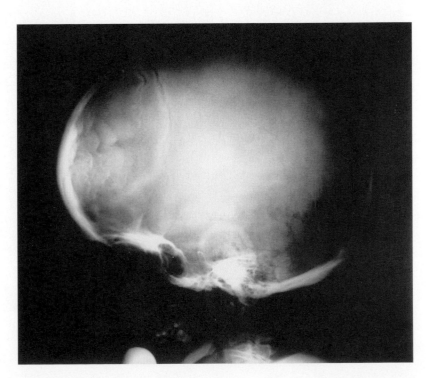

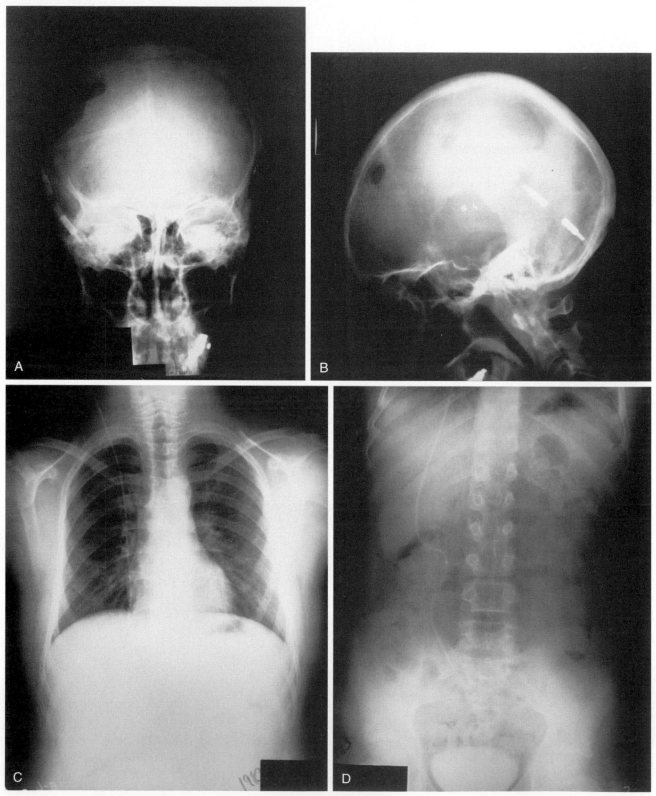

Figure 10–10. Hydrocephaly. *A*, Anteroposterior view of the skull showing a shunt in right parietal region. The shunt passes down the mandible. *B*, Lateral view showing the shunt's position in the neck area. *C*, The shunt's position in the chest. *D*, The shunt finally ends in the bladder.

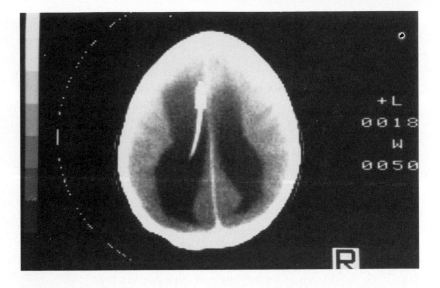

Figure 10–11. Computed tomographic scan showing shunt placement in the enlarged ventricles of hydrocephaly.

The disorder has several forms that affect its victims in varying degrees. It may be an isolated abnormality limited to a defect in the neural arch of a vertebra known as **spina bifida occulta** (Fig. 10–12). Depending on the severity of the defect, various pathologies may coexist. Large defects in the lumbar or cervical spine may be accompanied by protrusion of the meninges, known as a **meningocele.** As a rule, neurologic complications with meningoceles are slight or even absent, since no nerve elements are involved in the sac. If only the cord protrudes through a defect in the meninges as well as the spine, the result is a **myelocele.** In this type of spina bifida, the neural tube has not closed. Myeloceles may not be compatible with life. Unfortunately, most babies with spina bifida are born with a **myelomeningocele,** in which both the meninges and the spinal cord herniate through the spinal defect. This is the most severe form for the surviving infant, as neurologic deficiencies in the control of the lower limbs, bladder, and rectum result. The severity of damage is determined by the location of the lesion. The higher up the spine, the more damage is manifested because spinal nerves are disrupted from the point of injury. As the central nervous system is freely exposed to the outside, there is risk of infection of the meninges. Some patients with myelomeningocele demonstrate **Arnold-Chiari** syndrome, which is a cause of congenital hydrocephalus. Arnold-Chiari syndrome is a defect of the hindbrain, with bony fusion of the occiput and the upper cervical vertebrae leading to a small posterior cranial fossa. The medulla is forced through the great foramen into the upper cervical canal, leading to obstruction of the flow of cerebrospinal fluid. Surgeons surgically implant a shunt to allow fluid to drain.

Most spina bifida patients have normal intelligence. Only about 3 to 5 percent are severely mentally disabled. Approximately 95 percent of children have bowel and bladder problems, since nerves that control these functions are located in the tail of the spinal cord. The bladder may be flaccid and constantly leak urine or may be spastic, causing urine to back up into the kidneys. With proper medical treatment, 90 percent of the victims can live a normal life span.

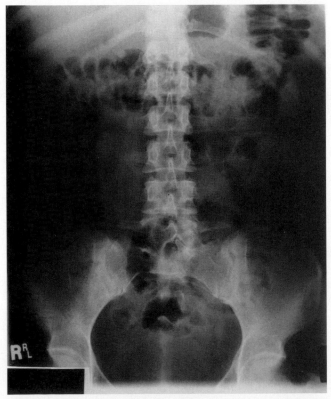

Figure 10–12. Spina bifida occulta occurring at L-5 and S-1.

Inflammatory Processes

Abscesses may either occur within the brain or be associated with the meninges. When the collection of pus is between the skull and the underlying dura mater, the abscess is known as an **epidural abscess.** All others are known simply as **brain abscesses.**

The microorganisms that cause abscess of the brain may come from a focus of infection in the skull, the most common being from the middle ear or the mastoid region. The infection spreads inward and causes abscess formation in the adjacent part of the brain. Another source of abscess is an infection in the frontal or other sinuses that communicate with the nasal cavity. These abscesses are likely to be in the frontal part of the brain. An infecting organism can come from a systemic infection or septic process in the lung also.

The symptoms of brain abscess are not easily manifested, as many parts of the brain where an abscess is likely to occur are "silent areas." That is, a lesion in this area of the brain does not produce any characteristic symptom. The clinical sign is gradually increasing intracranial pressure, which however, may also suggest a tumor. Increased pressure coupled with an existing middle ear, mastoid, or sinus infection should be highly indicative of abscess.

Computed tomography is the best imaging modality for the demonstration of abscesses. It can also show the underlying mastoiditis or sinusitis, thus eliminating the need for plain skull radiography. An untreated brain abscess eventually will rupture into the subarachnoid space or into the ventricular system. This often fatal rupture, as well as the increased intracranial pressure, is well documented on computed tomography.

Small saccular **aneurysms** may occur on the intracranial vessels. Congenital "berry" aneurysms may result in intraparenchymal hemorrhages. Many aneurysms appear in middle life as a result of atheroma and hypertension. They are symptomless until they rupture and cause a subarachnoid hemorrhage. Blood is spilled into the subarachnoid space and can be detected in the cerebrospinal fluid. Most aneurysms involve the circle of Willis, in particular the anterior communicating artery and the major subdivisions of the middle cerebral artery. In most patients, the ruptured aneurysm is characterized by sudden onset of pain, which may be around the orbit. Headaches are also a common symptom.

Not all aneurysms of the brain are the small, berry type. Figure 10–13 shows a subtraction image of a large cavernous carotid aneurysm. Noncontrast computed tomography and magnetic resonance im-

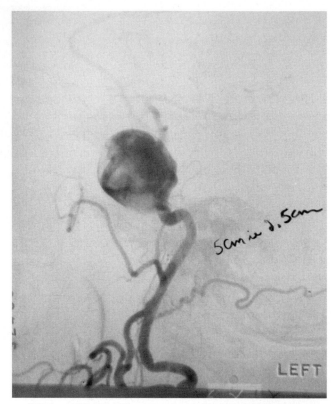

Figure 10–13. Giant cavernous carotid aneurysm.

aging are now the modalities used to diagnose this condition.

Cerebrovascular accidents are commonly referred to as **strokes.** Strokes are the third leading cause of death in the United States. Thrombosis, embolism, and hemorrhage are all possible causes of a stroke. A thrombosis affects the extra cerebral arteries of the elderly more often than young to middle-aged adults. However, the risk of a stroke caused by thrombosis increases with other factors such as smoking, obesity, and the use of oral contraceptives. A middle-aged woman with all three of these factors runs a higher risk of suffering from a cerebrovascular accident than an elderly man who is a nonsmoker and within a normal weight range.

The majority of cerebrovascular accidents are caused by emboli, which occur by separating from a thrombus in a large vessel such as the carotid artery. The embolus then travels until it lodges in a smaller brain vessel and results in an infarct. This accounts for 60 percent of all strokes. Most thrombi initially form because the vessel in which they occur has been damaged by atherosclerosis. This is why cerebrovascular accidents become increasingly prevalent in the elderly.

Whether from emboli or thrombi, vascular occlusions result in the sudden impairment of circulation in the cerebral blood vessels (known as **ischemia**).

This results in decreased oxygen in the brain tissue supplied by the affected vessel. The damaged brain tissue loses function within minutes and becomes soft and necrotic within a few days. This area of ischemic necrosis is known as an **infarct.**

Cerebrovascular accidents are also caused by rupture of vessels and bleeding into the brain. The ruptured vessel has usually been weakened by arteriosclerosis in a patient with hypertension. While the signs and symptoms of a brain hemorrhage depend on its location and size, almost half of the patients with large brain hemorrhages die within hours because the accumulation of blood displaces adjacent tissue, rapidly elevating the intracranial pressure.

In many cases of stroke, there is no need for imaging studies because the history of sudden onset of neurologic problems is indicative of a vascular process. However, computed tomography can be utilized to demonstrate an acute hemorrhagic infarct, edema, and necrosis.

Immediately following a cerebral infarct, the computed tomographic scan shows no abnormality, as does a static radionuclide brain scan. This information is not necessarily negative, since it rules out other causes of the patient's symptoms. Thirty-six to 48 hours following the stroke, the involved areas becomes lucent on the computed tomography.

Transient ischemic attacks (**TIA**) often precede a cerebrovascular accident. These "mini" strokes are a temporary interruption of circulation usually caused by arteriosclerotic plaque. TIAs are characterized by fleeting attacks of faintness, localized paralysis, and aphasia (loss of speech). Manifestations of TIAs completely resolve within 24 hours. The patient who presents with an obvious TIA may undergo a duplex ultrasonographic examination of the carotid arteries to determine the extent of any further arteriosclerotic disease. If warranted, the patient may undergo angiography to study the carotid arteries. These TIAs should be considered as a "warning" sign that a major stroke may be imminent: as many as 80 percent of people who have a TIA later suffer a stroke.

A suppurative process in the space between the dura mater and the arachnoid is known as a **subdural empyema.** It is most commonly caused by spread of infection from the frontal or ethmoid sinuses. Other causes may be from middle ear infection or mastoiditis, although this is less common than sinusitis. Subdural empyema is usually bilateral over the upper cerebral area. Computed tomography is best for demonstrating the involvement of the parenchyma. A skull radiograph may show diffuse areas of osteolytic destruction if the empyema has led to osteomyelitis. Even with proper treatment, a subdural empyema is associated with a high mortality rate.

Encephalitis is inflammation of the brain. This uncommon infection is almost always caused by a virus. Many of the viruses that cause encephalitis are spread by mosquitoes. Patients with this type present with symptoms of irritability, drowsiness, and headache. Herpes simplex 1 can also cause encephalitis. Although it is rare, the virus can invade the brain in a susceptible person and result in severe destruction of large areas of the temporal or frontal lobes of the brain. Computed tomography is important in the clinical diagnosis of encephalitis by ruling out abscess or tumor. Computed tomography will also show the best area for biopsy in herpetic encephalitis.

Bleeding from a ruptured artery or vein into the brain tissue can be caused by disease as well as the obvious head trauma that causes injury. Cerebrovascular diseases such as hemorrhagic neoplasm, hemorrhagic infarct, or a ruptured aneurysm can cause hemorrhage. **Cerebral hemorrhage,** also known as **hematoma,** is the escape of blood from the vessels into the cerebrum. Those hemorrhages not commonly related to injury are discussed in the following paragraphs. Two other types are discussed under the section on head injuries.

A **subarachnoid hemorrhage** is caused most commonly by rupture of a berry aneurysm in the circle of Willis. The hemorrhage is into the subarachnoid space between the arachnoid and the pia mater. As the cerebrospinal fluid is contained in this space, blood will be found in the fluid upon lumbar puncture. Clinically, the subarachnoid hemorrhage is characterized by a history of sudden headache, clouding of vision, and blood in the cerebral spinal fluid. The radiographic procedure that most readily displays blood in the subarachnoid space is computed tomography.

Hypertensive vascular disease is the main cause of an **intracerebral,** or **intraparenchymal,** hemorrhage. However, if the patient is young, rupture from an arteriovenous malformation is usually the cause. Hypertensive intracerebral hematoma can cause a stroke, as the hemorrhage results in blood collections within the tissue that displaces the surrounding brain. Intracerebral hematomas may occur anywhere within the brain; however, they are more often found in the basal ganglia, cerebellar hemispheres, or pons. MRI or an unenhanced computed tomographic scan will best define the area of accumulated blood.

Meningitis means inflammation of the leptomeninges. It most often occurs by itself but may be associated with other infections such as pneumonia. This bacteria-caused infection has an abrupt onset, with the patient experiencing fever, headache, and muscle pain. The patient often complains of a stiff neck. The types of meningitis are named for the types of bacteria that cause them. The streptococcus and pneumococcus bacteria reach the meninges from the middle ear or the frontal sinus. The blood may carry the bacteria from the lung. The meningococcus comes from the nose or throat. These three organisms are pyogenic so that the meningitis they produce, streptococcal meningitis, pneumococcal meningitis, and meningococcal meningitis, are acute and violent. Treatment by antibiotic therapy must be immediate to avoid alterations in the blood-brain barrier, which leads to edema, increasing cranial pressure, and subsequent death of the patient.

The tubercle bacillus–induced meningitis is in a class by itself. It has none of the acuteness of the other forms of meningitis. This is a chronic form of meningitis. The infection is carried by the blood stream from some other tuberculous lesion. The disease often sits at the base of the brain for an extended period of time as it gradually affects more and more cranial nerves. If the patient survives meningitis, there is the danger of developing hydrocephalus. Since the inflammation is in the subarachnoid space, fibrous adhesions may develop that block the flow of cerebrospinal fluid.

Although bacterial infection is the most common cause of meningitis, there is a **viral** form that may be caused by mumps, polio, or herpes simplex. **Chemical meningitis** can be caused by the introduction of a foreign substance into the subarachnoid space, such as a contrast medium for myelography.

Meningitis is diagnosed clinically by evaluation of the cerebrospinal fluid. Radiography plays a small role in this inflammatory process; however, bacterial and viral meningitis are best demonstrated on computed tomography. Plain-film radiography shows the underlying cause of the meningitis, such as sinusitis, mastoiditis, or pneumonia.

Osteomyelitis of the skull is most often caused by pyogenic bacteria from the sinuses or mastoid air cells. Osteomyelitis is a common complication of an empyema. Skull radiographs demonstrate changes that are like osteomyelitis in other parts of the skeleton. The radiographs first demonstrate many small, poorly defined areas of lucency. As the weeks progress, the lucencies enlarge and unite in a central area of the skull. Osteomyelitis of the skull must not be confused with multiple myeloma, which presents a similar radiographic pattern.

Head Injuries

Normally, the brain is well protected by the skull. However, when sufficient force is applied to the head, the brain can be damaged. The major cause of head injuries today is traffic accidents. The more common among the injuries are concussion, contusion, hemorrhage, and fracture. Over one fourth of all people who suffer fatal head wounds demonstrate no skull fracture. Trauma to the brain and brain stem is of primary concern to the emergency medical team. Because injury to the brain can occur without skull fractures, computed tomography has replaced plain-film skull radiography in major trauma cases so that the brain tissue and brain stem can be visualized. If skull radiographs are taken, a cross table lateral projection should be done to visualize any air within the brain or fluid levels within the sphenoid sinus. Another indication of severe trauma to the brain is the "halo sign." This occurs when there is a tear in the dura mater, which is common in fractures of the cranial base. The sign is so named because of a pink blood stain surrounded by leaking yellow cerebrospinal fluid.

The most common head injury is a **concussion.** A concussion occurs when there has been a violent blow or jar to the head. This causes the brain to strike the opposite side of the cranium, resulting in momentary loss of consciousness. There may be transient amnesia, vertigo, nausea, weak pulse, and slow respiration. The patient may experience a headache, but normally recovery occurs within 24 to 48 hours with no structural damage detected in the brain.

A **contusion** is more serious than a concussion. Contusions are bruises on the surface of the brain and are the result of the brain shifting inside the skull during acceleration and rapid deceleration such as a "whiplash" reaction received from a rear-end type of auto accident. When the bruise occurs on the same side of the brain as the trauma, it is known as a coup lesion. Contrecoup lesions are contusions that occur on the opposite side of the head. Contusions result in hemorrhages from small blood vessels, which cause further vessel occlusion and edema. All of these may lead to increased intracranial pressure, which must be closely watched for.

When sufficient force is applied to the skull, **fractures** of various type occur. Three of the common types of skull fractures include linear, comminuted, and depressed. Fractures of the cranium are classified according to their location. Sutures and vascular grooves of the skull can appear as fractures; therefore, a thorough knowledge of the anatomy of the skull is required. Fractures are often difficult to differentiate from suture lines or vascular grooves, but if the radiographer bears in mind the location of the serrated sutures and the fact that vascular markings are smooth, faint lines as seen on a radiograph, fracture should be more readily identifiable.

A **linear fracture** appears on a radiograph as an irregular or jagged radiolucent line (Fig. 10–14). The location of a linear fracture is important, as complications may occur. Pneumocephalus and epidural hematoma are two complications that can occur if the fracture is in the mastoid air cell area or if a vessel is lacerated.

In more severe trauma, the skull may break into three or more fragments, thus becoming a **comminuted fracture.** If any one fragment is depressed into the cranial cavity, thereby becoming known as a **depressed fracture** (Fig. 10–15), the dura mater is often torn, causing hemorrhage. If the force is sufficient to cause penetration of the cranial vault by the fragment, air and foreign material may also enter the cranial cavity and even possibly the brain.

Basilar skull fractures are often difficult to diagnose on skull radiography, as the fracture may be hidden by the dense, complex anatomic structures of the temporal and mastoid areas. Air-fluid levels identified in the sphenoid sinus on the cross table lateral film is an indication of this type of skull fracture. Computed tomography is a better modality to determine the presence of blood in the basilar cisterns as well as demonstrate any basilar skull fractures that may not be visible on a radiograph.

As stated in the previous section, hematomas (hemorrhages) can be caused by injury. These collections of blood manifest in exactly the same manner as those caused by atraumatic rupture of a vessel.

An **epidural hemorrhage,** also known as an **extradural hematoma,** is caused by a tear in the middle meningeal vessels, which causes bleeding between the bone and the dura mater. This type of hemorrhage is associated with severe trauma in which the skull has usually been fractured at the temporal area. Because of the location of the tear and bleed, the blood accumulates very rapidly. The outcome is fatal within several hours if the condition is not diagnosed and the hematoma removed surgically. Because of the rapid deterioration of the patient, radiography often plays a minor role in the diagnosis of this condition, as the patient will go straight to CT for unenhanced scans of the head. CT will demonstrate any skull fractures, thus eliminating the need for plain-film skull radiography and saving the patient valuable time for treatment.

A **subdural hematoma,** a common complication of injury, is the result of a tear of the veins between the dura mater and the arachnoid. Because it is venous in origin, bleeding is slow, taking hours or even days for the accumulation of blood to become large enough to cause compression of the underlying brain. Although a subdural hematoma is not as life-threatening as an epidural hematoma, surgery must still be performed to remove the blood to prevent the compression of brain tissue. Subdural hematomas are often found in patients who have a history of trauma to the frontal or occipital lobes caused by falling. However, these patients usually have no fractures.

Neoplasms

Neoplasms of the brain and spinal cord are not as neatly separated into benign and malignant categories as tumors found elsewhere in the body. Although the tumor itself may be benign, it may disrupt vital functions such as might be found in the brain stem, killing the patient.

Neoplasms of the brain are the second most common tumors occurring in children. (Leukemia occurs more often than neoplasms.) Patients most often present with increased pressure and accompanying edema. Because of the increased cranial pressure, patients may experience headaches, vomiting, blurred vision, and seizures. Surgery is almost always necessary for treatment.

Radiographic diagnosis of neoplasms is made by computed tomography, magnetic resonance imaging, and, in some cases, angiography. Magnetic resonance imaging is excellent for evaluating the

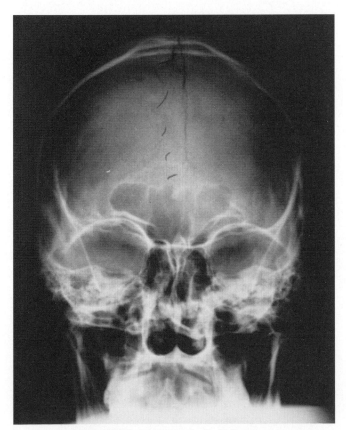

Figure 10–14. Linear skull fracture.

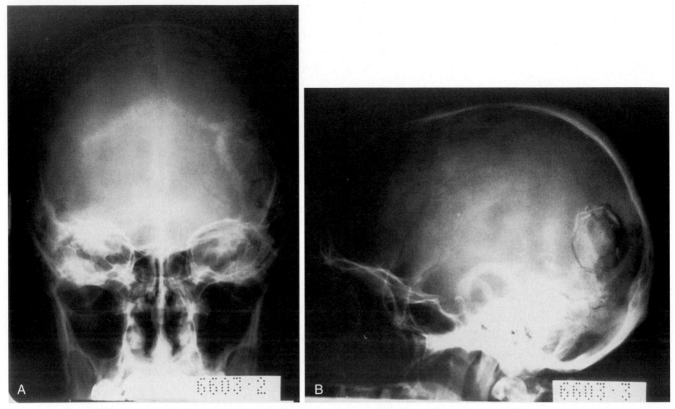

Figure 10–15. Depressed skull fracture. Anteroposterior *(A)* and lateral *(B)* views of a posterior parietal fracture.

brain stem, while computed tomography is better for detecting calcifications within the tumor. Because these two modalities are beyond the level of a student radiographer, the appearance of neoplasms on computed tomography or magnetic resonance imaging will not be discussed. Rather, only definitions and manifestations of the tumors will be presented. The neoplasms are described in order from most common to least common.

The most common primary brain tumor is the **glioma.** This tumor has a neurologic origin and occurs in the cerebral hemispheres and the posterior fossa. Benign forms of gliomas are known as **astrocytomas.** The malignant variety is the fast-growing **glioblastoma multiforme** (Fig. 10–16). It is the most common malignant brain tumor in adults, comprising 50 to 60 percent of all gliomas. Prognosis is very poor. Death usually results within 1 to 2 years of early diagnosis, less time if the diagnosis is made in the late stages of the neoplasm. Another highly malignant tumor with a very poor prognosis is the **medulloblastoma** (Fig. 10–17). This neoplasm occurs in the roof of the fourth ventricle in the midline of the cerebellum. Its victims are usually children between the ages of 9 and 12 years, but they may be as young as 5 or as old as 15. Males are twice as likely to be affected. These fast-growing tumors invade the fourth ventricle and rapidly cause death.

Meningiomas are the next most common brain tumor, accounting for about 20 percent of all brain tumors. This is a slow-growing benign neoplasm that occurs in the meninges, in particular the arachnoid and dura mater. Since the tumor does grow out of the meninges, it may also occur in the covering of the spinal cord. Although this is a benign tumor, it will eventually kill the patient as it exerts pressure on the brain. The tumor is a round, well-circumscribed lesion that usually does not invade the surrounding brain tissue, thus making excision easier and prognosis good. Calcifications within the meningioma may be seen on plain-film skull radiography, but is best identified by computed tomography. Angiography is used to demonstrate the vascularity of the tumor, which is essential before surgical removal is attempted.

Pituitary adenomas are also common (about 15 percent of all tumors). The tumor grows within the sella turcica where the pituitary gland is located. As it increases in size, the sella turcica becomes eroded and pressure is exerted on the optic chiasm, creating problems with vision. A lateral skull radiograph will demonstrate the deformity of the sella and erosion of the posterior clinoid processes (Fig.

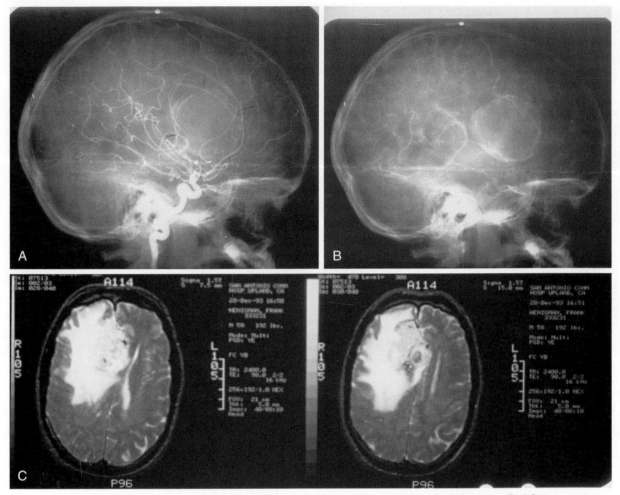

Figure 10–16. Glioblastoma multiforma. *A,* Mass seen on cerebral angiogram. *B,* After the venous phase is completed, the mass is highlighted more clearly. *C,* Computed tomographic scans show the glioblastoma in the right anterior surface of the brain.

10–18). Some types of pituitary adenomas secrete growth hormones, causing acromegaly in adults or gigantism in children. Other hormones that may be secreted in excess are adrenocorticotropic hormone, causing symptoms of Cushing disease; thyroid-stimulating hormone, resulting in hyperthyroidism; and prolactin, leading to amenorrhea. A full discussion of these hormones is found in Chapter XI.

Another benign tumor that originates *above* the sella turcica is the **craniopharyngioma.** This tumor is more commonly found in children between the ages of 5 and 18, whereas the pituitary adenoma is more likely found in the adult. Because this tumor is above the sella, as it enlarges, it depresses the optic chiasm, creating vision problems. Craniopharyngiomas contain both cystic and solid components and most have calcifications that can be seen on the skull radiograph and computed tomographic scan.

Tumors that are more common in children are those that occur in the pineal gland. **Teratomas** and **germinomas** are two types of pineal tumors that occur more often in males under the age of 25. These tumors may compress the ventricular system causing hydrocephalus and an enlarged ventricular system. Calcification within the adult pineal gland is common and a normal finding. However, calcification seen within the pineal region of a child should be suspect for teratomas, as these tumors often contain teeth.

Metastatic tumors of the brain are common, accounting for another 10 percent of all intracranial neoplasms. Metastases are usually multiple neoplasms, whereas primary brain neoplasms are usually a solitary tumor. Usually, the primary carcinoma is located in the lung or the breast, and is spread to the brain by the blood stream. Less commonly, the metastasis comes from the kidney and the gastrointestinal tract. Single metastatic tumors may be difficult to distinguish from primary tumors

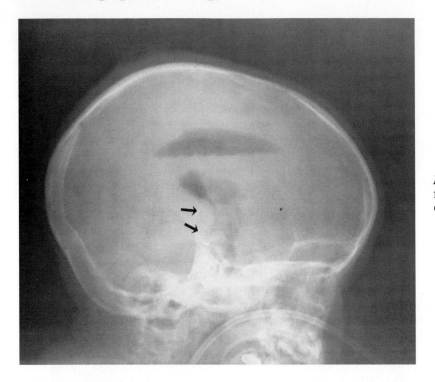

Figure 10–17. Anterior displacement of the fourth ventricle and obstruction of the aqueduct of Sylvius because of medulloblastoma.

on the computed tomographic scan, however, since single tumors in the adult are rare, metastasis should be considered.

A tumor that is usually found at the clivus of the skull is a **chordoma.** This locally invasive tumor does not usually metastasize. On plain-film radiog-

raphy, the destruction of the dorsum sellae and clivus, along with cloudlike calcification, can be seen. Computed tomography can demonstrate the mass, calcifications, and bony destruction.

Acoustic neuromas are uncommon benign tumors with a very slow rate of growth. These neo-

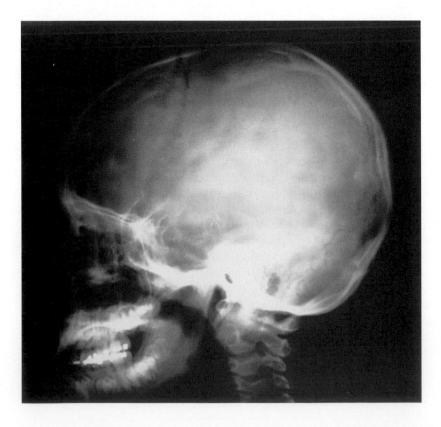

Figure 10–18. Erosion of the sella turcica caused by a pituitary adenoma.

Table 10-1.
Clinical and Radiographic Characteristics of Common Pathologies

Pathologic Condition	Causal Factors*	Manifestations	Radiographic Appearance
Congenital hydrocephaly	Newborn, stenosis of aqueduct of Sylvius	Enlarged ventricles, enlarged head	CT or MRI show enlarged ventricles
Hydrocephaly	Children and adults, tumors or reabsorption problems	Pressure atrophy of brain	CT and MRI show smaller brain due to atrophy and increased fluid
Spina bifida	Newborn, congenital, genetic, and environmental	Meningocele Myelocele Myelomeningocele Arnold-Chiari syndrome Bladder and bowel problems	Defect of posterior arches of the spine
Abscesses	Infection in sinuses, middle ear, or mastoids	Intracranial pressure	CT with contrast shows a radiodense area
Cerebrovascular accident	Thrombus, embolism, or hemorrhage	Sudden onset of neurologic problems	CT shows lucencies in 36–48 hours
Osteomyelitis	Pyogenic bacteria, complication of empyema		Small, poorly defined areas of lucency similar to multiple myeloma

*Includes age, if relevant.
CT, computed tomography; MRI, magnetic resonance imaging.

plasms are more common in adults and are associated with tinnitus and deafness. The origin at the eighth cranial nerve causes the tumor to destroy the internal auditory meatus. These tumors do not invade other parts of the body.

Spinal Cord Disease

Although intracranial neoplasms are more common than spinal cord tumors, the latter cannot be overlooked. Primary spinal neoplasms include **meningiomas** (previously discussed) and **neurofibromas.** Neurofibromas occur with equal frequency among men and women. They may occur at any point in the spinal canal and are hallmarked by foraminal widening.

A frequent lesion of the spinal canal is herniation of the pulpy nucleus into the body of a vertebra, usually caused by degeneration or tearing of the

cartilage plate that separates the nucleus from the vertebral body.

An intervertebral disc may be protruded or herniated into the vertebral canal and press on the spinal cord or stretch the nerves. This is the condition known popularly as **slipped disc.** The most common cause of the protrusion is trauma, and manifestations include lower back pain, weakness, and sciatica. Besides computed tomography and magnetic resonance imaging, myelography is used to demonstrate the location of the slipped disc or tumor.

Table 10–1 summarizes the clinical and radiographic characteristics of common pathologies of the nervous system.

Review Questions

1. List the different parts of the brain and the functions of each part.
2. Describe how the sympathetic and parasympa-

thetic systems of the autonomic nervous system work together to maintain balanced activity in the body.

3. What will a discogram demonstrate that can not be demonstrated on a myelogram?

4. Spina bifida is characterized by what abnormality of the spine? What pathologies may coexist with this congenital abnormality?

5. Why is it so important to take notice of TIAs?

6. Describe the appearance of a linear fracture of the calvarium. How does this compare with the vascular markings of the skull?

7. What are causes of increased intracranial pressure? Why is increased intracranial pressure dangerous?

8. Compare and contrast meningitis and encephalitis in terms of pathogenesis, location of lesion, and clinical manifestations.

9. What is the relationship between cerebrovascular accidents and atherosclerosis? Explain.

10. What are the differences between epidural, subdural, subarachnoid, and intracerebral hematomas in terms of pathogenesis and development of symptoms?

11. How does congenital hydrocephalus differ from acquired hydrocephalus in terms of pathogenesis and clinical expression?

12. Subarachnoid and epidural myelograms are indicated for different reasons. List when each is more desirous. What are contraindications for either type of myelogram?

13. Compare lumbar and cervical areas as puncture sites for myelography.

14. For the following terms, provide the definition, location, and complication.

Anencephaly	Myelomeningocele
Spina bifida	Astrocytoma
Glioblastoma	Medulloblastoma
Craniopharyngioma	Chordoma
Pituitary adenoma	Meningioma

15. Explain the difference between internal and external hydrocephalus.

16. Explain the difference between concussion and contusion.

17. What is the halo sign? What causes it?

18. List the ventricles and the connections between each.

CHAPTER XI

Endocrine System

Goals

1. To review the basic anatomy and physiology of the endocrine system.
2. To become acquainted with the pathophysiology of the endocrine system.
3. To become familiar with all of the common pathologic conditions of the endocrine system.

Objectives

At the completion of the chapter, the radiographer will be able to:

1. List the different endocrine glands and the hormones they secrete.
2. Describe the physiology of the endocrine system.
3. Define terminology relating to the endocrine system.
4. Describe the various pathologic conditions affecting the endocrine system.
5. List the special imaging modalities utilized to demonstrate the various pathologic conditions.

The complex activities of the body are carried out jointly by the endocrine system and the central nervous system. Through nerve impulses, the central nervous system is keyed to act instantaneously. The action of the endocrine system, however, is more subtle; the endocrine glands slowly discharge their secretions into the bloodstream, controlling organs from a distance.

The endocrine system is made up of the ductless glands of internal secretion. They are called ductless because they have no ducts to carry away their secretions and must depend on the capillaries and, to a certain extent, the lymph vessels for this function. The substances secreted by these glands are called hormones. Although most hormones are excitatory in function, some are inhibitory.

The secretion of hormones is controlled by a feedback mechanism. The presence and amount of the hormone, or the substances released by the tissue that is excited by the hormone, regulate further secretion of the hormone by the gland. This ensures that the right amount, no more and no less, of the hormone will maintain proper balance of bodily functions.

The endocrine glands that secrete hormones are the pituitary, thyroid, parathyroid, adrenals, ovaries, testes, pineal body, and pancreas. The ovaries and testes were discussed in Chapter VII and the pancreas was discussed in Chapter IV. Therefore, these areas will only be reviewed briefly.

ANATOMY, PHYSIOLOGY, AND FUNCTION

Pituitary Gland

The pituitary gland, or hypophysis, has been called the "orchestra leader" and "master gland" because it exerts control over all other glands. Despite its important function, it is no larger than a garden pea. Even though the pituitary is the most important gland of the endocrine system, it is controlled by the hypothalamus.

The pituitary gland lies protected within the sphenoid bone in the sella turcica. It is further protected by an extension of the dura mater called the pituitary diaphragm. A stem-like portion of the pituitary, the pituitary stalk, extends through the diaphragm and provides a connection to the hypothalamus on the underside of the brain.

The pituitary gland is actually made up of two separate glands with different embryonic origins and functions; the anterior lobe develops as an upward extension of the pharynx, while the posterior lobe develops as a downward extension of the brain.

The master role is played by the anterior lobe, with its numerous anterior pituitary hormones influencing the actions of other endocrine organs. This internal regulation is further coordinated by action of the hypothalamus on the anterior lobe, which actually controls the release of the anterior pituitary hormones, which are of six major types.

Somatropin (a **growth hormone**) promotes bodily growth of both bone and soft tissues. By increasing the rate at which amino acids enter cells and their ability to convert molecules into proteins, somatropin stimulates the growth and multiplication of body cells, especially those of the bones and skeletal muscles.

A **thyrotropic (thyroid-stimulating)** hormone of the anterior pituitary lobe influences the thyroid and causes secretion of the thyroid hormone. Two **gonadotropic** hormones influence the ovaries and testes and are necessary for the proper development and function of the reproductive system. A **follicle-stimulating** hormone stimulates the growth of graafian follicles and the secretion of estrogen in the female and the development of the seminiferous tubules and sperm cells in the male. A **luteinizing** hormone stimulates the formation of the corpus luteum and secretion of estrogen and progesterone in the female, while in the male it stimulates development and secretion of testosterone in the interstitial cells of the testes.

Prolactin, a lactogenic hormone, is responsible for breast development during pregnancy and, as its name implies, for production of milk.

Growth of the adrenal glands is under the influence of the adrenotropic hormone, **adrenocorticotropic** hormone (ACTH), which also stimulates the adrenal cortex to synthesize and release corticosteroids. ACTH also appears to have a function in relation to pigmentation of the skin, which is primarily a function of the last of the anterior pituitary hormones, **melanocyte-stimulating** hormone.

The posterior lobe secretes two hormones, which are actually made in the hypothalamus and pass through the pituitary stalk into the posterior lobe where they are secreted into the blood stream. The first of these, an antidiuretic hormone called **vasopressin,** limits the development of large volumes of urine by stimulating water reabsorption by the distal and collecting tubules of the kidneys. The second hormone, **oxytocin,** stimulates both the ejection of breast milk and the uterine contractions in pregnancy.

Thyroid Gland

The thyroid gland is composed of two pear-shaped lobes separated by a middle strip of tissue called the isthmus, which crosses in front of the second and third tracheal cartilages. The thyroid gland perches like a butterfly with wings extended on the front part of the neck below the larynx. The lobes are molded to the trachea and esophagus down as far as the sixth tracheal cartilage, and they extend upward to the sides of the cricoid and thyroid carti-

lages. The thyroid may be felt slightly and may even be visible as a swelling in some diseases of the gland.

The thyroid consists of tiny sacs, or follicles, that are filled with a gelatinous yellow fluid called colloid. The colloid contains the hormone secreted by the thyroid.

The main function of the thyroid is the secretion of two iodine-laden hormones, **thyroxine** and **triiodothyronine,** which together are referred to as **thyroid hormone.** This hormone is high in iodine and vital for growth and metabolism. Thyroid hormone maintains the metabolism at a higher rate than would be maintained otherwise, and through variations in the gland activities, it alters the metabolic rate in accordance with changing physiologic demands. This hormone also helps regulate growth and differentiation of tissue during fetal development.

A secondary function of the thyroid gland is the secretion of **calcitonin,** which produces a decrease in the concentration of calcium in blood serum. It helps to maintain the balance of calcium in the blood, which is necessary for a variety of bodily processes. The balance is achieved in conjunction with the functioning of the parathyroid glands.

Parathyroid Glands

The parathyroid glands are small, round glands, usually two on each side, that lie behind the thyroid gland and are usually embedded in its surface. The superior pair is located approximately at the middle lobe of the thyroid gland; the inferior pair is at the lower end of the thyroid lobe. They are not always found at these locations, and they may vary in number. They have been found implanted within the thyroid gland itself, behind the pharynx, and even in the thorax, embedded with the thymus.

Parathyroid hormone regulates the calcium and phosphorus content of the blood and bones. The regulation of calcium content is very important in certain tissue activities such as blood formation, coagulation of blood, milk production in pregnant women, and maintenance of normal and neuromuscular excitability.

Parathyroid hormone promotes calcium absorption in the blood, increasing its calcium concentration. It suppresses the concentration of calcium in the bones. This mechanism is opposite that of the hormone calcitonin from the thyroid gland. These two hormones together maintain calcium balance.

Adrenal Glands

The adrenal glands, also known as the suprarenal glands, resemble small caps perched on the top of each kidney (see Fig. 6–2). They are composed of two distinct parts, the cortex and the medulla, each with a different function. The cortex is indispensable to life, but the medulla is not.

All of the known adrenal hormones of the cortex are steroids, many of which can be manufactured synthetically. They are classified as **glucocorticoids,** secreted mainly by the middle zone of the cortex; **mineralocorticoids,** secreted by the outer zone of the cortex; and sex hormones, secreted by the inner zone of the cortex. The glucocorticoids include **cortisol (hydrocortisone), cortisone,** and **corticosterone** and affect literally all cells in the body. Their general effect, however, is in the metabolism of carbohydrates, fats, and proteins; resistance to stress; antibody function; lymphatic functioning; and recovery from injury and inflammation. The mineralocorticoids are concerned with the regulation of sodium and potassium and their excretion. The principal one is **aldosterone,** which acts on the kidneys to maintain the homeostasis of potassium and sodium ions, conserve water, and decrease urine output.

The adrenal cortex in both sexes secretes large amounts of male hormone **androgen** and small amounts of female hormone **estrogen.** These hormones are produced not only by the adrenals, but also by the testes in the male and the ovaries in the female, and are responsible for secondary sex characteristics, such as hair growth and pitch of voice. They also affect the growth of muscles and bones, accounting in part for observed sexual differences. The presence of ACTH in the blood supply is necessary for the anatomic integrity of the adrenal cortex and its functions in secreting androgens and cortisol.

The adrenal medulla secretes **epinephrine (adrenaline)** and **norepinephrine (noradrenaline).** Epinephrine makes approximately 80 percent of the total secretions of the adrenal medulla and is considered more potent than norepinephrine. It aids the body in meeting stressful situations, such as defense flight, attack, or pursuit. By stimulating or boosting the sympathetic nervous system, epinephrine aids in coping with stress. The effects of these hormones are increased heart rate, blood pressure, blood glucose level, respiratory rate, and airway size.

Pancreas

The pancreas was described as a part of the hepatobiliary system in Chapter IV. In brief, the specialized cells, called the islets of Langerhans, secrete **insulin** and **glucagon** into the bloodstream. Insulin is necessary for the use and storage of carbohydrates and plays a role in reducing the amount of glucose in the blood by accelerating its transport into body cells. Insulin decreases blood glucose levels, and glucagon acts to increase them. Glucagon causes the liver to convert glycogen to glucose. Blood glucose levels are also dependent on the action of many of the other endocrine secretions, such as the pituitary growth hormone, epinephrine, ACTH, and the glucocorticoids, which increase it, and the thyroid hormone, which decreases it.

Gonads

The male and female sex glands were discussed in Chapter VII. The female ovaries and the male testes produce hormones important to the functioning of the reproductive system. These glands become active at puberty under the influence of the anterior pituitary gland and produce the secondary sex characteristics of pubic and axillary hair in both sexes, deep voice and beard in the male, and breast development and onset of menses in the female. The hormones secreted are **estrogen** and **progesterone** in the female and **testosterone** in the male.

Pineal Gland

The pineal gland is a small, firm, oval body located near the base of the brain. Although exact functions have not been established, it is postulated that it secretes **melatonin** (skin-lightening agent), which inhibits secretion of the luteinizing hormone of the pituitary.

Table 11–1 summarizes the endocrine glands, the hormones that they secrete, and the functions of those hormones.

SPECIAL IMAGING PROCEDURES

Imaging modalities are used to diagnose both the underlying endocrine disorders and the secondary changes that may occur in various areas of the body. Disorders of the endocrine glands themselves are usually evaluated by ultrasonography, **computed tomography** (CT), magnetic resonance imaging, and radionuclide scanning. Secondary pathologic manifestations elsewhere in the body are generally evaluated on plain radiographs. For areas that are not encased in bone, computed tomography is often of more value because the abundance of fat may prevent an optimal ultrasonographic examination. Ultrasonography is unable to study the glands that are embedded in bone (ie, the pituitary and the pineal); therefore, computed tomography and magnetic resonance imaging are the best modalities for demonstrating abnormalities in these areas.

Table 11–1.
The Endocrine Glands and Hormones

Gland	Hormone	Function
Pituitary		
Anterior Lobe	Growth hormone (somatotropin)	Bone and soft-tissue growth
	Thyrotropic hormone	Causes thyroid to produce thyroid hormone
	Gonadotropic hormones	
	Follicle-stimulating hormone	Stimulates
		Graafian follicle growth
		Secretion of estrogen in ovaries
		Development of seminiferous tubules
		Production of sperm cells
	Luteinizing hormone	Stimulates
		Ovulation
		Secretion of estrogen and progesterone
		Development of testicle interstitial cells
		Secretion of testosterone
	Lactogenic hormone (prolactin)	Causes breasts to develop and produce milk
	Adrenocorticotropin hormone	Causes adrenals to release corticosteroids
		Affects skin pigmentation
	Melanocyte-stimulating hormone	Forms the melanin pigment in the skin
Posterior Lobe	Antidiuretic hormone (vasopressin)	Causes kidney to reabsorb water
	Oxytocin	Causes uterine contractions and breast milk ejection
Thyroid	Thyroid hormone (thyroxine, triiodothyronine)	Regulates growth, development, and metabolism
	Calcitonin	Promotes calcium absorption in bones
		Reduces calcium content in blood
Parathyroid	Parathyroid hormone	Controls phosphorus content in blood and bone
		Promotes calcium content in blood
		Reduces calcium absorption in bones
Adrenal		
Cortex	Glucocorticoids (hydrocortisone, cortisone, and corticosterone)	Causes metabolism of carbohydrates, fats, and proteins
		Causes lymphatic functions
		Antibody formation
		Recovery of injury and inflammation
	Mineralocorticoids	Regulates sodium and potassium
	Sex hormones (androgen, estrogen)	Promotes secondary sex characteristics
Medulla	Epinephrine (adrenaline)	Stimulate sympathetic nervous system responses
	Norepinephrine (noradrenaline)	
Gonads		
Ovaries	Estrogenic hormones (estradiol, estrone)	Promote secondary sex development after puberty
Testes	Testosterone	Promotes secondary sex development
Pineal	Melatonin	Skin-lightening agent
		Inhibits secretion of luteinizing hormone
Pancreas		
Islets of Langerhans	Insulin	Regulates use of carbohydrates
		Reduces glucose in blood
	Glucagon	Promotes glucose in blood

Ultrasonography can visualize the adrenal glands, but it does present a challenge to the sonographer. High resolution computed tomography can reliably image the normal adrenal glands as well as any tumors or masses, particularly in the obese individual. Biopsy procedures utilizing computed tomographic guidance can also be performed. The procedure cannot always reliably differentiate between benign and malignant tumors; the presence of metastatic deposits can help substantiate the diagnosis.

The thyroid gland is best seen either by ultrasonography or by **nuclear medicine** after the administration of radioactive iodine. The thyroid uptake test for the study of thyroid function has remained a routine diagnostic tool even though more sophisticated procedures are available. The procedure is simple and easily performed and gives a useful clinical index of thyroid function. Although ultrasonography can demonstrate the gland itself and identify masses or other abnormalities in structure, it can not demonstrate the functioning aspect of the thyroid.

PATHOLOGY

Pituitary Gland

Hyperpituitarism results from an excessive secretion of the growth hormone. The causative factor is usually a tumor (Fig. 11–1) or hyperplasia of the anterior lobe of the pituitary gland. When too much growth hormone is secreted before the bone growth has ceased, a condition known as **gigantism** results. People with this condition may reach a stature of 7 or 8 feet and have long limbs. The patients may have normal or retarded mental development. Sexual development and muscular strength are below normal. The epiphyseal plate of the long bones is delayed by several years, thereby increasing the length of the long bones. The vertebral bodies show wedging. Acromegalic characteristics may develop in these patients if hypersecretion of the growth hormone continues after the epiphyseal plates close.

If the adenoma develops after growth is completed and overactivity of the hormone occurs, it may produce a condition called **acromegaly.** Once the epiphyseal lines are closed at puberty, no further longitudinal growth can take place. Thus, if excessive amounts of growth hormone are secreted, appositional enlargement occurs in the bones, but all the tissues share in the overgrowth. Acromegalics are unable to increase in stature but have large hands and prominent coarse facial features. The lips and nose are particularly large, as are the mandible, hands, and feet (Fig. 11–2). Overgrowth of

bones causes a curvature of the spine, and the joints are more susceptible to degenerative lesions.

The pituitary gland controls the level of secretion of gonadal and thyroid hormones as well as the production of growth hormone. When there is decreased function of the pituitary gland, disturbances in bone growth and maturation are widely manifested. **Hypopituitarism** is insufficient production and secretion of the growth hormone of the pituitary gland. The most common cause of hypopituitarism is an adenoma of the pituitary gland.

In children, hypopituitarism causes **dwarfism.** Dwarfism caused by pituitary insufficiency is rare and may result from tumors of the anterior lobe. Because there is insufficient growth hormone to stimulate the growth of the bones in length or in width, the result is a person who is small in stature. The skeleton is small and delicately formed. This may be accompanied by thyroid, adrenocortical, and gonadal insufficiency. In true pituitary dwarfism, the children fail to develop sexually as well, but they are not mentally deficient.

Simmonds syndrome is a result of chronic pituitary insufficiency and is an example of **progeria,** or premature senility. The syndrome can occur both in children and in adolescents. Growth ceases and the patient presents as an aged person. The patient will die of old age or its complications while still a chronologically young person.

Diabetes insipidus is a rare type of diabetes caused by infiltrative processes such as neoplasms, head injury, or in some cases, surgery. A patient with this type of diabetes presents with an abnormal increase in the amount of urine output. It contains no sugar and is therefore insipid, or tasteless.

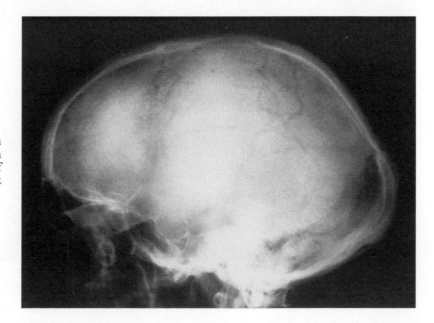

Figure 11–1. A 72-year-old man with an expanding sella turcica, which suggests an intrasellar tumor, as does progressive loss of vision. Pituitary tumor was confirmed at surgery.

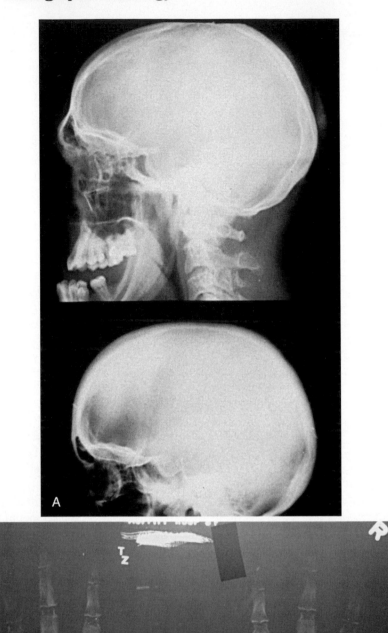

Figure 11–2. *A,* Top, Lateral view of a 31-year-old man with acromegaly, showing enlargement of the sella turcica caused by pituitary adenoma. Note the prominent glabella and elongated mandible. Bottom, Lateral view of a 31-year-old woman with enlargement of the sella turcica caused by pituitary adenoma. *B,* Radiograph of hands showing enlargement (acromegaly) caused by hyperpituitarism.

The excessive urination is due to failure of water reabsorption in the kidney, resulting from deficiency of antidiuretic hormone. This polyuria leads to excessive thirst.

Thyroid Gland

Iodine is the essential element of thyroid hormone. Most disorders of the thyroid gland are caused by either overproduction or underproduction of the thyroid hormone and its iodine-containing substance. The iodine in the thyroid hormone is combined with a protein in the blood, which is then referred to as protein-bound iodine. However, when the hormone enters the tissue, the separate components become unbound from the protein.

In the condition called **hyperthyroidism,** there is overdevelopment, or enlargement of the thyroid gland with excessive secretion of the thyroid hormone. This is called **Graves disease.** Graves disease most often develops in the third and fourth decades of life and affects females more often than males. In Graves disease, the thyroid gland undergoes hyperplasia and there is an associated lymphocytic infiltration. **Exophthalmos,** a protrusion of the eyes caused by fatty tissue edema behind the eyes, is a prominent symptom of this condition. The major clinical symptoms include nervousness, emotional instability, an inability to sleep, tremors, rapid pulse rate, palpitations, excessive sweating, and heat intolerance. Weight loss is frequent, despite an increased appetite. Muscular wasting is most apparent in the muscles of the shoulder girdle. Patients with hyperthyroidism have a variety of cardiac symptoms and signs. Enlargement of the heart, however, is unusual.

In **hypothyroidism** there is underdevelopment of the thyroid gland and a deficiency of thyroid hormone. During the early growth and development years, undersecretion of thyroid hormone produces dwarfism, with significant physical malformations and often mental retardation. This condition is known as **cretinism.** Cretinism is characterized by retarded mental, physical, and sexual development. Children with cretinism typically have a short, stocky build, with short legs and muscular incoordination. Development of the head is abnormal, with a short forehead, broad nose, wideset eyes, and a short, thick neck. The eyelids are puffy and wrinkled. The mouth is open, with thick lips and a protruding tongue. The major radiographic abnormalities include a delay in the appearance and subsequent growth of ossification centers and retarded bone age. Skull changes are common and include an increase in the thickness of the cranial vault, underpneumatization of the air cells of the sinuses and mastoids, and widened sutures with delayed closure.

In older individuals, thyroid deficiency produces **myxedema,** with low metabolic functioning. Childhood or juvenile myxedema occurs because of thyroid dysfunction after birth. These children are usually spared the serious mental retardation of the cretin. Adult myxedema is a form of hypothyroidism that occurs most frequently in adults between the ages of 30 and 60. It is four times more common in females. There is characteristic reduced intellectual and motor functioning and weight gain. The face and eyelids are edematous. The edema is quite viscous and adds firmness to the skin, which does not pit when pressed as in other types of edema. Patients with this condition will have bags under the eyes. The speech is slow or slurred. The skin is coarse, dry, scaling, and cold. On radiographs, the heart will be noted to be enlarged, which is usually caused by pericardial effusion. Because of the edema, soft-tissue swelling on the films of the extremities may be seen.

Generalized enlargement of the thyroid with normal or low thyroid function is termed **nontoxic goiter.** It results when one or more factors occur that inhibit the ability of the thyroid gland to secrete the quantities of active thyroid hormone necessary to meet the needs of the body. Among these causes are iodine deficiency, enzymatic defects, and antithyroid compounds. By far the most common type of goiter is caused by iodine deficiency. Goiters were once common in endemic form in inland geographic areas such as the Great Lakes region and in mountainous regions, where the iodine content of the soil and water is very low. The addition of iodine to table salt has now eliminated this cause.

Thyroid adenoma is a benign neoplasm. It is a solitary nodule of thyroid cells surrounded by a fibrous tissue capsule. These tumors are rarely symptomatic. They usually first present as a palpable mass in the thyroid gland if they are over 1 cm in size. Usually located within the neck, these tumors will be surrounded by a thin zone of compressed thyroid tissue.

Thyroid carcinoma is twice as common in females as in males and can occur at any age. Radiation therapy during childhood, such as for an enlarged thymus, increases the risk for thyroid carcinoma.

There are three major classifications for thyroid carcinoma: papillary adenocarcinoma, follicular adenocarcinoma, and medullary adenocarcinoma. Thyroid carcinoma differs from most other carcinomas in that it is well differentiated, with a papillary growth pattern. The most common type of carcinoma is the **papillary** type. This slow-growing tumor metastasizes through the lymph nodes. **Follic-**

ular carcinoma is more difficult to determine, as its appearance is close to that of normal thyroid tissue. A rare type of thyroid carcinoma, **medullary** carcinoma, is so called because the cells occur in solid masses rather than producing glands. Medullary carcinoma arises from the calcitonin-secreting cells of the thyroid.

Parathyroid Glands

Hyperparathyroidism is a relatively common and important disease that may be mild and go undetected for a long time. **Primary hyperparathyroidism** occurs when the cause of increased parathyroid hormone production lies in the parathyroid glands, and production is not controlled by normal feedback mechanism. The causes are adenoma, hyperplasia, and carcinoma. **Secondary hyperparathyroidism** occurs with conditions associated with low serum calcium, most often chronic renal failure or vitamin D deficiency. The metabolic changes in secondary hyperparathyroidism are quite complex and will not be discussed further.

In primary hyperparathyroidism, the excess parathyroid hormone causes increased breakdown of bone, increased absorption of calcium by the intestine, and increased reabsorption of calcium by the kidney. Urine calcium is also increased because the increase in glomerular filtration of calcium is greater than the increase in reabsorption by the renal tubules.

Bone destruction with pathologic fracture is a less common presentation and is associated with more advanced stages of the disease. As osteoblasts attempt to repair the bone destruction, increased amounts of the enzyme alkaline phosphatase are released into the serum. When the cause of hyperparathyroidism is renal failure, there is often an associated increase in bone density known as osteosclerosis. When osteosclerosis occurs along the superior and inferior margins of the vertebral bodies, it produces the classic appearance of "rugger jersey" spine.

The bone lesions are characterized by the presence of giant multinucleated osteoclasts and fibrosis, sometimes with cyst formation (giant cell tumors). The bone resorption is commonly detected by x-rays of the hands and teeth. A ground glass appearance is present when there has been an overall loss of bone density. Patients with hyperparathyroidism are also prone to repeat bouts of acute pancreatitis.

In **hypoparathyroidism,** functioning of the parathyroid glands is decreased. Most cases of hypoparathyroidism result from surgical removal of all four parathyroid glands, an uncommon complication of the treatment of hyperparathyroidism or of surgical removal of the thyroid gland. In rare instances it occurs idiopathically, with replacement of the parathyroids by fat. Hypoparathyroidism leads to decreased serum calcium and increased serum phosphorus, which in turn is manifested by increased irritability of muscles and convulsions. Little or no calcium is excreted by the kidneys in the urine.

Adrenal Glands

Cushing syndrome is produced by excessive production of glucocorticoids. The most common cause is iatrogenic from the use of corticosteroids in the treatment of other diseases. Noniatrogenic Cushing syndrome may be caused by adrenal hyperplasia resulting from production of ACTH by pituitary hyperplasia or, less commonly, by corticosteroid-secreting adenomas or carcinomas of the adrenal cortex or by ACTH-secreting carcinomas such as bronchogenic carcinoma.

The most obvious effect of Cushing syndrome is a peculiar obesity limited to the face and trunk. The patient has a protuberant abdomen, a "moon" face, and thin extremities. Other common findings include sexual impotence, purple striae on the skin, easy bruising, hypertension, hirsutism, muscle weakness, and hyperglycemia. Cushing syndrome produces radiographic changes in multiple systems. Osteoporosis can be found throughout the body in a diffuse form. The demineralization of the vertebral bodies may cause them to suffer compression fractures (Fig. 11–3). The femur and the humerus are common places to find a spontaneous fracture. Elevated steroid levels increase the levels of calcium in the urine, which may lead to renal calculi or nephrocalcinosis.

Addison disease, also known as **adrenocortical insufficiency,** is an uncommon condition characterized by insufficient production of adrenocortical hormones. In about 70 percent of the cases, it is the result of an autoimmune process that slowly destroys the cortex of the adrenal glands. In the remaining cases, destruction may be caused by tuberculosis, tumor growth, or inflammatory necrosis. Another cause of adrenal insufficiency is the excessive administration of steroids.

Addison disease may strike at any age, affects men and women equally, and frequently is noticed for the first time after a period of stress or trauma. Symptoms include anemia, fatigue, anorexia, nausea, weight loss, and fainting due to hypotension or hypoglycemia, loss of body hair, and depression. The deficient production of corticosteroids leads to increased release of the hormone ACTH. ACTH

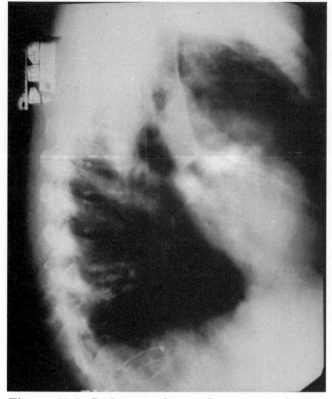

Figure 11–3. Cushing syndrome. Compression fracture caused by excessive production of steroids.

cause a melatonin-stimulating hormone-like effect, which accounts for the increased skin pigmentation characteristic of Addison disease.

The diagnosis is made by a number of laboratory tests that search for the levels of circulating hormones in the blood or the lack of response of the adrenal gland to certain tests that normally stimulate the action of the gland. The treatment of Addison disease requires replacing the missing hormone.

A **pheochromocytoma** is a tumor that most commonly arises in the adrenal medulla. It is usually a benign neoplasm, but a small percentage of tumors may be malignant. Pheochromocytomas arise in the abdomen. The tumor may be located anywhere along the sympathetic nervous system. Even though it is a rare cause of hypertension, the diagnosis of this as a cause is important because removal of the pheochromocytoma will cure the hypertension. As in Addison disease, "pheos" are diagnosed mainly by laboratory tests. However, radiography, computed tomography, and ultrasonography play an important role in confirming the location of the neoplasm. Masses may displace the ureter or kidney, or may appear as filling defects in the bladder on the intravenous pyelogram.

Neuroblastoma is a tumor of the adrenal medulla and is the second most common malignancy in children under the age of 5 years. Recall that nephroblastoma (Wilms) tumor is the most common malignancy found in children. About 10 percent of neuroblastomas arise outside the adrenal gland retroperitoneally. The tumor is highly malignant and metastasizes early and fast either by permeation or embolic spread to regional lymph nodes and abdominal organs. Computed tomography is the best modality to show metastasis through the lymph nodes. Neuroblastomas tend to become quite large before detection. By that time, metastasis has occurred, and the patient has a dismal prognosis. One type of neuroblastoma (Hutchinson syndrome) is characterized by profuse osseous metastases, particularly to the skull and the orbit. Another type (Pepper syndrome) is characterized by hepatic metastases.

Features that differentiate the neuroblastoma from a Wilms tumor bear looking at. The neuroblastoma frequently has calcification, while this is an uncommon finding in a Wilms tumor. Since the neuroblastoma arises from the adrenal gland, which sits superior to the kidney, this neoplasm tends to cause the entire kidney and ureter to be displaced downward. The intravenous pyelogram demonstrates downward and lateral renal displacement. A Wilms tumor, on the other hand, has an intrarenal origin and distorts and widens the pelvocalyceal system from within.

Pancreas

Diabetes mellitus is a generalized chronic disease resulting from a disorder of carbohydrate metabolism. It is believed to be caused by inadequate secretion of insulin by the beta cells of the islets of Langerhans in the pancreas. Without insulin, glucose can not enter the cells to provide them with their major energy-producing nutrient.

The American Diabetes Association has recommended that the course of diabetes be divided into the four stages of prediabetes, suspected diabetes, chemical or latent diabetes, and overt diabetes. The prediabetics are offspring of diabetic parents, and it is assumed that these individuals will subsequently develop diabetes. Suspected diabetics are patients who have abnormal glucose tolerance test results or diabetic symptoms influenced by obesity, pregnancy, infections, trauma, or pharmaceutical and hormonal agents. These patients are normal in all respects, and when the causative agent is removed, the metabolism returns to normal. The chemical or latent diabetics have no signs or symptoms of the disease, but have abnormal glucose tolerance test results or an elevated fasting blood glucose level independent of stress. The overt diabetics have symptoms of diabetes.

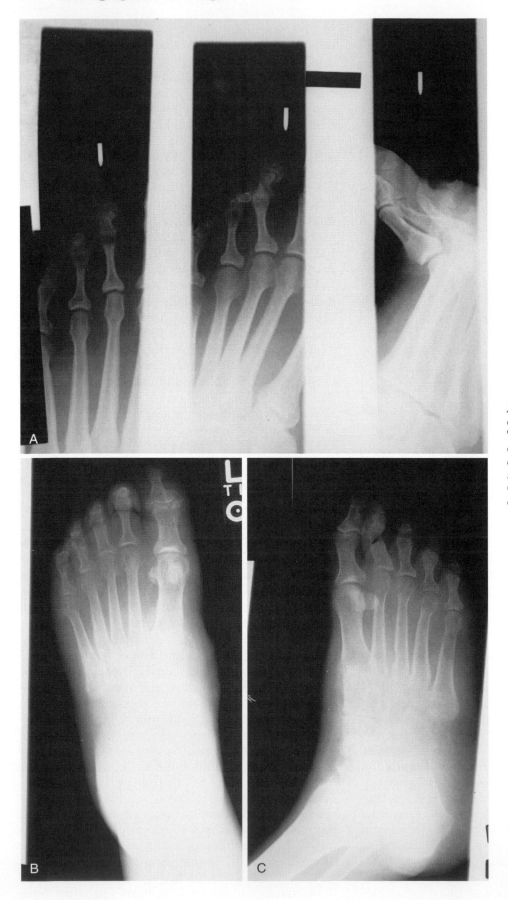

Figure 11–4. Osteomyelitis caused by diabetes mellitus. *A,* The distal phalanx of the second toe is almost obliterated because of osteomyelitis. *B* and *C* are from the same patient. Complications included severe osteomyelitis and anemia.

Table 11–2.
Endocrine-Related Diseases Resulting from Deficient or Excess Hormone Secretion

Hormone	Hormone-Deficient Diseases	Hormone-Excess Diseases
Adrenocorticotropin hormone	Addison disease	Cushing syndrome
Growth hormone	Dwarfism, Simmonds syndrome	Gigantism, acromegaly
Antidiuretic	Diabetes insipidus	Inappropriate antidiuretic hormone secretion syndrome
Thyroid hormone	Cretinism, hypothyroidism	Hyperthyroidism
Parathyroid hormone	Hypoparathyroidism	Hyperparathyroidism
Glucocorticoids	Addison disease	Cushing syndrome
Mineralocorticoids	Addison disease	Conn syndrome
Insulin	Diabetes mellitus	Insulin shock

Table 11–3.
Clinical and Radiographic Characteristics of Common Pathologies

Pathologic Condition	Causal Factors*	Manifestations	Radiographic Appearance
Hyperpituitarism	Excess growth hormone		
	Children	Gigantism	Delayed epiphyseal closing
	Adults	Acromegaly	Thick skull table, enlarged mandible and hands
Hypopituitarism	Deficient growth hormone		
	Children	Dwarfism	Small skeletal features
	Young adults	Simmonds syndrome	Early closure of epiphyseal plates
Hyperthyroidism	30–40 years, females, excess thyroid hormone	Graves disease, exophthalmos	Atrophy of shoulder muscles
Hypothyroidism	Children	Cretinism	Thick diploë of skull, underpneumatization of sinus and mastoids
	Adults	Myxedema	Soft-tissue swelling due to edema
Hyperparathyroidism			
Primary	Increased hormone	Breakdown of bone, increased absorption of calcium	Pathologic fractures, rugger jersey spine, ground glass appearance
Secondary	Chronic renal failure	Too complex for this text	
Hypoparathyroidism	Surgical removal of all parathyroid glands	Low serum calcium, high serum phosphorus	
Cushing syndrome	Use of steroids	Moon face, hypertension, hirsutism	Diffuse osteoporosis, pathologic fractures, renal calculi
Addison disease	Low adrenocortical hormone	Anemia, fatigue	—
Diabetes mellitus	Faulty carbohydrate metabolism	Polyuria, increased thirst, appetite	Arteriosclerosis, osteomyelitis

*Includes age, if relevant.

Although diabetes may develop at any time in life from a few months old to over 80 years of age, researchers have subdivided diabetes into two types—the juvenile and the maturity-onset diabetes. These are based from the time of the onset of diabetes. Patients under the age of 25 years are classified as having juvenile diabetes. Patients over the age of 25 have maturity-onset. However, maturity-onset diabetes is found more frequently in obese people over the age of 40.

The most common characteristics of diabetes mellitus are polyuria, increased thirst, excessive appetite, and loss of weight and strength. Increased urine output occurs because large amounts of water are taken from the body's tissues to dilute the large amounts of sugar in order to eliminate it from the body. The body is unable to utilize the carbohydrates in the sugar, and the patient becomes weak or loses strength. The loss of nutrients for energy causes the excessive appetite.

Complications of diabetes mellitus involve the vascular, endocrine, and nervous systems. Arteriosclerosis is likely to be more progressive in a diabetic patient because lipids are deposited within the walls of the blood vessels. Coronary artery disease may also develop. Gangrene is frequently the result of infection when there are circulatory disturbances of the lower extremities. Bone destruction due to osteomyelitis can be seen on the radiographs (Fig. 11–4). The retina may be damaged, with impaired vision and sometimes blindness. Kidney symptoms are edema and hypertension. The cause of death is often renal failure as a complication of diabetes.

Hypoglycemia is a condition in which the blood sugar falls below normal levels. A person who is a known diabetic must always be watchful for the signs of hypoglycemic shock, which include lightheadedness, sweaty face and hands, and nervousness. Hypoglycemia occurs more often in juvenile diabetes mellitus than in the adult type.

One of the most serious complications of diabetes mellitus is diabetic acidosis or coma. It usually occurs when there is poor control of diabetes. The diabetic coma may range from drowsiness to deep unconsciousness. If the process is not reversed, the blood pressure falls and there is circulatory collapse and renal failure leading to death.

Table 11–2 summarizes the endocrine-related diseases that result from either deficient or excessive secretion of the various hormones.

Table 11–3 summarizes the clinical and radiographic characteristics of common pathologies of the endocrine system.

Review Questions

1. Describe the functions of the thyroid gland. What do its hormone secretions regulate? What will overactivity of the thyroid gland produce?
2. What diagnostic modality will best demonstrate enlargement of the adrenal gland? What are the hormones produced by this gland? What is adrenal insufficiency and what causes it?
3. Explain how exophthalmos is produced. What is it associated with?
4. What is hypothyroidism? What two processes does hypothyroidism cause?
5. Hyperparathyroidism creates what two radiographic appearances caused by osteosclerosis and general loss of bone density?
6. For each of the following hormones, list the gland that produces it and what the function of that hormone is:

Growth hormone	ACTH
Oxytocin	Calcitonin
Epinephrine	Prolactin
Insulin	Mineralocorticoids
Luteinizing hormone	Glucocorticoids
Glucagon	Androgen

7. For each of the following diseases, list what causes it, what gland it is associated with, and what the manifestations are:

Graves disease	Cretinism
Myxedema	Goiters
Cushing syndrome	Addison disease
Diabetes mellitus	Diabetes insipidus
Gigantism	Acromegaly
Dwarfism	Simmonds syndrome

8. Compare and contrast neuroblastoma with Wilms tumor. Where does each occur, what are the manifestations, what is common—or uncommon—with each, what does the intravenous pyelogram show with each, and how does each effect the anatomy of the kidney?
9. What gland is associated with diabetes insipidus? What gland is responsible for diabetes mellitus? Which of these types of diabetes is more common? What are the complications of diabetes mellitus?
10. What is hypoglycemia? How is hypoglycemia associated with diabetes mellitus?

Glossary

Abscess – localized collection of pus

Achalasia – failure of the esophagogastric junction sphincter to relax, resulting in dilation of the esophagus (also called megaesophagus)

Achondroplasia – congenital disorder of cartilage formation resulting in a form of dwarfism

Acromegaly – abnormal enlargement of the extremities caused by hypersecretion of the growth hormone after adulthood

Addison disease – produces symptoms of fatigue, anemia, and weight loss, among others; caused by inadequate secretion of adrenocortical hormone (also known as adrenocortical insufficiency)

Adenocarcinoma – carcinoma derived from glandular tissues

Adenoma – benign epithelial neoplasm that grows in a gland-like pattern

Adenomyosis – benign ingrowth of the endometrium into the uterine musculature

Adrenocorticotropic hormone – secreted by the pituitary gland, stimulates the adrenal cortex to synthesize and release corticosteroids; also called corticotropin

Adynamic ileus – *see* ileus

Aganglionic megacolon – dilation and hypertrophy of the colon due to congenital absence of the ganglion cells in the distal segment of the large bowel (also called Hirschsprung disease)

Anencephaly – severe congenital malformation in which the cranial vault is absent

Aneurysm – dilatation of an artery due to a weakening in the wall

Angioma – tumor composed of blood vessels

Ankylosis – immobility and consolidation of a joint due to disease (*see also* spondylosis)

Annular lesions – lesions that are ring-shaped, that is, annular lesions of the colon with the apple core or napkin ring appearance

Anoxia – lack of oxygen

Anuria – without urine

Aplasia – lack of development of an organ

Arteriosclerosis – group of diseases characterized by thickening and loss of elasticity of the arterial walls

Arthritis – inflammation of the joint

Asthma – recurring attacks of dyspnea with wheezing

Astrocytoma – a tumor composed of neuroglial cells of ectodermal origin

Atelectasis – incomplete expansion of the lung at birth or collapse of the adult lung

Atherosclerosis – a form of arteriosclerosis in which lipids are deposited within the artery wall

Atresia – congenital absence or closure of an organ

Atrophy – progressive wasting away of any part of the body, resulting in impaired function or loss of function

Autoimmune disease – disease in which the body attacks itself

Barrett esophagus – ulcerative areas of the lower esophagus caused by reflux esophagitis

Benign – referring to neoplams, those which are localized, limited in growth, not malignant, and have a favorable prognosis for recovery

Bicornuate – having two horns or cornua

Bright disease – *see* glomerulonephritis

Bronchiectasis – chronic dilation of one or more bronchi

Bronchitis – inflammation of one or more bronchi

Cachexia – marked ill health in general; weakness and emaciation

Calcitonin – hormone secreted by the thyroid gland, decreases the concentration of calcium in the blood serum

Calculus (plural, calculi) – abnormal concentration of mineral salts occurring within a body part

Callus – unorganized network of woven bone formed about the ends of a fractured bone

Carcinoma – malignant neoplasm made up of epithelial cells

Cathartic colon – a colon that can only be evacuated through the use of cathartics

Cauda equina – end of the spinal cord, which is shaped like a horse's tail

Celiac disease – *see* sprue

Cerebral hemorrhage – escape of blood from the vessels into the cerebrum

Cholangitis – inflammation of the bile ducts

Cholecystitis – inflammation of the gallbladder

Choledochal cyst – rare congenital cyst of the common bile duct

Cholelithiasis – presence or formation of gallstones

Chondroma – a tumor or tumor-like growth of cartilage cells

Chondrosarcoma – malignant tumor derived from cartilage cells

Chordoma – malignant tumor found at the clivus of the skull

Cirrhosis – interstitial changes that occur within the liver as a result of chronic disease

Coarctation – narrowing

Colitis – inflammation of the colon

Concussion – condition resulting from a violent jar to the head

Congenital – deformities present at birth

Congestion – capillary filling

Congestive heart failure – condition in which the heart cannot supply enough blood at a sufficient rate to meet the metabolic requirements of tissue

Contrecoup – denoting an injury occurring at a site opposite to the point of impact

Contusion – bruising of the brain

Corkscrew esophagus – asynchrony of peristalsis of the esophagus, resulting in a curled appearance

Craniopharyngioma – benign tumor that originates above the sella turcica

Cretinism – arrested physical and mental development due to hypothyroidism

Crohn's disease – inflammation of the intestine, usually the terminal ileum

Croup – condition of infants and children caused by obstruction of the larynx by allergy, foreign body, or infection

Cryptorchidism – failure of one or both testes to descend into the scrotum

Cushing syndrome – condition produced by excessive intake of glucocorticoids; produces common findings such as "moon face," thin extremities, and sexual impotence

Cyanosis – bluish discoloration of the skin due to reduced oxygen in the blood

Cystadenocarcinoma – adenocarcinoma with cyst formation, usually of the ovary

Cystadenoma – large cystic mass

Cystic fibrosis – inherited disease involving lungs, pancreas, and sweat glands; abnormally thick mucus clogs the bronchi and pancreatic duct, leading to repeated bouts of infection

Cystitis – inflammation of the bladder

Degeneration – initial cellular response following injury; also refers to sublethal cell injury caused by exogenous and endogenous agents

Degenerative joint disease – *see* osteoarthritis

Dermoid – *see* teratoma

Dextrocardia – describes anatomy in which the heart is on the right side of the body

Dextro-rotated – describes the axis of an organ being turned to the right

Diagnosis – determination of the disease that an individual has

Diaphysis – shaft of a long bone

Didelphia – the condition of having a double uterus

Differentiation – the process of determining the difference between tissues; the more like normal tissue a neoplasm is, the less likely the chance of malignancy

Disease process – abnormal change that takes place in the body

Dislocation – displacement of a part

Diverticulosis – presence of diverticula without inflammation

Diverticulum (plural, diverticula) – a circumscribed pouch or sac of lining membrane that protrudes from a weakened area of a wall of an organ

> **Esophageal d., pulsion type** – narrow neck with a round head; a *Zenker* type is located in the upper esophagus, *epiphrenic* above the hemidiaphragm, and *pharyngeal pouch* at the cricopharyngeal junction

> **Esophageal d., traction type** – occurs at the tracheal bifurcation or middle one third; caused by disease; triangular in shape with a broad base

> **Meckel's d.** – congenital diverticulum found in the ileum

Dwarfism – condition resulting from insufficient growth hormone secreted during the growing years to stimulate bone growth

Dysplasia – abnormal development of tissue characterized by loss of normal uniformity of individual cells

Dyspnea – shortness of breath

Edema – accumulation of abnormal amounts of fluid in tissue spaces

Embolus – any particulate matter that is traveling through a vessel

Emphysema – overinflation of the lungs associated with partial obstruction of the bronchus that interferes with exhalation

Empyema – pus-filled body cavity, such as the pleural cavity

Encephalitis – inflammation of the brain

Enchondroma – benign growth of cartilage arising in the metaphysis of a bone

Endocarditis – inflammation of the heart valves, usually caused by bacteria

Endogenous – anything that is internal in nature, referring to disease-causing agents

Endometriosis – occurrence in abnormal location within the pelvic cavity of tissue that resembles the endometrial lining of the uterus

Enzymatic necrosis – autodigestion of the pancreas caused by escaping enzymes from the acinar cells of the pancreas

Epididymitis – inflammation of the epididymis

Etiology – study of causes of disease

Ewing sarcoma – most common primary malignant bone tumor in children 5 to 15 years of age; occurs in the diaphysis of long bones

Exogenous – anything that is external in nature; usually refers to disease-causing agents

Exophthalmos – protrusion of the eyes, caused by edema associated with hyperthyroidism

Exostosis – benign growth projecting from a bone

surface characteristically capped by cartilage (also called osteochondroma)

Exudate – thick cloudy fluid created by decreased hydrostatic pressure and increased osmotic pressure

Fibrous dysplasia – fibrous displacement of osseous tissue

Fistula – abnormal communication between two internal organs

Fracture – breaking or discontinuity of a bone

> **Avulsion f.** – separation of a small fragment of bone at the site of ligament attachment
>
> **Bennett f.** – fracture of the base of the first metacarpal
>
> **Bimalleolar f.** – fracture of the lateral and medial malleoli of the ankle
>
> **Boxer's f.** – fracture at the neck of the fifth metacarpal
>
> **Colles f.** – fracture of the lower end of the radius with backward displacement
>
> **Comminuted f.** – fracture of three or more fragments
>
> **Complete f.** – fracture involving both cortices, across the entire bone
>
> **Compound f.** – fracture that breaks the skin (open)
>
> **Compression f.** – fracture in which both ends of the bone fragment are compressed toward each other
>
> **Epiphyseal f.** – fracture that occurs through the ununited areas of the epiphyses
>
> **Fatigue f.** – fracture that occurs through areas of maximum stress or fatigue
>
> **Fissure f.** – a crack into the cortex that does not break into the bone
>
> **Galeazzi f.** – fracture of radial shaft with dislocation of the ulna
>
> **Greenstick f.** – fracture of one side of the bone while the other side is bent
>
> **Impacted f.** – fracture in which one fragment of the bone is firmly driven into the other
>
> **Incomplete f.** – a fracture that does not break across the complete section of bone
>
> **Monteggia f.** – fracture of the proximal half of the ulna with dislocation of the head of the radius
>
> **Pathologic f.** – fracture caused by weakening of the bone from pathology
>
> **Plastic f.** – bending of the bone that does not result in an actual break
>
> **Pott f.** – fracture of the distal tibia
>
> **Smith f.** – reversed Colles fracture
>
> **Torus f.** – type of greenstick fracture in which the cortex folds back onto itself
>
> **Trimalleolar f.** – fracture of the lateral, medial, and posterior malleoli of the ankle

Frequency – rate of occurrence of a pathologic process that is measured over a given period of time

Functional disease – function of the organ is impaired but the structural elements are unchanged

Gangrene – death of a large mass of tissue because the blood supply to that tissue is completely obstructed

Gastritis – inflammation of the mucosa of the stomach

Germinoma – a neoplasm of the germ cells of the pituitary gland

Gigantism – condition resulting from excess growth hormone secreted prior to cessation of bone growth

Glioblastoma multiforme – malignant astrocytoma

Glioma – a tumor composed of neuroglia

Glomerulonephritis – inflammation of the capillary loops of the renal glomeruli

Goiter – enlargement of the thyroid gland, causing a swelling in the front of the neck

Gout – inherited type of arthritis characterized by tophi; usually affecting the big toes of males

Grading – the process of determining degree of differentiation or malignancy of tissue

Granulation tissue – scar tissue

Granuloma – localized area of chronic inflammation with central necrosis

Granulomatous colitis – inflammation of the colon with formation of granulomas

Grawitz tumor – *see* hypernephroma

Growth disturbance – the presence of any type of lesion or tissue mass that is related to the reproductive capability of the cell

Gynecomastia – enlargement of the male breast

Hamartoma – benign tumor-like nodule composed of an overgrowth of mature cells

Hematuria – blood in the urine

Hemorrhage – rupture of a blood vessel

Hemothorax – blood within the pleural cavity

Hepatitis – inflammation of the liver

> **Deficiency h.** – caused by malnutrition from deficient diet, usually as a result of alcoholism
>
> **Toxic h.** – necrosis of the liver due to certain drug ingestion
>
> **Viral h.** – A, benign form, rarely fatal, spread by fecal contamination; B, serious form, may be fatal, spread by infected body fluids; C, serious, may become chronic, contracted through parenteral drug abuse, a cause of post-transfusion hepatitis; Delta, seen superimposed or in conjunction with hepatitis B; E, very rare in the U.S., spread by fecal-oral route

Hepatoma – any tumor of the liver, but most often refers to a malignant tumor of the liver, especially hepatocellular carcinoma

Hereditary – that which is derived from ancestors, refers to diseases that result from developmental disorders genetically transmitted from either parent

Hiatal hernia – protrusion of any structure through the esophageal hiatus of the diaphragm

Paraesophageal h. – part or almost all of the stomach protrudes through the hiatus into the thorax to the left of the esophagus, with the gastroesophageal junction remaining in place

Sliding h. – the upper stomach and the cardioesophageal junction protrude upward into the posterior mediastinum; the protrusion, which may be fixed or intermittent, is partially covered by peritoneum

Hirschsprung disease – *see* aganglionic megacolon

History – written description of symptoms in a patient's record

Hydatid disease – cysts growing in a body organ

Hydrocele – collection of fluid in the testes or along the spermatic cord

Hydrocephaly – fluid within the ventricles and connecting spaces of the brain

Hydronephrosis – distention of the renal pelvis and calices caused by obstruction

Hydrops – abnormal accumulation of serous fluid in an organ

Hydrothorax – *see* pleural effusion

Hyperemia – increased blood to a part

Hypernephroma – renal cell carcinoma (also called Grawitz tumor)

Hyperpituitarism – excessive secretion of the growth hormone

Hyperplasia – abnormal increase in the number of normal cells in normal arrangement in an organ or tissue

Hypertension – persistently high arterial blood pressure

Hypertrophic arthritis – *see* osteoarthritis

Hypertrophy – abnormal increase in the size of cells

Hypopituitarism – insufficient production and secretion of the growth hormone

Hypoplasia – incomplete development or underdevelopment of an organ or tissue

Hypoxia – reduced oxygen

Iatrogenic – adverse reactions while under the care of a physician

Icterus – *see* jaundice

Idiopathic – describes disease of unknown cause

Ileus – intestinal obstruction

Adynamic i. – caused by inhibition of bowel motility (also called paralytic)

Mechanical i. – caused by mechanical obstructions such as hernia, adhesions, volvulus

Imperforate anus – absence of opening at the end of the anal canal

Incidence – number of newly diagnosed cases of a disease in 1 year

Infarct – area of dead or necrotic tissue

Infection – microbiologic injuries in body tissues caused by invasion and multiplication of microrganisms

Inflammation – protective tissue response to injury or destruction

Intussusception – prolapse of a portion of intestine into a portion that is immediately adjacent

Invasion – the attack or onset of a disease

Involution – progressive degeneration occurring naturally with age

Ischemia – deficiency of blood in the muscle

Jaundice – yellowness of the skin and sclera of the eye due to excess bilirubin in the blood (also called icterus)

Medical j. – hepatitis that is not caused by obstruction, ie, hemolytic (associated with hemolytic anemia) or hepatic (also called hepatocellular and caused by injury to or disease of liver cells)

Surgical j. – hepatitis that is caused by blocking of the bile flow (also called obstructive)

Legg-Calvé-Perthes disease – ischemic necrosis of the femoral head resulting in the fragmentation and flattening of the head of the femur

Leiomyoma – benign tumor derived from smooth muscle

Leptomeninges – two meninges, the arachnoid and pia mater, referred to as one

Lesion – physical or biochemical changes within a cell

Leukemia – progressive, malignant disease of the blood-forming organs

Libo-rotated – describes the axis of an organ being turned to the left

Linitis plastica – diffuse fibrous proliferation of the submucous connective tissue of the stomach resulting in thickening and febrosis so that the lining is rigid, like a "leather bottle" (infiltrating adenocarcinoma)

Lipoma – soft fatty tumor

Lymphadenitis – inflammation of the lymph nodes

Lymphangitis – inflammation of lymphatic channels

Lymphedema – chronic dilation of a part due to obstruction of lymph fluid

Lymphoma – any neoplastic formation of the lymphoid tissue

Lymphostasis – obstruction of the flow of lymph

Malignant – refers to tumors that have the potential to metastasize, become worse, and cause death

Manifestations – observed changes caused by disease

Mechanical ileus – *see* ileus

Medulloblastoma – malignant neoplasm occurring in the roof of the fourth ventricle in the midline of the cerebellum

Megacolon – *see* aganglionic megacolon

Megaesophagus – *see* achalasia

Meningioma – benign, slow-growing neoplasm that occurs in the meninges

Meningitis – inflammation of the leptomeninges

Meningocele – protrusion of the meninges through a defect in the vertebral column

Metaplasia – change in cell from normal to abnormal

Metastasis – transplantation of cells to a new site

Microcephaly – severe congenital abnormality wherein the infant is born with an exceedingly small head

Miscibility – ability of a substance to mix with other fluids

Morbidity rate – ratio of sick to well persons in a given area

Mortality rate – ratio of actual deaths to expected deaths from a given disease

Multiple myeloma – most common primary malignant bone tumor of any age group; a malignant neoplasm of the plasma cells usually arising in the bone marrow, manifested by skeletal destruction

Myelocele – protrusion of the spinal cord through a defect in the spinal canal

Myelomeningocele – protrusion of the spinal cord and meninges through a defect in the spinal cord

Myocardial infarct – lack of sufficient oxygen and blood in the heart muscles, causing an area of necrosis

Myocarditis – inflammation of the myocardium of the heart

Myoma – muscle tumor

Myxedema – condition of nonpitting edema associated with hypothyroidism

Necrosis – death of cells

Neoplasm – tumor resulting from any new and abnormal growth in which there is uncontrolled and progressive cell multiplication

Nephroblastoma – most common renal malignancy in children under 5 years of age (also called Wilms tumor)

Nephrocalcinosis – numerous irregular spots of calcium contained in the renal parenchyma

Nephroptosis – downward displacement of a kidney

Nephrosis – any kidney disease marked by degenerative lesions of the renal tubules

Neuroblastoma – malignant tumor of the adrenal medulla

Neurofibroma – tumor made up of peripheral nerves within the spinal cord

Neuroglia – supporting structure of the nervous tissue in the central nervous system

Neuroma – a tumor or new growth largely made up of nerve cells

Nidus – center or point of origin of a morbid process, ie, the center of an osteoid osteoma

Nosocomial disease – acquired from hospital environment

Oliguria – decreased amount of urine secreted in relation to the amount of fluid taken in

Orchiectomy – excision of one or both testes

Orchiopexy – fixation of undescended testes in the scrotum

Organic disease – involves physical and biochemical changes within the cell

Osmolality – the concentration of a solution; the amount of solute substances that dissociates in solution

Ossification – process of bone replacing hyaline membrane cartilage

Osteitis – inflammation of the bone

Osteitis deformans – inflammation of bone resulting in weakened deformed bones of increased mass, which leads to bowing of long bones and deformation of flat bones (also called Paget disease)

Osteoarthritis – noninflammatory degenerative joint disease causing degeneration of the articular cartilage (also called, degenerative joint disease, hypertrophic arthritis)

Osteoblasts – cells associated with the production of bone

Osteochondroma – *see* exostosis

Osteoclastoma – giant cell tumor of the bone

Osteoclasts – cells associated with the absorption and removal of bone

Osteodystrophy – abnormal development of bone

Osteogenesis imperfecta – hereditary disease involving defective synthesis of collagen and characterized by brittle, osteoporotic, easily fractured bones

Osteogenic sarcoma – malignant tumor of the connective tissue of the bone (also called osteosarcoma)

Osteoid osteoma – a small, painful, well-circumscribed tumor of spongy bone occurring in the long bones and vertebrae of young people

Osteomalacia – softening of bones due to lack of calcium, phosphorus, or vitamin D

Osteomyelitis – inflammation of the bone and bone marrow due to a pyogenic infection

Osteopetrosis – hereditary disease marked by abnormally dense bones

Osteoporosis – abnormal decrease in density of bone

Osteosarcoma – *see* osteogenic sarcoma

Paget disease – *see* osteitis deformans

Pancreatitis – inflammation of the pancreas

Paralytic ileus – *see* ileus

Patent arterial duct – failure of the arterial duct to close after birth, resulting in a left-to-right shunt

Pathogenesis – sequence of events that renders the disease apparant

Pathology – study of disease

Pathophysiology – the physiology of disordered function; the change that occurs as a result of functional disease

Pelvic inflammatory disease – inflammation of the uterine tubes

Pericardial effusion – fluid in the pericardial sac

Pericarditis – inflammation of the pericardium of the heart

Phagocytosis – digestion of bacteria by leukocytes

Pheochromocytoma – benign neoplasm arising in the adrenal medulla

Phrygian gallbladder – common anomaly in which the fundus of the gallbladder folds over the body

Phytobezoar – a mass within the stomach composed of vegetable matter

Pleural effusion – fluid in the pleural cavity (also called hydrothorax)

Pleurisy – inflammation of the pleura

Pneumoconiosis – any lung disease caused by permanent deposition of substantial amounts of particulate matter in the lungs, ie, silica, asbestos, beryllium

Pneumomediastinum – air within the mediastinal space

Pneumonia – inflammation of the lungs

Pneumothorax – air in the pleural cavity

Polycystic ovaries – an endocrine disorder resulting from long-term anovulation, in which the enlarged ovaries contain many follicles that fail to reach maturity and rupture

Polycystic renal disease – inherited renal cystic disease characterized by multiple cysts replacing the normal parenchyma of the kidney

Polyps – a growth or mass from a membrane protruding into the lumen of a vessel or organ

Polyuria – excessive excretion of urine

Prevalence – number of cases of any given disease at any given point in time

Procedure – a manipulation the patient is put through for evaluation

Progeria – premature old age

Prognosis – predicted course of a disease and the prospects for recovery

Prolactin – lactogenic hormone secreted by the pituitary gland

Prolapse – falling down or downward displacement of a body part or viscus

Pseudotumor – phantom tumor

Pulmonary edema – fluid in the lung caused by congestive heart failure; a transudate

Pulmonary emboli – embolus found within the lung, often fatal

Pyelitis – inflammation of the renal pelvis

Pyelonephritis – inflammation of the kidney and its pelvis

Pyosalpinx – accumulation of pus in the uterine tube

Reflux esophagitis – inflammation of the mucosa and submucosa of the lower esophagus caused by reflux of the gastric contents into the esophagus

Regeneration – a type of repair in which normal parenchymal cells that are identical to the original cells are produced

Regional enteritis – *see* Crohn's disease

Reiter syndrome – arthritis commonly found in young males that affects the lower extremities

Repair – the body's attempt to return to normal

Rheumatic heart disease – inflammation of the heart valves leading to scarring deformity and caused by one or more episodes of rheumatic fever

Rheumatoid arthritis – chronic and progressive inflammation of the small joints characterized by atrophy of the muscles

Rheumatoid spondylitis – rheumatoid arthritis of the spine affecting predominately young males

Rickets – a type of osteomalacia found in children, caused by vitamin D deficiency

Sacralization – anomalous fusion of the fifth lumbar vertebrae with the sacrum

Sarcoma – malignant neoplasm made up of connective tissue

Seminoma – malignant neoplasm of the testis

Septal defects – small openings in the septum of the heart

Sequestrum – dead bone

Sign – objective manifestation of a disease that is physically observed by the health examiner

Situs inversus – a condition in which all organs are found on the opposite side of the body than normal

Somatropin – growth hormone

Spermatocele – cystic dilation of the epididymis containing spermatozoa

Spina bifida – development anomaly marked by the defective closure of the vertebrae to protect the spinal cord

Spondylitis – inflammation of the vertebrae

Spondylolisthesis – forward displacement of one vertebra on top of another

Spondylosis – condition of the spine characterized by fixation and stiffness (see also ankylosis)

Sprue – malabsorption syndrome caused by the ingestion of gluten-containing foods and characterized by frothy, foul-smelling stools (also called celiac disease)

Subluxation – partial dislocation

Staging – the determination of distinct phases in the course of a disease

Stein-Leventhal syndrome – comprising the constellation of obesity, oligomenorrhea, and hirsutism with polycystic ovarian disease

Stenosis – narrowing or contraction of a body passage or opening

Stricture – abnormal narrowing of a duct or organ

Structural disease – *see* organic disease

Sublethal cell injury – any injury to a cell that does not cause it to die (*see also* degeneration)

Suppurative – inflammation associated with pus

Symptom – a patient's perception of a disease, eg, headache or abdominal pain

Syndrome – cluster of findings that characterize a specific abnormal disturbance

Teratoma – a true neoplasm, either benign or malignant, made up of different types of tissue, none of which is native to the area in which it occurs; usually found in an ovary or testes (also called dermoid)

Test – analysis of specimens taken from a patient

Tetralogy of Fallot – most common cause of cynosis at birth, resulting from the simultaneous occurance of pulmonary stenosis, ventricular septal defect, right ventricle enlargement, and over-riding of the aorta

Thrombus – mass (blood clot) adhering to the wall of a vessel; it is a common cause of infarct

Thymoma – tumor derived from the epithelial elements of the thymus

Thyrotrophin – thyroid stimulating hormone

Thyroxine – one of two of the iodine-laden hormones that make up the thyroid-stimulating hormone

Transitional vertebra – a vertebra that takes on the characteristics of the vertebrae on either side of it

Transudate – serum fluid that, because of either increased hydrostatic pressure or decreased osmotic pressure in the vascular system, passes through a membrane or tissue

Trauma – direct physical injury

Trichobezoar – mass within the stomach composed of hair (hairball)

Triiodothyronin – one of two of the iodine-laden hormones that make up the thyroid-stimulating hormone

Tuberculosis – any infectious disease caused by mycobacterium tuberculosis

Ulcer – excavation of the surface of an organ or tissue

Ulcerative colitis – chronic ulceration of the mucosa and submucosa of the colon

Unicornuate – having only one horn or cornua

Uremia – presence of toxic wastes in the blood

Ureterocele – intravesical ballooning of the lower end of a ureter

Varix (plural, varices) – enlarged tortuous vein, artery, or lymph vessel

Vasopressin – antidiuretic hormone

Viscosity – resistance to flow

Volvulus – torsion of a loop of bowel, causing obstruction

Wilms tumor – *see* nephroblastoma

Zollinger-Ellison syndrome – thickening of the gastric folds of the fundus of the stomach as a result of tumors in the pancreas caused by hypersecretion of acids

Index

Note: Page numbers in *italics* refer to illustrations; page numbers followed by t refer to tables.

Monteggia fracture(s), 53, *56*
Müllerian duct(s), congenital anomalies of, 168, *171–172*
Multiple myeloma, 42, *43*, 64t
Muscle tissue, 6
Myelography, 257–258, *258*
Myeloma, multiple, 42, *43*, 64t
Myelomeningocele(s), 263
Myocardial infarction, 231
Myxedema, 281

N

Negative contrast agent(s), characteristics of, 12
Neonate(s), respiratory distress syndrome in, 194, 218t
Neoplasm(s), classification of, 7
  definition of, 4
Nephroblastoma(s), *153*, 156
Nephrocalcinosis, 148, *150*, 156t
Nephrography, 134
Nephroptosis, 137, 140
Nephrostomy, percutaneous, 135–136
Nervous system, anatomy of, 251–256, *253–255*
  central, 251–254, *253–255*, 256
  congenital anomalies of, 259–260, *260–263*, 263
  inflammatory diseases of, *264*, 264–265
  neoplasms of, 267–271, *269–270*
  peripheral, 254
  physiology of, 256
  radiographic procedures for, 256–258, *258–259*
Nervous tissue(s), 6
Neuroblastoma(s), 283
Neurologic imaging, contrast agents for, 17
Neuroma(s), acoustic, 270–271
Nodular metastatic lung cancer, 215, *216*, 219t
Noncommunicating hydrocephalus, 259–260, *261–263*
Nonionic contrast agent(s), vs. ionic contrast agents, 12–15, *13–14*, 14t
Nontoxic goiter, 281
Norepinephrine, 277
Nuclear medicine study(ies), of gallbladder, 77
  of liver, 77
  of skeletal system, 29

O

Oblique fracture(s), 46, *47, 49*
Obstructive jaundice, 84
Omnipaque (iohexal), for neurologic imaging, 17
Open fracture(s), 46
Operative cholangiography, 77, *78–79*
Oragrafin (sodium/calcium ipodate), for biliary imaging, 15
Oral cholecystography, 78–79, *80–81*
Osmolality, of contrast agents, 14t, 14–15
Osteitis deformans, 34, *36*, 64t
Osteoarthritis, 57, *60*, 64t
Osteoblast(s), activity of, 24
Osteochondroma(s), 39, *40*, 64t
Osteoclastoma(s), 39, *41*, 64t
Osteodystrophy, 34, *35*, 64t
Osteogenesis imperfecta, 30, *31*, 64t

Osteogenic sarcoma, 42, *44*
Osteoma(s), osteoid, 39, *42*, 64t
Osteomalacia, 31, 34, *34*, 64t
Osteomyelitis, 34, *36*, 64t
  from diabetes mellitus, *284*, 285t, 286
  of skull, 266, 271t
Osteopetrosis, 30, *31*, 64t
Osteoporosis, *33*, 64t
Osteosarcoma(s), 64t
Ovary(ies), abscesses of, 172, *175*
  anatomy of, 162, *163*
  carcinoma of, 179–180, *181*
  cysts of, 177, *178*
Oxytocin, 276

P

Paget disease, 34, *36*, 64t
Pancreas, anatomy of, 74, *75*
  computed tomography of, 79
  congenital anomalies of, 91
  hormones secreted by, 278t
  neoplasms of, *92*, 93, 93t
  pathologic conditions of, 283–284, *285*
  physiology of, 76, 277
  pseudocysts of, *84, 92*, 93
  ultrasonography of, 80–82
Pancreatitis, 90–91, *92*, 93t
Pancreatography, endoscopic retrograde cholangiographic, 82, *83*
Pantopaque (iophendylate), for neurologic imaging, 17
PAP (percutaneous antegrade pyelography), 135
Papillary adenocarcinoma, gastric, 114
Paraesophageal hiatal hernia(s), 103, *106*
Paralytic ileus, 115, 117, *117–118*, 127t
Parasympathetic nervous system, 254, 256
Parathyroid gland(s), pathologic conditions of, 282
  physiology of, 276
Parathyroid hormone(s), 278t
Patent arterial duct, 234–235, 247t
Pathologic fracture(s), *40*, 50
Pelvic inflammatory disease (PID), 172, 183t
Pelvis, Paget disease of, *36*
Percutaneous antegrade pyelography (PAP), 135
Percutaneous nephrostomy, 135–136
Percutaneous transhepatic cholangiography (PTC), 78, *79*
Percutaneous transluminal angioplasty, gastrointestinal, 101–102
Perfusion, physiology of, 188
Pericardial effusion, 241, *242*, 247t
Peripheral nervous system, 254
Pheochromocytoma(s), 283
Phrygian cap gallbladder, 85, *86*
Phytobezoar(s), 111, *112*
PID (pelvic inflammatory disease), 172, 183t
Pineal gland, hormones secreted by, 278t
  physiology of, 277
Pituitary gland, adenomas of, 268–269, *270*
  pathologic conditions of, 279, *279–280*, 281
  physiology of, 275–276
Pituitary hormone(s), 276, 278t
Pivot joint(s), structure of, 24, *27*
Plastic fracture(s), 50, *51*
Pleura, anatomy of, 188, *189*

ISBN 0-7216-4129-6